ECG Interpretation

ECG Interpretation
The Self-Assessment Approach

Zainul Abedin, MD, FRCP (C), FHRS
Associate Professor of Clinical Medicine
Texas Tech University Health Sciences Center
El Paso, TX
Adjunct Associate Professor of Electrical Engineering and Computer Science
University of Texas at El Paso

Robert Conner, RN

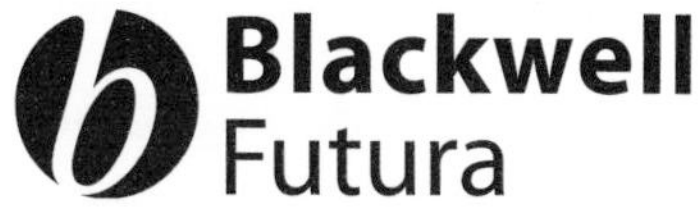

Published by Blackwell Publishing

Blackwell Futura is an imprint of Blackwell Publishing
Blackwell Publishing, Inc., 350 Main Street, Malden, Massachusetts 02148-5020, USA
Blackwell Publishing Ltd, 9600 Garsington Road, Oxford OX4 2DQ, UK
Blackwell Science Asia Pty Ltd, 550 Swanston Street, Carlton, Victoria 3053, Australia

First published as *12Lead ECG Interpretation* © W.B. Saunders Company 1989
Second edition published 2008

1 2008

ISBN: 978-1-4051-6749-9

Library of Congress Cataloging-in-Publication Data

Abedin, Zainul, MD.
ECG interpretation : the self-assessment approach / Zainul Abedin & Robert Conner.
— 2nd ed.
p. ; cm.
Rev. ed. of: 12 lead ECG interpretation. 1989.
Includes bibliographical references and index.
ISBN 978-1-4051-6749-9 (pbk. : alk. paper) 1. Electrocardiography—Examinations, questions, etc. 2. Electrocardiography—Programmed instruction. I. Conner, Robert P. II. Abedin, Zainul, MD. 12 lead ECG interpretation. III. Title.
[DNLM: 1. Electrocardiography—methods—Programmed Instruction. 2. Arrhythmia—diagnosis—Programmed Instruction. WG 18.2 A138e 2008]

RC683.5.E5A24 2008
616.1′2075470076—dc22

2007011252

A catalogue record for this title is available from the British Library

Commissioning Editor: Gina Almond
Development Editor: Lauren Brindley
Editorial Assistant: Victoria Pittman
Production Controller: Debbie Wyer

Set in 9.5/12pt Minion by Graphicraft Limited, Hong Kong
Printed and bound in Singapore by Fabulous Printers Pte Ltd

For further information on Blackwell Publishing, visit our website:
www.blackwellcardiology.com

Contents

CHAPTER 1

Complexes and intervals

An *electrocardiogram* (ECG) is a recording of cardiac electrical activity made from the body surface and displayed on graph paper scored horizontally and vertically in 1 millimeter (mm) increments. Each millimeter on the horizontal axis represents 40 milliseconds (0.04 second) of elapsed time and each millimeter on the vertical axis represents 0.1 millivolt (mV) of electrical force. Each 5 millimeter mark on the paper is scored with a heavier line representing 200 milliseconds (msec) or 0.20 seconds on the horizontal axis or time line and 0.5 millivolt on the vertical axis or amplitude line. Recordings of electrical activity made from within the cardiac chambers are called intracardiac *electrograms*.

Paper used for routine cardiac monitoring is marked across the top by small vertical lines placed at 3-second intervals. Heart rate per minute can be rapidly estimated by counting the number of beats in a 6-second recording and multiplying that number by 10, or can be precisely calculated by counting the number of small squares between complexes and dividing that number into 1500. All monitoring systems currently marketed display the heart rate both on screen and on paper recordings.

The complexes

An electrocardiogram consists of only two elements: *complexes* and *intervals*. The normal complexes are (1) the P wave, (2) QRS complex, (3) T wave, and (4) U wave (Figure 1.1).

The *P wave* represents depolarization of the atrial myocardium. Normal P waves are rounded, do not exceed 0.25 mV (2.5 mm) in amplitude in any lead or exceed 110 milliseconds (0.11 second) in duration. Normal P wave axis is +15 to +75 degrees in the frontal plane leads. The amplitude of the P wave is measured from the baseline or *isoelectric line* to the top of the waveform. Because the right atrium is depolarized slightly before the left atrium, the first half of the P wave represents right atrial depolarization and the last half left atrial depolarization, but normally these events overlap, producing a single deflection.

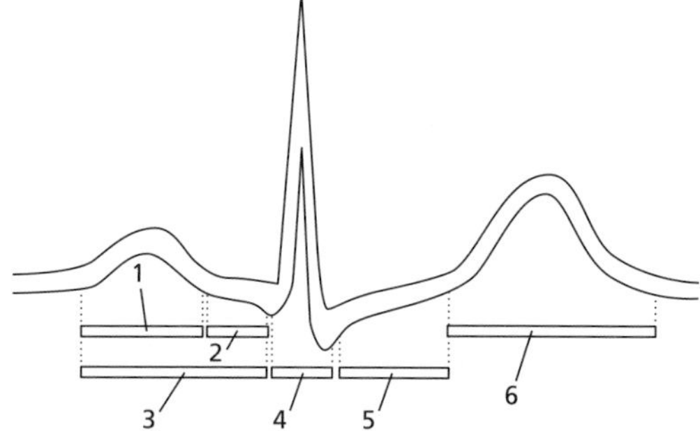

Figure 1.1 1: P wave, 2: PR segment, 3: PR interval, 4: QRS complex, 5: ST segment, 6: T wave.

Figure 1.2 correlates the features of the surface ECG with cardiac electrical events. It is essential to note that sinus node discharge (1) is *electrocardiographically silent* on surface tracings, as is conduction through the atrioventricular node (4), the bundle of His and bundle branches (5).

The recovery sequence can be divided into three phases: (1) the *absolute refractory period* (7), during which the conduction structures are unresponsive to any stimulus; the *supernormal period* (8), and the *relative refractory period* (9), during which the conduction tissues will transmit an impulse, but typically at a slower rate than is normally observed. Refractory periods shorten and lengthen incrementally as the heart rate accelerates or slows, i.e. as the cycle length changes. Therefore the exact length of the refractory periods will vary according to the heart rate and the health of the conduction system.

The so-called *supernormal period* (8) is one of medicine's great misnomers. In fact, the phenomenon of *supernormal conduction* is nearly always observed

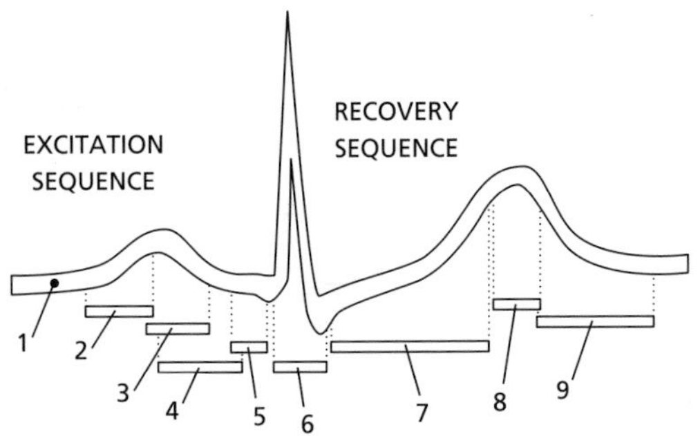

Figure 1.2

EXCITATION SEQUENCE	ECG
1. Sinus node depolarization	Silent
2. Right atrial activation	1st half of P wave
3. Left atrial activation	2nd half of P wave
4. Atrioventricular node	Silent
5. His bundle/bundle branches	Silent
6. Ventricular activation	QRS complex
RECOVERY SEQUENCE	**ECG**
7. Absolute refractory period	ST segment
8. Supernormal period	Peak of T wave
9. Relative refractory period	T wave.

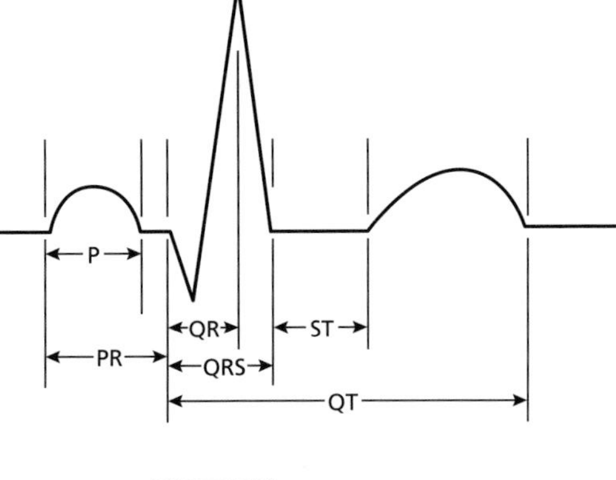

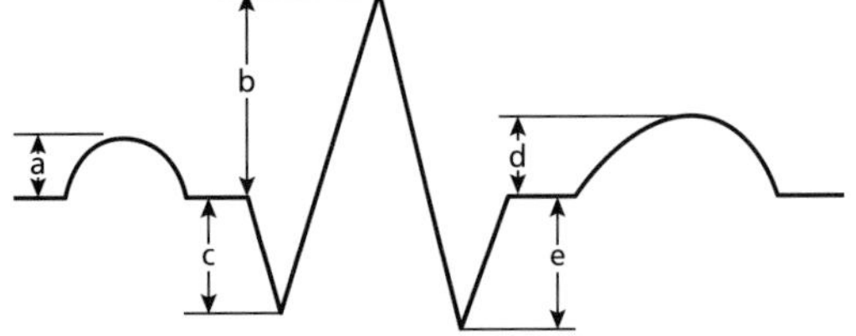

Figure 1.3 Complexes and intervals. a: P wave amplitude, b: R wave amplitude, c: Q wave amplitude, d: T wave amplitude, e: S wave amplitude.

in the setting of severe conduction impairment when conduction is *subnormal*, not 'supernormal.' Supernormal conduction is a function of timing: impulses that fall on the peak of the T wave are conducted whereas impulses arriving earlier or later are not. Supernormality is therefore characterized by (1) conduction that is better than expected and (2) better earlier than later.

The *QRS complex* represents ventricular myocardial depolarization. The QRS amplitude exhibits a wide range of normal values, but an amplitude greater than 1.1 mV (11 mm) in lead aVL, greater than 2.0 mV (20 mm) in lead aVF in the frontal plane leads, or greater than 3 mV (30 mm) in the horizontal plane (precordial) leads is considered abnormally high. The duration of the normal QRS complex ranges from 50 to 100 msec (0.05 to 0.10 sec).

The positive and negative deflections of the QRS complex are named according to universal conventions. The first deflection of the QRS complex, if *negative*, is called a *Q wave*. The Q wave amplitude is measured from the baseline to the deepest point of the written waveform (Figure 1.3). Small, narrow Q waves are expected findings in leads I, III, aVL, aVF, V5 and V6. Normal Q waves do not exceed 30 msec (0.03 sec) duration in any lead. The Q wave may be represented by a lower case (*q*) or upper case (*Q*) letter according to its size in relation to the other QRS deflections. Completely negative QRS complexes or QRS complexes in which no positive deflection reaches more than 1 mm above the baseline are called *QS complexes* (Figure 1.4).

The first *positive* deflection of the QRS complex, whether preceded by a negative deflection (Q wave) or not, is called the *R wave*. The R wave amplitude is measured from the baseline to the peak of the written waveform (Figure 1.3). In the case of polyphasic QRS complexes, subsequent positive deflections are labeled R′. The R wave may be represented by an upper or lower case letter according to its relative size (Figure 1.4).

A *negative* deflection following an R wave is called an *S wave*. The S wave amplitude is measured from the baseline to the deepest point of the written waveform. In the case of polyphasic QRS complexes, a subsequent negative deflection following the first S wave is called an S′ wave. Like Q waves

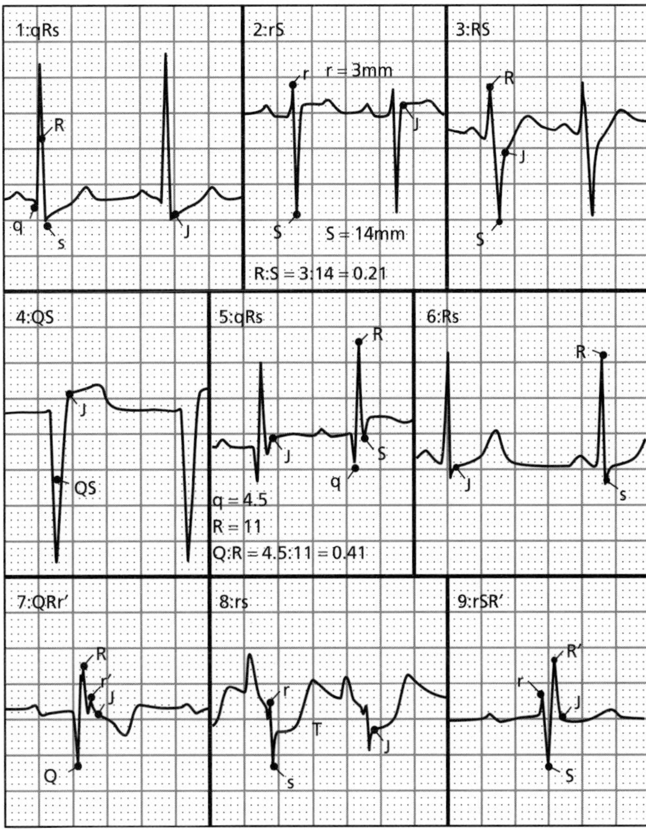

Figure 1.4 Waveform nomenclature.

and R waves, an S wave may be represented by a lower or upper case letter according to its size.

The *T wave* represents ventricular myocardial repolarization. Its amplitude, which is measured from the baseline to the highest point of the written waveform, does not normally exceed 0.5 mV (5 mm) in any frontal plane lead or 1.0 mV (10 mm) in any horizontal plane (precordial) lead. The proximal limb of a normal T wave exhibits a gentle upward slope, while the distal limb, the descending component, has a steeper slope as it returns to the baseline (compare 1a to 3a in Figure 1.6). In other words, normal T waves are not sharply pointed ('tented'), nor are they symmetrical. T wave polarity varies according to the lead, being normally positive (upright) in leads I, II, and V3–V6 in adults, negative (inverted) in lead aVR, and variable in leads III, aVL, aVF, and V1–V2.

The *U wave*, a low-voltage deflection that probably represents repolarization of the Purkinje fibers, is sometimes seen following the T wave (Figure 1.5). Its polarity is usually the same as the preceding T wave. The U wave begins *after* the T wave has reached the isoelectric base line. The second component of a bifid T wave should not be mistaken for a U wave. The presence of a U wave may be attributed to electrolyte imbalance (particularly hypokalemia), drug effects, and myocardial ischemia. Bradycardia tends to accentuate the U wave.

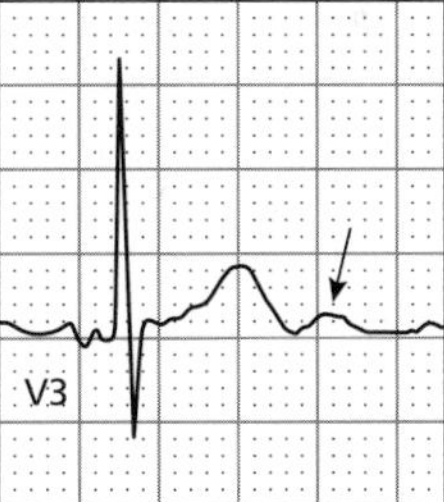

Figure 1.5 The U wave.

The intervals

The clinically relevant ECG intervals are shown in Figure 1.3.

The *PR interval* consists of two components: (1) the P wave and (2) the PR segment. The duration of the PR interval, measured from the beginning of the P wave to the first deflection of the QRS complex, is typically 120 to 200 msec (0.12 to 0.20 sec) in adults. A PR interval greater than 180 msec (0.18 sec) in children or 200 msec (0.20 sec) in adults is considered *first-degree atrioventricular block.*

The *QR interval,* measured from the beginning of the QRS complex to the highest point of the R wave, is an indirect reflection of ventricular activation time. Its clinical importance and applications are discussed in subsequent chapters.

The *QRS interval,* measured from beginning to end of the total QRS complex, normally ranges from 50 to 100 msec (0.05 to 0.10 sec) in duration. If the QRS interval is 120 msec (0.12 sec) or more, *intraventricular conduction delay* is present.

The *ST segment* is measured from the end of the QRS complex to the beginning of the T wave. The junction of the QRS complex and the ST segment is called the *J point* (Figure 1.4). The ST segment is normally *isoelectric* at the J point (in the same plane as the baseline) but may be normally elevated up to 1 mm in the frontal plane leads and up to 2 mm in the horizontal plane leads. Any ST segment depression greater than 0.5 mm is regarded as abnormal.

The *QT interval,* measured from the beginning of the QRS complex to the end of the T wave, normally varies with heart rate and to a lesser extent with the sex and age of the subject. The QT interval adjusted for rate is called the *corrected QT interval* (QTc). The upper limits of normal QT intervals, adjusted for rate, are shown in Table 1.1. Prolongation of the QT interval is seen in congenital long QT syndromes (Romano–Ward, Jervell and Lange–Nielson), myocarditis, myocardial ischemia, acute cerebrovascular disease, electrolyte imbalance, and as an effect of a rather long list of drugs. Polymorphic ventricular tachycardia, known as *torsade de pointes* (TDP), is often associated with QT prolongation. Since women normally have longer QT intervals, they are more susceptible to torsade than males.

Table 1.1 Upper limits of the QTc interval.

Rate	*QTc interval (sec)*
40	0.49–0.50
50	0.45–0.46
60	0.42–0.43
70	0.39–0.40
80	0.37–0.38
90	0.35–0.36
100	0.33–0.34
110	0.32–0.33
120	0.31–0.32

A word of caution is in order about the measurement of intervals. It is often the case that the inscription of a wave is not crisply demarcated, leaving some doubt about exactly when a complex begins or ends. Exact measurement may be particularly problematic if the complex is of low voltage or if the ascent from or return to the baseline is slurred. It is often difficult to determine when T waves end, for example. Exact measurement of the PR interval may be difficult if the beginning of the P wave or the QRS complex is not clearly inscribed. In such cases, clear delineation of the complexes must be sought by examining different leads. A tracing in which baseline wander or artifact obscures the complexes is of little or no diagnostic value.

Two other commonly used intervals are the *P to P interval* (P–P), the time in seconds from one P wave to the following P wave, used to indicate atrial rate and/or regularity, and the *R to R interval* (R–R), the time in seconds from one QRS complex to the next QRS complex, used to indicate ventricular rate and/or regularity.

Slurring, notching and splintering

As shown in Figure 1.6, the normal QRS complex is narrow and displays deflections that are crisply inscribed. In the presence of intraventricular conduction delay, the QRS widens and the initial deflection tends to drift, a finding known as *slurring.* In addition, *notching* may be noted on the initial deflection, whether it is positive or negative. Notches are localized deformities that do not extend downward or upward to the baseline, i.e. they are

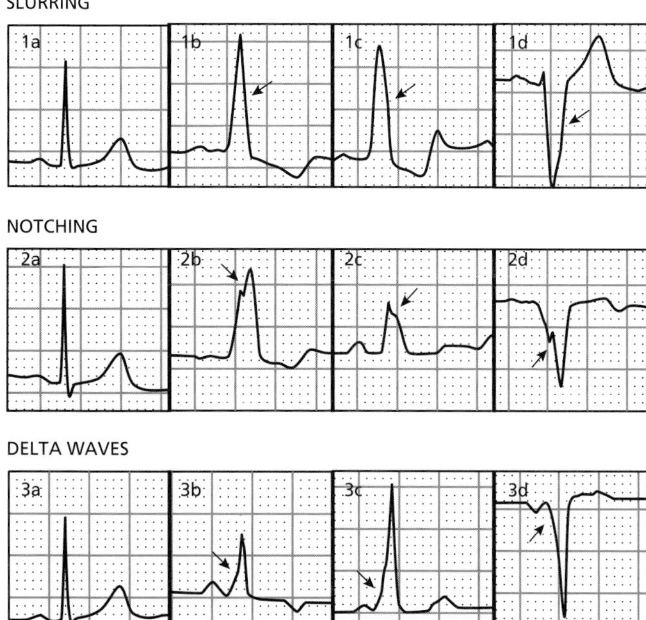

Figure 1.6 Slurring, notching and delta waves.

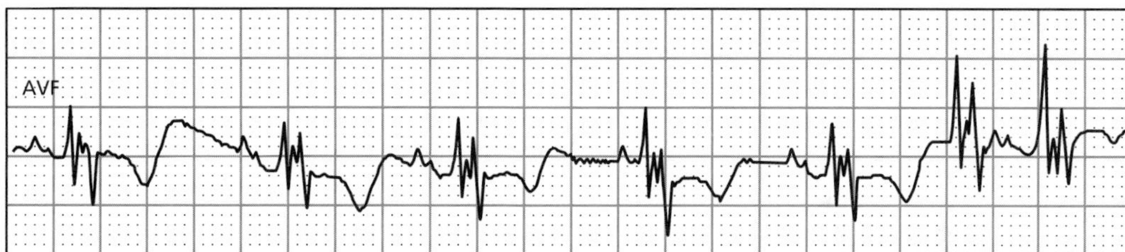

Figure 1.7 Splintering of the QRS complex.

not discrete waves. Very occasionally a QRS deformity known as *splintering* is encountered (Figure 1.7). Splintering of the QRS complex is associated with advanced, severe myocardial disease.

Several QRS deformities are associated with specific conditions: *delta waves* are the result of ventricular fusion due to pre-excitation and are one of the hallmarks of the Wolff–Parkinson–White syndrome. They are described in the chapter devoted to that syndrome. *Osborne waves* or *J waves*, hump-shaped depressions noted at the J point, are most often noted in extremely hypothermic subjects. They are described in the chapter on myocardial ischemia.

2

CHAPTER 2

Mean QRS axis determination

Depolarization of the myocardial cells generates electrical forces that move in three dimensions, changing direction continuously over the course of each heart beat. These forces collectively exhibit both magnitude and direction, constituting a vector. Clearly all the minute electrical forces generated by the myocardial syncytium cannot be considered individually, but they can be averaged together at any given moment during systole to identify a single net amplitude and direction called the *instantaneous vector*. Combining all the instantaneous vectors during systole into a single vector that represents the entire depolarization process results in the *net* or *mean cardiac vector*. To further simplify the process, the mean vector is calculated for only one plane in three-dimensional space. The resulting vector is the *mean QRS axis*.

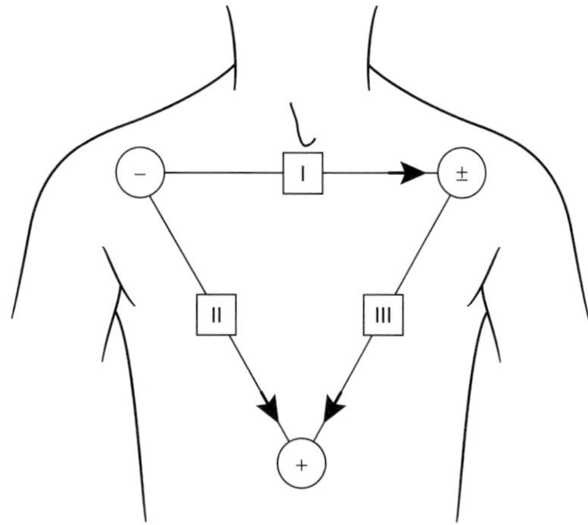

Figure 2.1 The orientation of the bipolar leads.

The frontal plane leads

The six *frontal plane leads* or *limb leads* consist of three bipolar leads (I, II and III) and three unipolar leads (aVR, aVL and aVF). The *bipolar leads* are so designated because each records the difference in electrical potential between two limbs (Figure 2.1). Lead I connects the right and left arms, with its positive pole to the left. Lead II connects the right arm and left leg, and its positive pole and orientation are downward and leftward. Lead III connects the left arm and right leg, and its positive pole and orientation are downward and rightward. The triangle formed by these leads is called *Einthoven's triangle*, and the relationship between the voltage of the complexes in the limb leads ('standard leads') is summarized by *Einthoven's law*, which states that the net voltage of the complex in lead II equals the algebraic sum of the voltage in leads I and III (L2 = L1 + L3).

The positive poles of the *unipolar leads* (aVR, aVL and aVF) are the corners of the Einthoven triangle and the negative pole (the *Wilson central terminal*) is the electrically neutral center of the heart. Unipolar leads are so called because the negative point of reference is the electrically silent central terminal. All unipolar leads are designated by the letter *V*. Because the deflections of the unipolar leads are small, they must be *augmented*. The designations are broken down as follows: *R*, *L* and *F* stand for *right* arm, *left* arm and *foot* respectively, *V* indicates that the leads are *unipolar*, and the letter *a* that they are *augmented* (Figure 2.2).

The hexaxial reference system

Electrical axis in the frontal plane is determined by reference to the six frontal plane leads. First, however, the limb leads must be arranged to form a reference system. To begin forming the hexaxial reference system, the bipolar leads are moved toward each other until they intersect, as shown in Figure 2.3. Note that the orientation of the leads (*arrows*) remains the same. Arranged in this manner, the bipolar leads divide the precordium into six segments of 60 degrees each.

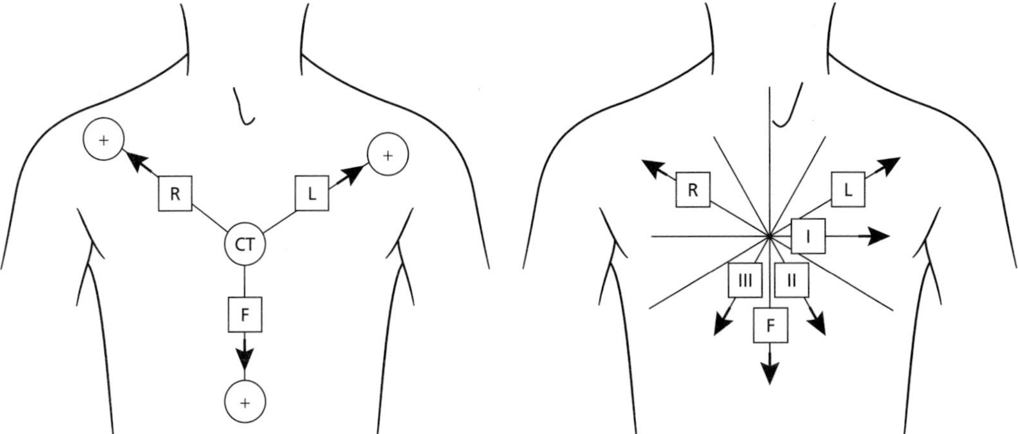

Figure 2.2 The orientation of the unipolar leads. CT: central terminal.

Figure 2.4 The hexaxial system.

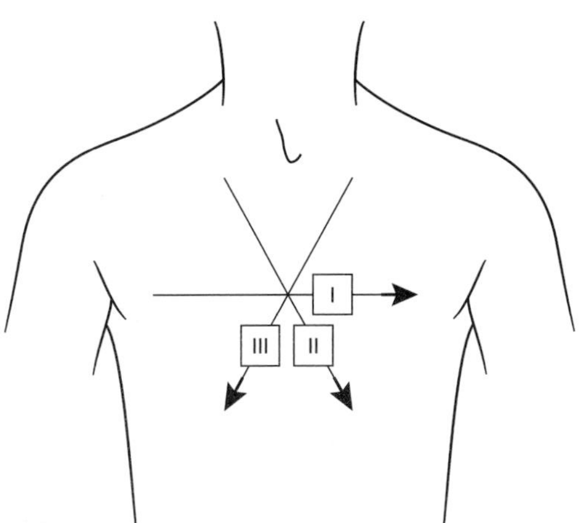

Figure 2.3 Orientation of the bipolar leads.

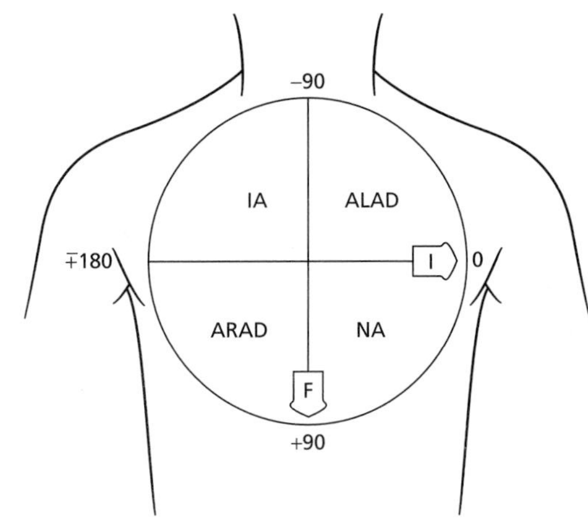

Figure 2.5 The quadrants of normal and abnormal axis. ALAD: abnormal left axis deviation, ARAD: abnormal right axis deviation, IA: indeterminate axis (usually considered extreme right axis deviation), NA: normal axis.

The next step is the addition of the unipolar leads, arranged so that they intersect the bipolar axes. The central point through which all six leads pass is the central terminal. The orientation of the unipolar leads remains the same; the precordium is now divided into 12 segments of 30 degrees each (Figure 2.4).

Leads I and aVF divide the precordium into four quadrants. Figure 2.5 illustrates the resulting quadrants of normal and abnormal axis. When the four quadrants thus formed are closed by a circle, each quadrant marks off an arc of 90 degrees.

The quadrant between the positive poles (*arrows*) of leads I and aVF is the *quadrant of normal axis* (NA). The quadrant to the right is the *quadrant of abnormal right axis deviation* (ARAD); above the quadrant of normal axis is the *quadrant of abnormal left axis deviation* (ALAD). The remaining quadrant is the *quadrant of indeterminate axis* (IA), sometimes called 'no man's land,' but considered by most authors to represent extreme right axis deviation.

Each 30-degree arc of the completed hexaxial system (Figure 2.6) is given a numerical value. Conventionally, the positive pole of lead I is designated as the zero point, the hemisphere above lead I is considered negative, the hemisphere below positive, and the positive poles of the other leads are

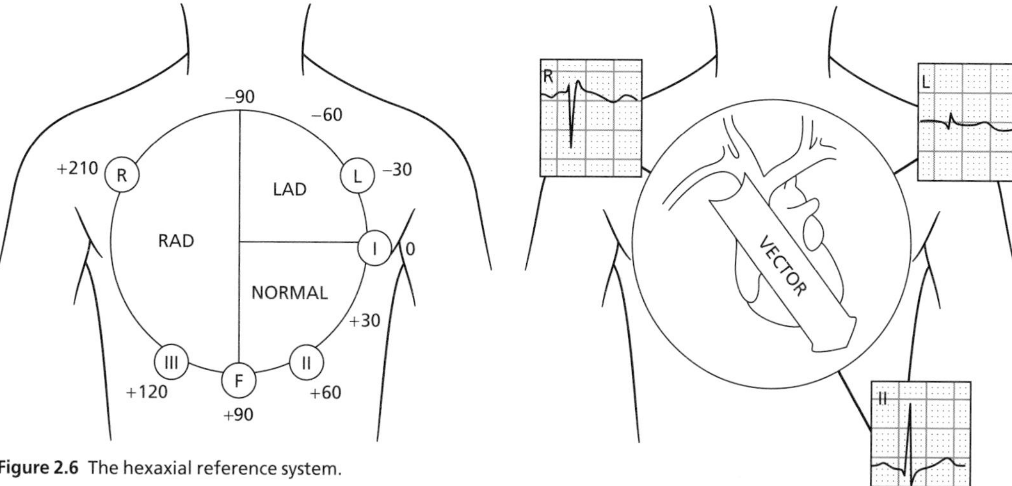

Figure 2.6 The hexaxial reference system.

Figure 2.7 The net cardiac vector.

numbered accordingly. In actual practice the quadrant of indeterminate axis ('northwest axis') is considered to represent extreme right axis deviation, and the positive numbers are therefore extended around to the positive pole of lead aVR, giving it a value of +210 degrees.

Normally the net direction of the electrical forces moves *downward and leftward.*

The three leads shown in Figure 2.7 and the complexes they record demonstrate three simple rules that must be clearly understood in order to determine the QRS axis.

(1) If the electrical forces are moving *toward* the positive pole of a lead, a *positive* complex (lead II in Figure 2.7) will be inscribed.

(2) Correspondingly, if the electrical forces are moving *away* from the positive pole of a lead, a *negative* complex (aVR, Figure 2.7) will be inscribed.

(3) If the electrical forces are moving *perpendicularly* to the positive pole of a lead, a *biphasic* or *flat* complex (aVL, Figure 2.7) will be inscribed.

The flattened or biphasic complex recorded by the lead perpendicular to the net electrical force is called a *transition complex* and marks the *null plane* at which the positive-to-negative transition occurs (Figure 2.8).

Because net electrical movement is normally downward and leftward, the P–QRS–T sequence is normally positive in lead II, and correspondingly negative in lead aVR. Based on the three rules given above, it is possible to formulate three questions that will assist in determining the QRS axis.

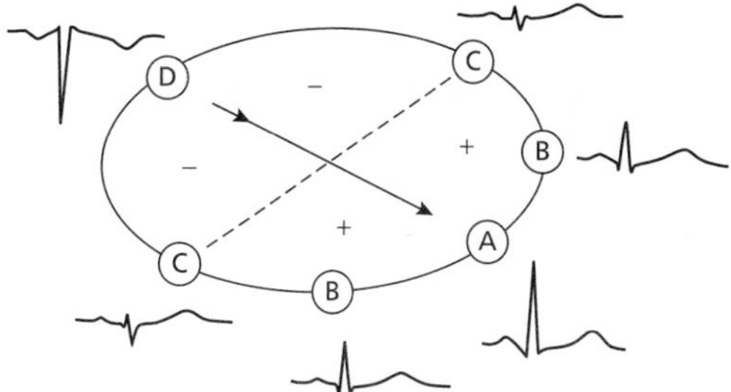

Figure 2.8 Complex size and polarity vis-à-vis the mean QRS vector. C - - -C marks the null plane.

(1) Which lead records the most positive (tallest) R wave? The answer will reveal which lead the electrical forces are going most directly toward.

(2) Which lead records the most negative (deepest) S wave? The answer will reveal which lead the electrical forces are moving most directly away from.

(3) Which lead records the smallest (flattest) QRS complex? The answer will reveal which lead is most nearly perpendicular to the movement of the net vector.

The student may be assisted in committing the hexaxial system to memory if the axis of lead I is considered to be the equator and the axis of lead aVF considered to mark the poles. The positive pole of lead aVF is the South Pole (F = *foot* = south). The inferior leads form a family: lead II is in the quadrant of normal axis, lead III in the quadrant of right

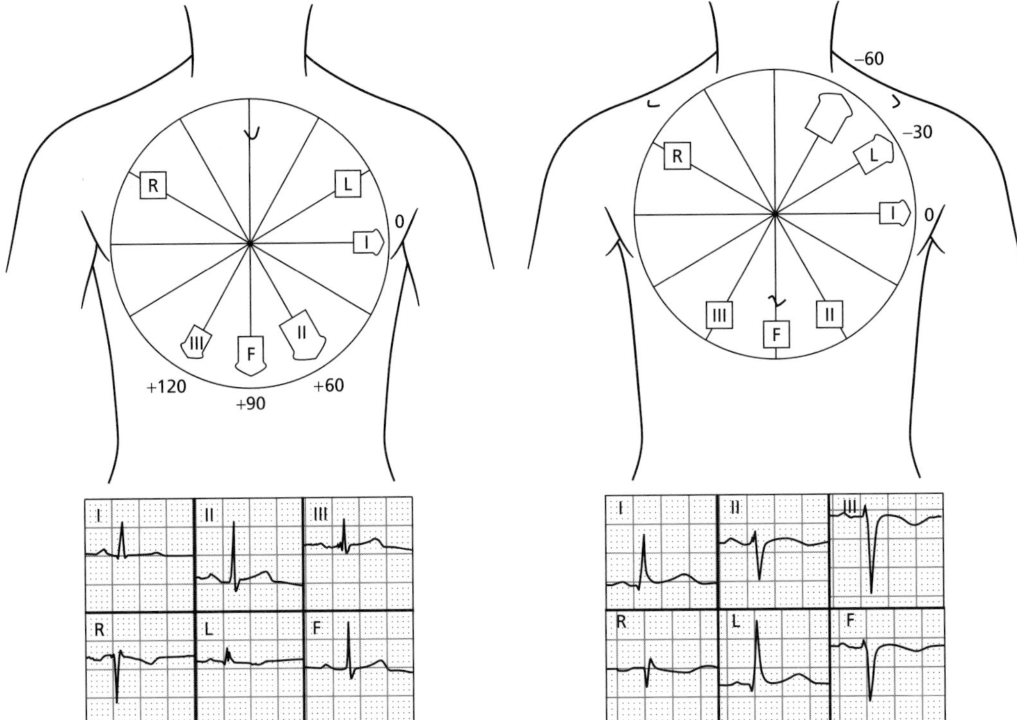

Figure 2.9 Normal axis.

Figure 2.10 Left axis deviation.

axis deviation, and lead aVF forms the boundary between the two quadrants (Figure 2.9).

An example of abnormal left axis deviation is shown in Figure 2.10. In this example the tallest R wave appears in lead aVL because the net electrical force is directed upward and leftward. The smallest QRS complex appears in lead aVR because the motion of the electrical forces is perpendicular to that lead. Note, however, that *the S wave in lead III is deeper than the R wave in lead aVL is tall.* This means that the net vector is more directly oriented *away* from the positive pole of lead III than it is *toward* the positive pole of lead aVL (the arrowheads in Figure 2.10 are sized to reflect this fact). The axis is more leftward than the positive pole of lead aVL (−30 degrees), i.e. in the −60 degree range. Leads I and aVL are both in the hemisphere toward which the electrical forces are moving, and write positive complexes. Leads II, III and aVF are in the hemisphere the forces are moving away from and therefore write negative complexes. Lead aVR, which is in the null plane, writes a small biphasic complex.

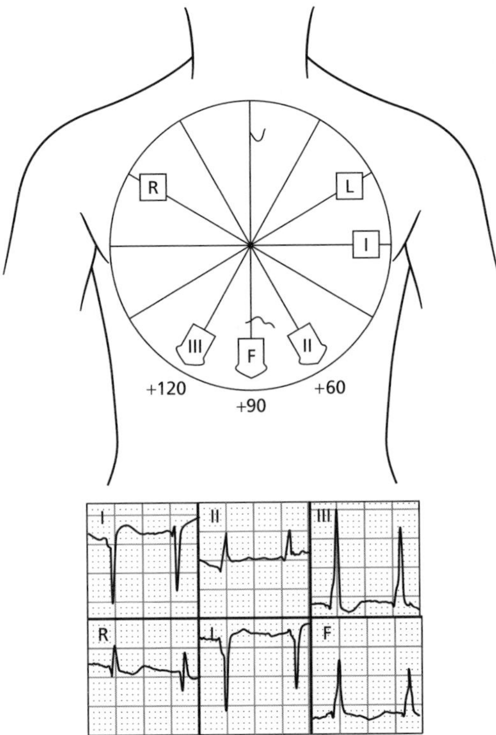

Figure 2.11 Right axis deviation.

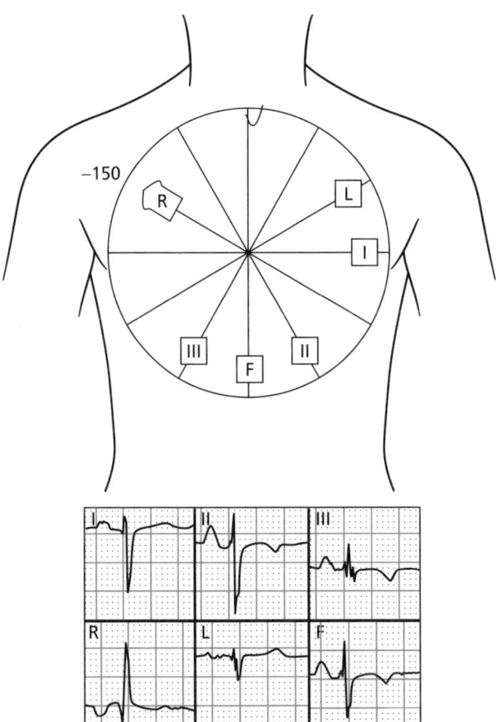

Figure 2.12 Extreme right axis deviation.

These principles may be confirmed by examining an example of right axis deviation (Figure 2.11) and extreme right axis deviation (Figure 2.12).

All ECG machines currently marketed calculate the axis of the P wave, QRS complex, and T wave each time a recording is made. In a small number of cases, truly indeterminate axis is encountered: axis which neither the ECG machine nor the electrocardiographer can determine. In these unusual cases, *every* QRS complex appears to be a transition complex (Figure 2.13).

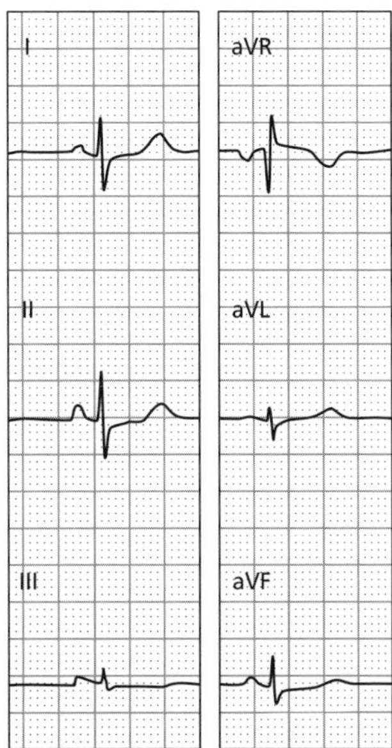

Figure 2.13 Indeterminate axis.

The essential skill is not to be able to calculate axis to within a degree, but to recognize abnormalities of axis and changes in axis at a glance. The clinician encounters as many examples of borderline axis as of borderline blood gases or serum electrolytes, and recognizes that axis deviation is not a diagnosis but a supportive finding associated with many of the ECG abnormalities to be discussed in the following chapters.

CHAPTER 3
The normal electrocardiogram

This chapter introduces the horizontal plane leads, describes the salient features of the normal ECG, and defines transition and low voltage and the sequence of ventricular activation and its relationship to the QRS complex.

The horizontal plane leads

The *horizontal plane* or *precordial leads* are unipolar (V) leads. The positive electrode is moved across the anterior chest wall and the indifferent electrode is the Wilson central terminal. *Lead V1* is located in the 4th intercostal space to the right of the sternum, *V2* in the 4th intercostal space to the left of the sternum, *V4* in the 5th intercostal space at the left midclavicular line, and *V3* midway between V2 and V4. Lead *V5* is located at the 5th intercostal space at the left anterior axillary line, and *V6* in the 5th intercostal space at the left midaxillary line. The spatial orientation of the precordial leads is shown in Figure 3.1. Placement of the precordial leads is always done using skeletal landmarks. Misplacement of the leads can create spurious abnormalities.

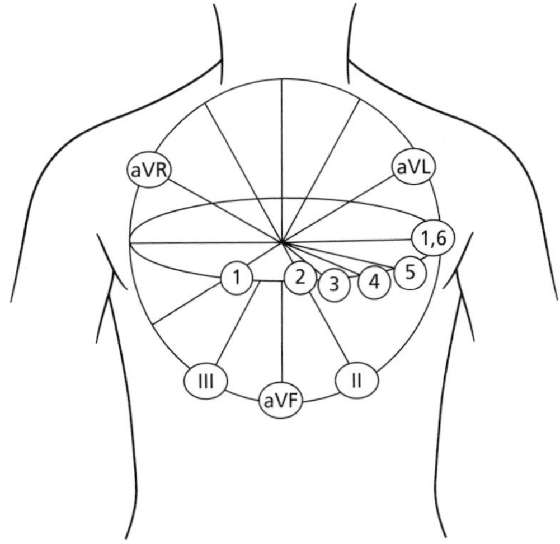

Figure 3.1 The vertical and horizontal planes and their leads.

Features of the normal electrocardiogram

Figure 3.2 shows a normal electrocardiogram. Those features of particular importance are numbered for ease of reference. All complexes (P–QRS–T) are normally positive in lead II (1, Figure 3.2). Correspondingly, the same complexes are all negative in lead aVR (2). The mean QRS axis of the tracing is normal: the tallest R wave in the frontal (vertical) plane is in lead II. Lead V1 exhibits a *small initial r wave* (3) and a *deeper S wave*. The T wave in lead V1 (4) may be positive, biphasic, or negative. The T waves in leads V2–V6 are normally positive in adults. Each T wave begins with a gradually upward sloping proximal limb (5) which then drops back to the baseline more abruptly in the distal limb. Sharp angles within the proximal limb of the ST segment are abnormal and should be regarded with suspicion.

The amplitude of the R waves in the precordial leads normally increases from V1 to V3 until an equiphasic (RS) complex is observed (6). This *transition complex* marks the *transition zone*, which is normally found in V3, V4, or between those leads. A transition complex (RS) in lead V1 or V2 indicates *early transition*; an equiphasic complex in V5 or V6 indicates *late transition*. The point at which the ST segment originates from the QRS complex is called the *J point* (7). Further attention to deformities of the J point will be given in the discussion of myocardial ischemia.

The QRS complex in lead V6 typically begins with a narrow *q wave* (8) followed by a large R wave. The sort of rS complex normally seen in V1 is called a *right ventricular pattern* by some authors and the qR complex of V6, a *left ventricular pattern*. It should be recalled, however, that any given QRS

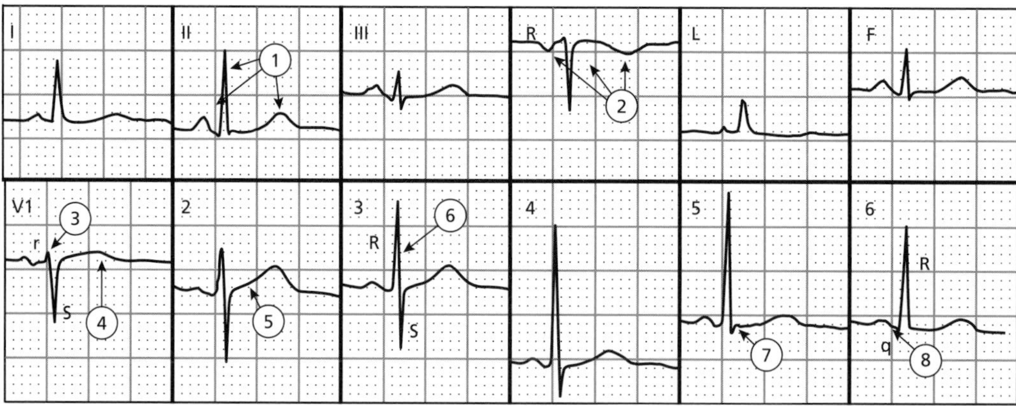

Figure 3.2 The normal electrocardiogram.

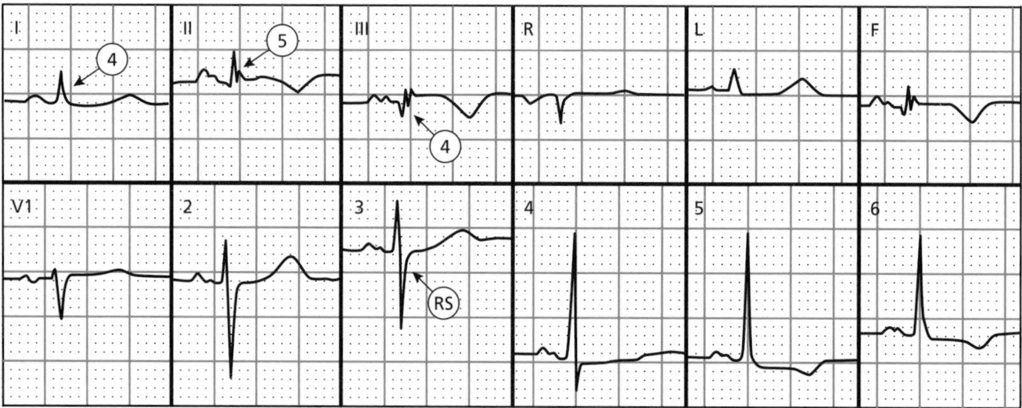

Figure 3.3 Low voltage.

complex is the sum of all cardiac electrical events and not just those generated near the positive pole of a particular lead.

Low voltage

Low voltage is diagnosed when the total of all positive and negative deflections in leads I, II and III is less than 15 mm. The tracing shown in Figure 3.3 is an example of low voltage. Low voltage is often seen in subjects with poorly conductive fluid or tissue between the myocardium and the skin (emphysema, obesity, pericardial effusion), myocardial loss due to infarction, or myocardial replacement (amyloidosis).

Poor R wave progression

Figure 3.4 illustrates poor R wave progression. The QRS complex in V1 exhibits an rSr configuration (1), a normal variant found in around 5% of the population. If the initial R wave in lead V3 is less than 2 mm in height, poor R wave progression is diagnosed. Poor progression is often seen in subjects with left ventricular hypertrophy, anterior wall myocardial infarction, emphysema, and left bundle branch block.

Ventricular activation and the QRS complex

All electrical forces that exist in the heart at any given moment during systole can be averaged together to obtain an instantaneous vector. The instantaneous vector, represented diagrammatically by an arrow (Figure 3.5), represents the average direction and amplitude of the total electrical forces in progress at any instant. The sequence of instantaneous vectors permits a description of the

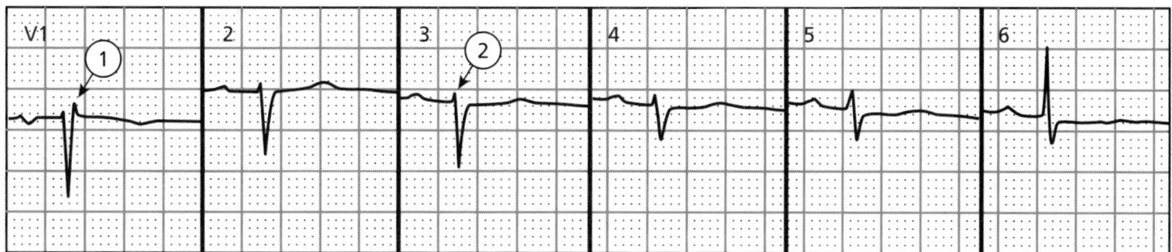

Figure 3.4 Delayed R wave progression.

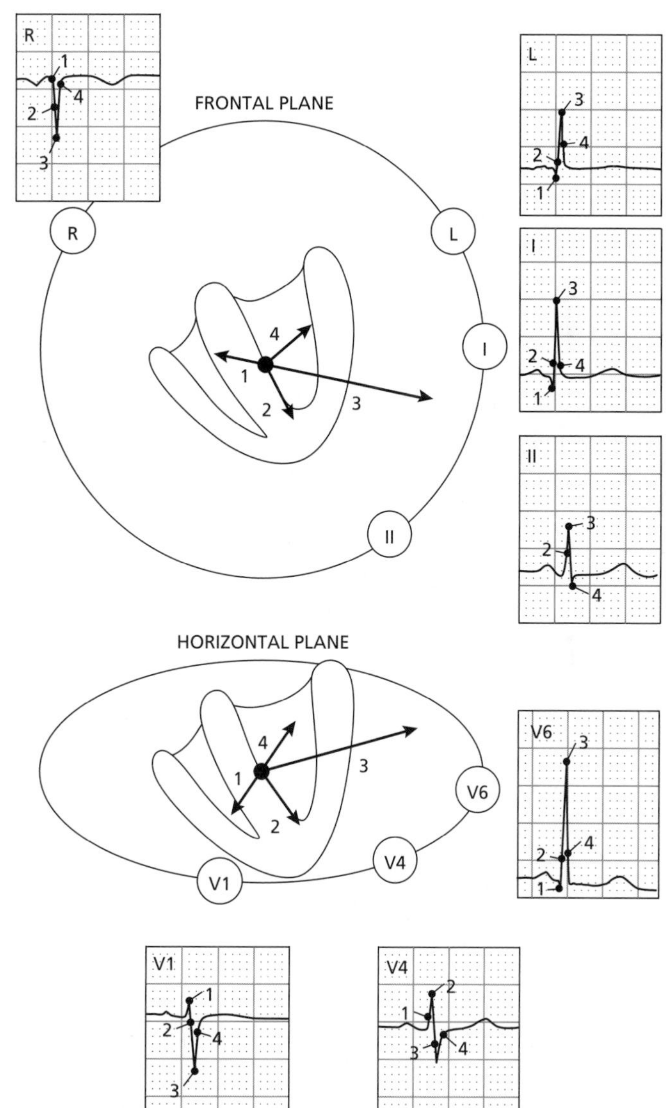

Figure 3.5 Normal ventricular activation.

activation of the ventricular muscle segment by segment.

Although the electrical wavefront represented by the instantaneous vectors is three-dimensional, the leads employed for routine ECG tracings record the vector in only two of many possible planes. The limb leads (I, II, III, aVR, aVL and aVF) detect electrical activity in the frontal or coronal plane, and the precordial leads (V1–V6) detect activity in the horizontal or transverse plane (Figure 3.1).

Depolarization of the sinoatrial node, the atrioventricular node, the bundle of His, and the bundle branches produces no deflection on a tracing taken from the body surface because the forces generated are too small to be detected at any distance. Depolarization of the ventricles begins on the surface of the left ventricular septum and results in an initial wave of depolarization that moves anteriorly and rightward, producing an instantaneous vector, the septal vector, represented by *arrow 1* in Figure 3.5. The septal vector results in the *small initial r wave* in V1 and the corresponding *small initial q wave* ('septal q waves') in leads I, aVL and V6.

From its septal origin the depolarization process spreads over the lower left and right sides of the septum and penetrates the apical region of the ventricles. This wavefront, represented by *arrow 2*, is oriented along the long axis of the septum, directed anteriorly and leftward toward the positive pole of lead II. Because this vector is approximately perpendicular to lead V1, the initial positive deflection in that lead drops back to the isoelectric baseline. Leads facing anteriorly or leftward or both now begin to record a positive deflection (R wave) in response to this vector. Lead aVR, facing away from the net movement of vector 2, begins the inscription of a negative complex.

The depolarization process next moves into the thick anterior and lateral walls of the left ventricle, a phase of activation represented by *arrow 3*, moving leftward, posteriorly, and inferiorly. Those leads facing away from this strong vector (aVR, V1) will now complete the inscription of a deeply negative S wave, while leads facing the movement of this left ventricular vector will complete the inscription of tall R waves, and the precordial lead most nearly perpendicular to the net movement of this vector will write an equiphasic (RS) transition complex.

Activation of the thick basal walls of the ventricles, the base of the left ventricular cone, marks the completion of the depolarization process and results in a final vector directed posteriorly, leftward and superiorly, the vector represented by *arrow 4*. Leads facing away from the net movement of this vector record the distal limb of a prominent S wave, while those facing the movement of vector 4 complete the descending limb of a prominent R wave or complete the inscription of a small terminal *s wave*.

If vector 3 is directed more anteriorly than normal, lead V1 or V2 will be more nearly perpendicular to its net movement and a transition complex will appear in those leads. The result, early transition, reflects anterior axis deviation in the horizontal plane. This may occur as a normal variant or may represent a reorientation of electrical forces due to right ventricular hypertrophy. If vector 3 is directed more posteriorly than usual, lead V5 or V6 will then be more nearly perpendicular to its movement and the transition complex (RS) will appear in those leads. The result, late transition, reflects posterior axis deviation in the horizontal plane, which may occur as a normal variant or in response to a shift in forces due to left ventricular hypertrophy.

Right ventricular forces are represented by vectors 1 and 2 but are quickly overshadowed by the much greater forces generated by the thicker walls of the left ventricle (vector 3). The four instantaneous vectors selected to represent the sequence of ventricular activation will be invoked again in the following chapter to illustrate the altered activation sequence due to bundle branch blocks and to explain the QRS alterations that result.

Self-Assessment Test One

1.1. An equiphasic (RS) complex seen in lead V2 is an indication of . . .
   a. early transition
   b. normal transition
   c. late transition

1.2. Depolarization of the left ventricular septum results in the inscription of . . . in lead V1 and the inscription of . . . in leads I and aVL.
   a. a small initial q wave
   b. a small initial r wave
   c. a transition (RS) complex

1.3. Is the electrocardiogram shown below normal? If not, why not?

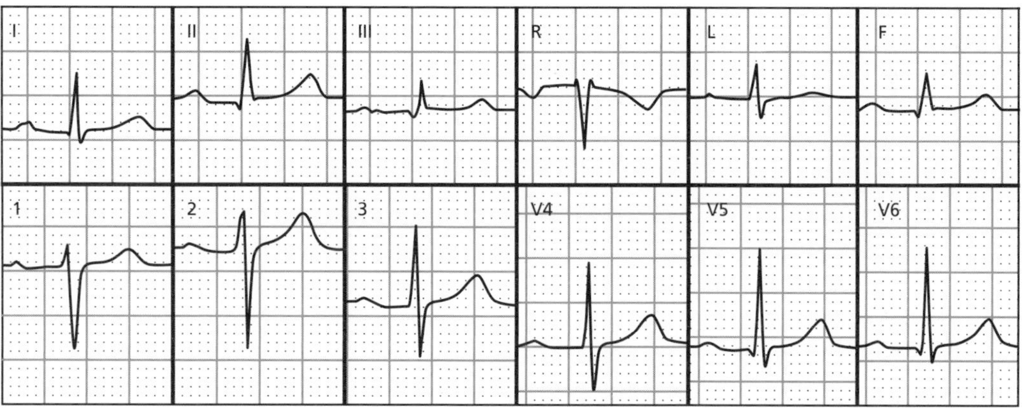

1.4. The sides of Einthoven's triangle are formed by which leads?
   a. II, III, aVF
   b. I, II, III
   c. aVR, aVL, aVF

1.5. Determine the frontal plane axis.

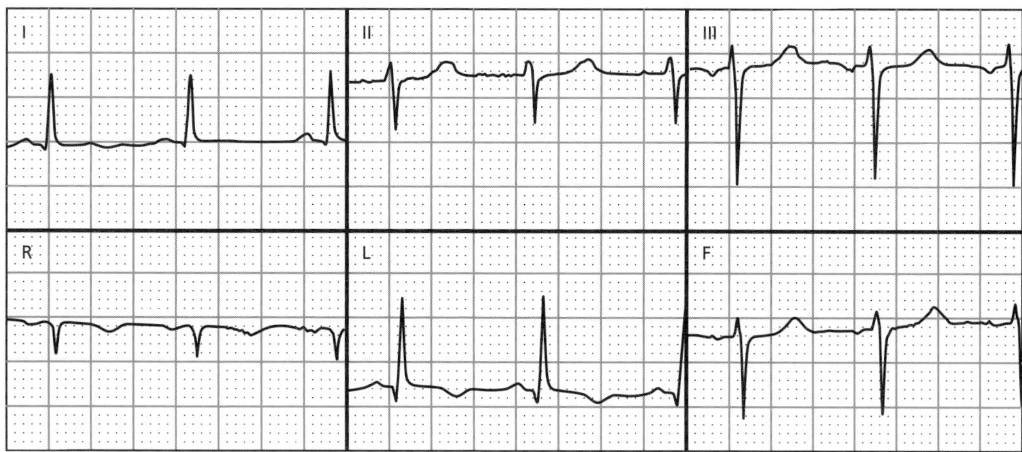

1.6. The positive pole of lead III is in the quadrant of . . .

a. normal axis
b. right axis deviation
c. left axis deviation

1.7. Determine the frontal plane axis.

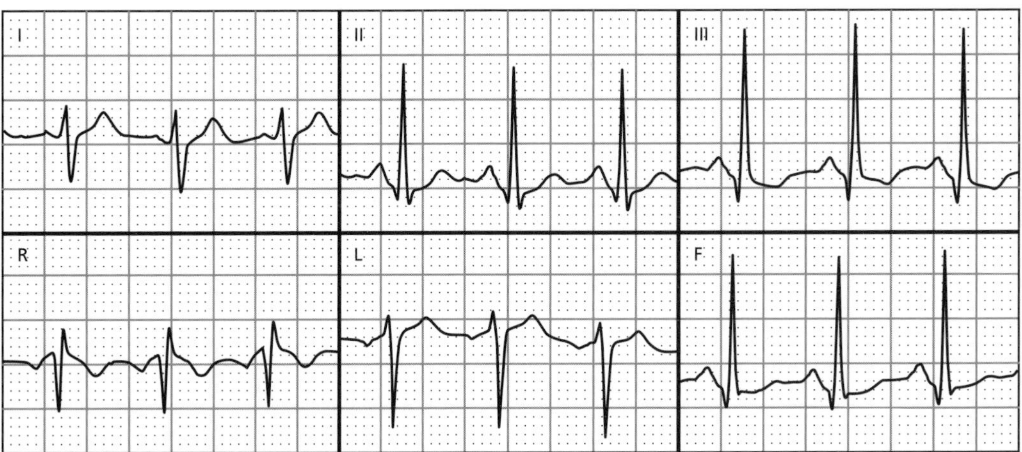

1.8. The T wave in lead V1 in adults may normally be . . .

a. positive only
b. positive or biphasic
c. positive, biphasic, or negative

1.9. The normal left ventricular pattern consists of . . .

a. a qR complex
b. an RS complex
c. an rS complex

1.10. Is this electrocardiogram normal? If not, why not?

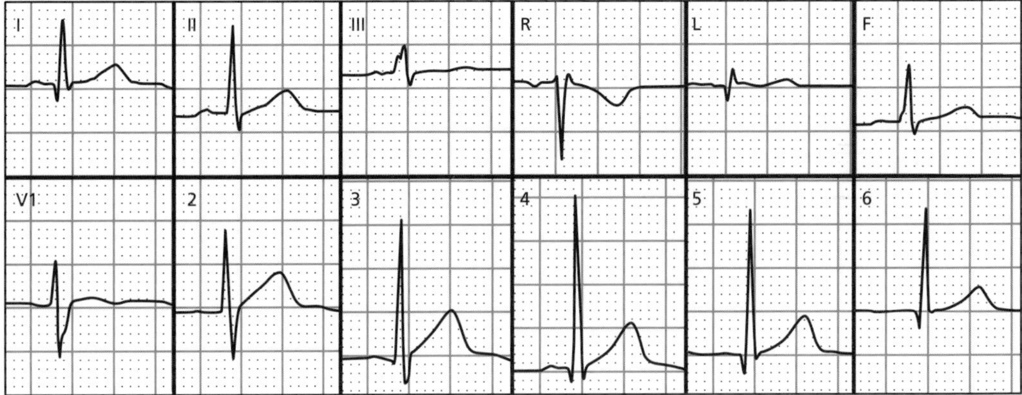

1.11. Determine the frontal plane axis.

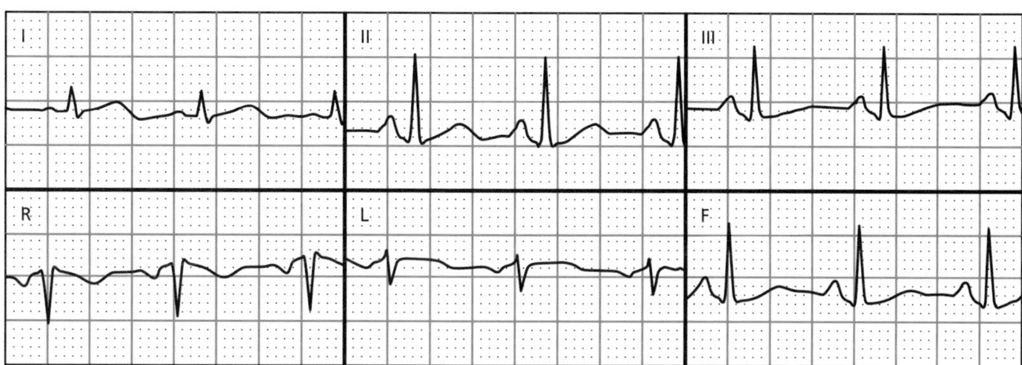

1.12. Determine the frontal plane axis.

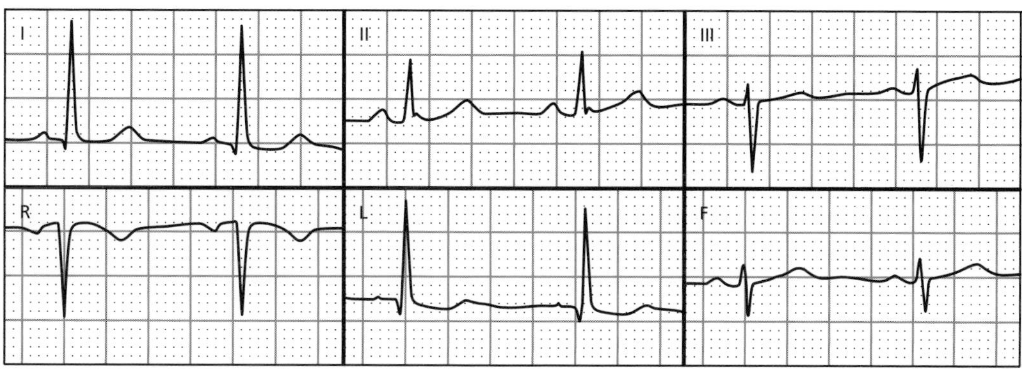

1.13. Determine the frontal plane axis.

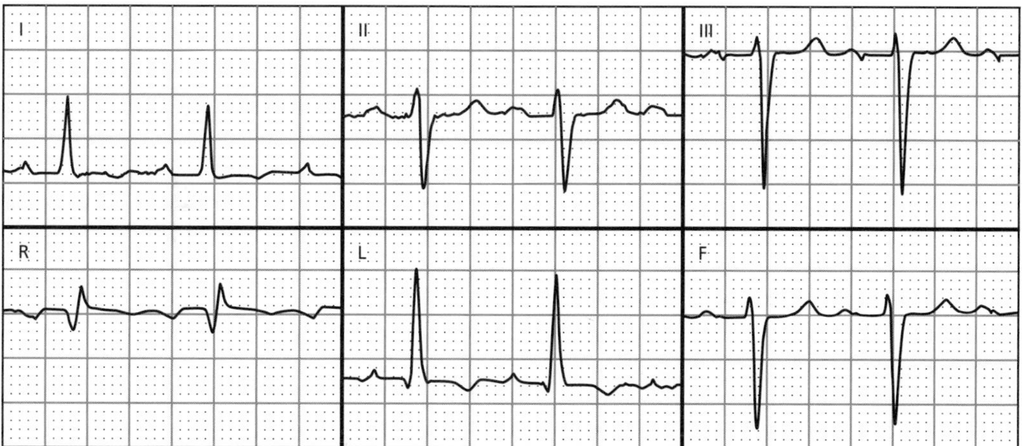

1.14. Determine the frontal plane axis.

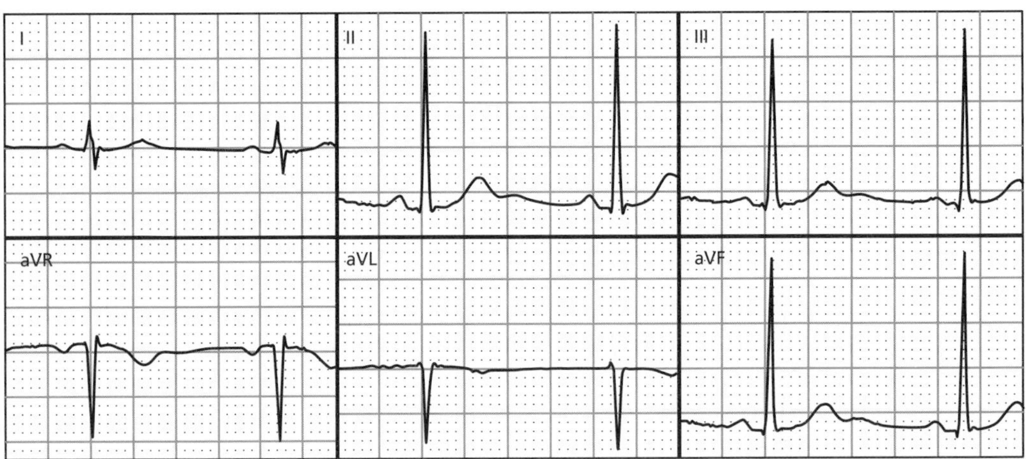

1.15. Determine the frontal plane axis.

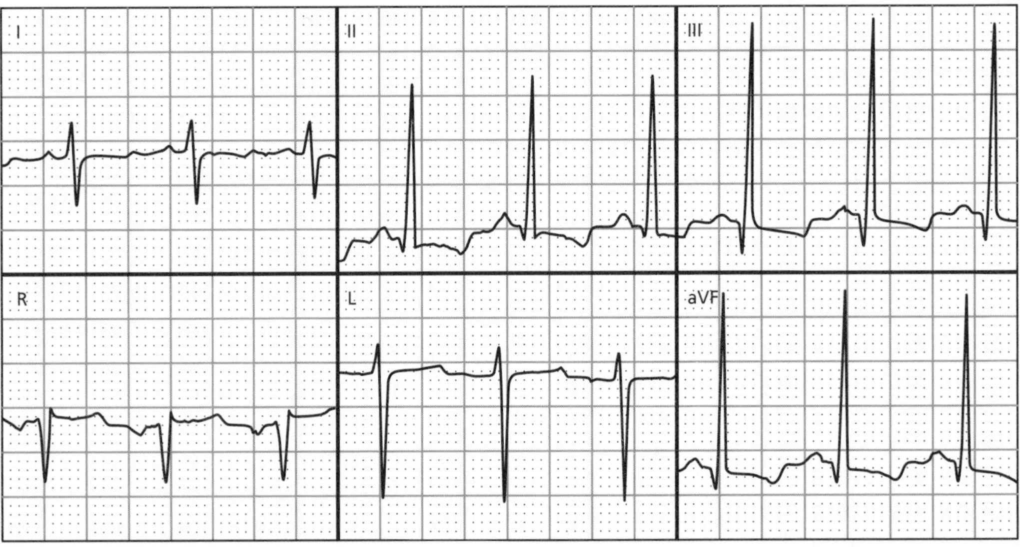

1.16. Determine the frontal plane axis.

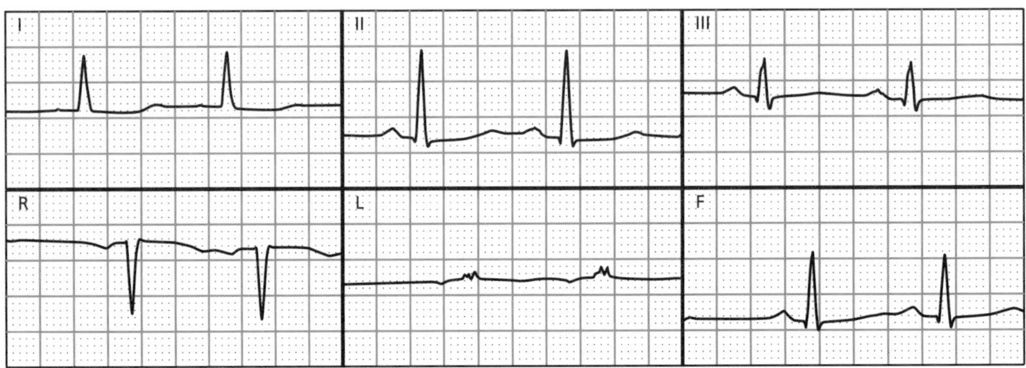

1.17. Is this electrocardiogram normal? If not, why not?

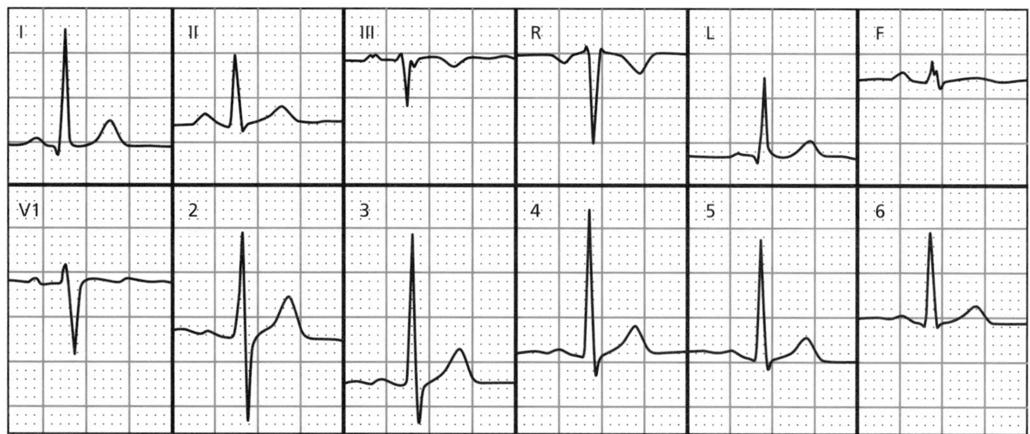

1.18. Determine the frontal plane axis.

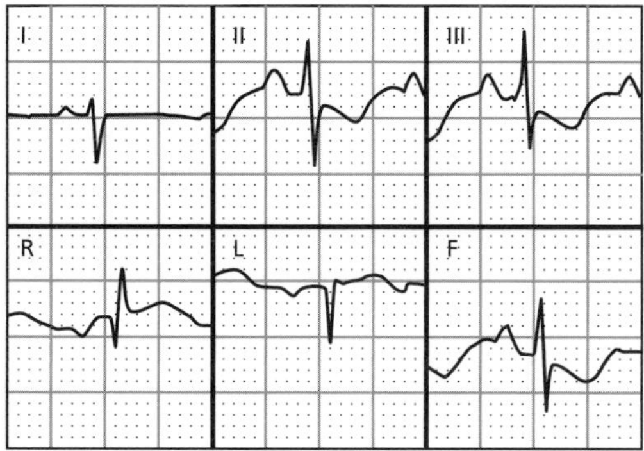

1.19. Is this electrocardiogram normal? If not, why not?

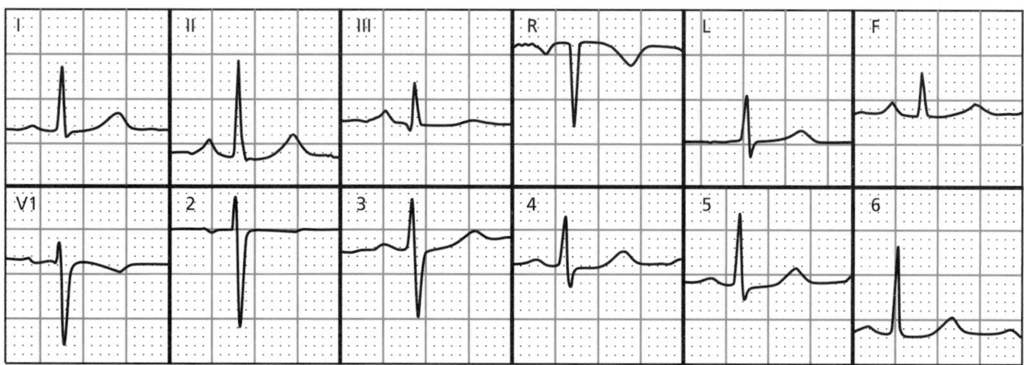

1.20. Is this QRS complex normal? If not, why not?

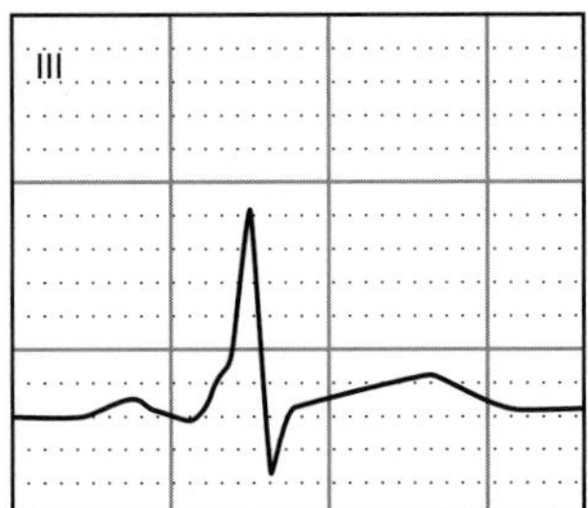

4

CHAPTER 4
Intraventricular conduction defects

The fibrous skeleton of the heart

Each of the four valves is encircled by a ring of fibrous tissue, the *annulus fibrosus*, which serves as a line of attachment for the fixed edges of the valve leaflets. The contiguous annuli are connected by dense tissue: the mitral and aortic annuli are fused at their left point of contact by a small triangular area of tissue, the *left fibrous trigone* (*lft* in Figure 4.1).

The mitral, tricuspid and aortic annuli are fused at their mutual point of contact by another core of connective tissue, the *right fibrous trigone* or *central fibrous body* (*cfb*, Figure 4.1). An extension of the central fibrous body and part of the aortic annulus projects downward as the *membranous interventricular septum* (*ms*), a thin, tough partition that separates the upper parts of the ventricular chambers. The membranous septum is continuous

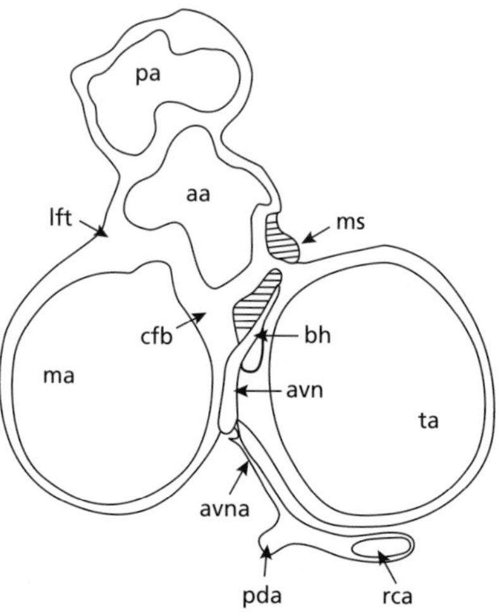

Figure 4.1 The fibrous skeleton of the heart. aa: aortic annulus, avn: atrioventricular node, avna: AV nodal artery, bh: bundle of His, cfb: central fibrous body, lft: left fibrous trigone, ma: mitral annulus, ms: membranous septum, pa: pulmonic annulus, pda: posterior descending artery, rca: right coronary artery, ta: tricuspid annulus.

below with the much thicker summit of the muscular interventricular septum.

There is a very close association between the structures of the fibrous skeleton and the distal conduction system. The atrioventricular node is situated adjacent to the mitral annulus, and the bundle of His penetrates the central fibrous body ('the penetrating bundle'), passes downward in the posterior edge of the membranous septum, and branches into the right and left bundle branches at the summit of the muscular septum. The fascicles of the left bundle branch are closely adjacent to the aortic annulus and the summit of the muscular septum. Congenital deformities of the valves, great vessels and atrial or ventricular septa are accompanied by derangements of the fibrous skeleton and sometimes by conduction disturbances. Pathologic changes in the central skeleton or valve rings due to hypertension or valvular disease are also associated with a significant increase in the incidence of distal conduction disturbances.

The distal conduction system

The *atrioventricular node* (*avn*, Figure 4.1) is situated in the lower atrial septum adjacent to the annulus of the mitral valve. Resting above the septal leaflet of the tricuspid valve, anterior to the ostium of the coronary sinus, it is supplied by the nodal branch of the right coronary artery in 90% of subjects and by a corresponding branch of the circumflex artery in the remaining 10%.

The *atrioventricular bundle of His* (*bh*) begins at the distal atrioventricular node, penetrates the midportion of the central fibrous body, and descends in the posterior margin of the membranous septum to the summit of the muscular septum. The posterior and septal fascicles of the left bundle branch arise as a continuous sheet from the His bundle along the crest of the septum. At its terminus, the His bundle bifurcates to form the anterior fascicle of the left bundle branch and the single slender fascicle of the right bundle branch. In about half the population there is a dual blood supply to the His bundle derived from the nodal branch of the right coronary artery and first septal perforating artery of the left anterior descending coronary artery. In the remainder, the bundle of His is supplied by the posterior descending branch of the right coronary artery alone.

The *right bundle branch* arises from the bifurcation of the bundle of His, its fibers diverging from those of the anterior fascicle of the left bundle branch. The right bundle branch is a long slender fascicle that travels beneath the endocardium or within the muscle of the ventricular septum and ends at the base of the anterior papillary muscle of the tricuspid valve. The blood supply of the right bundle branch is derived from the nodal branch of the right coronary artery and the first septal perforator of the anterior descending artery in 50% of the population and from the first septal perforator alone in the rest.

The initial portion of the *left bundle branch* is related to the non-coronary and right coronary cusps of the aortic valve. Its fibers fan out from the length of the His bundle along the crest of the muscular septum and are organized into three recognized fascicles.

The *left anterior fascicle* of the left bundle, the longest and thinnest of the fiber tracts, diverges from the rest to reach the base of the anterior papillary muscle of the mitral valve. This fascicle receives its blood supply from the septal perforating branches of the left anterior descending coronary artery. Anatomically and physiologically the left anterior fascicle and the right bundle branch are bilateral complements of each other: they are structurally similar, share a common blood supply, and are the two fascicles most subject to conduction block. In fact, right bundle branch block with left anterior fascicular block is a commonly encountered form of bifascicular block.

The *middle* or *centroseptal fascicle* arises from the angle between the anterior and posterior fascicles of the left bundle branch or occasionally from one or both of the other fascicles. Interconnections normally exist between the three major fascicles. Block of the middle fascicle produces no generally recognized ECG pattern. The distal conduction system is therefore quadrifascicular in nature.

The *left posterior fascicle* is a short, fan-shaped tract of fibers directed toward the base of the posterior papillary muscle of the left ventricle. Its blood supply is derived from both the nodal branch of the right coronary artery and the septal perforating branches of the anterior descending artery in 50% of the population and from the nodal branch alone in the rest.

The fascicles of the bundle branches end in a subendocardial network of specialized myofibrils, the *Purkinje fibers*, which spread the impulse over the myocardium.

Electrocardiographic criteria and anatomic correlations

Certain QRS changes emerge when conduction slows or is lost in either of the main bundle branches or in the anterior or posterior fascicles of the left bundle branch. The QRS changes are called *bundle branch blocks* and *fascicular blocks*, respectively. An older terminology for fascicular block was *hemiblock*, a term still occasionally encountered. 'Hemiblock' implies 'half a block,' appropriate terminology only if the left bundle branch is conceived of as divided into two equal halves.

Left anterior fascicular block

Left anterior fascicular block, conduction delay or complete loss in the left anterior fascicle of the left bundle branch (*LAFB*, Figure 4.2), is the most common of the intraventricular conduction defects. This block reorients the mean vector superiorly and leftward, producing *left axis deviation* (–30 to –90 degrees) and characteristic changes in the QRS complex: *small initial q waves* (1, Figure 4.3) and *tall R waves* (2) appear in the lateral leads (I and aVL), *small initial r waves* (3) and *deep S waves* (4) appear in the inferior leads (II, III and aVF). *Notching* (5) is sometimes observed in the terminal portion of the QRS in lead aVR. *Late transition* (6) is commonly noted, and the *septal r waves* usually seen in leads V5 and V6 are often replaced by terminal *S waves* (7).

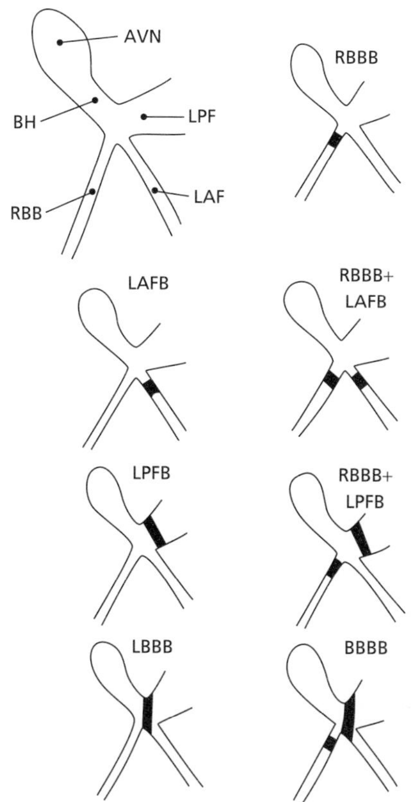

Figure 4.2 Left anterior fascicular block.

Left posterior fascicular block

Left posterior fascicular block (*LPFB*, Figure 4.2), conduction loss or delay in the left posterior fascicle of the left bundle branch, is the least common of the intraventricular conduction defects. This block reorients the mean vector inferiorly and to the right, producing *right axis deviation* (+100 to +180 degrees) and characteristic changes in the QRS complex: *small initial r waves* (1, Figure 4.4) and *deep S waves* (2) appear in the lateral leads (I and aVL), *small initial q waves* (3) and *tall R waves* (4) appear in the inferior leads (II, III and aVF). Left posterior fascicular block nearly always appears in conjunction with right bundle branch block as is shown in Figure 4.4. A rare case of isolated LPFB is shown in Figure 4.5.

Right bundle branch block

Delay or loss of conduction in the right bundle branch results in *right bundle branch block* (*RBBB* in Figure 4.2) and the appearance of characteristic QRS deformities, which include: (1) *QRS complex prolongation* to 120 msec (0.12 sec) or more, (2) an *rSR′ pattern* in lead V1, (3) a *wide S wave* in the lateral leads (I, aVL and V6), (4) *increased ventricular activation time*, and (5) *T wave inversion* in

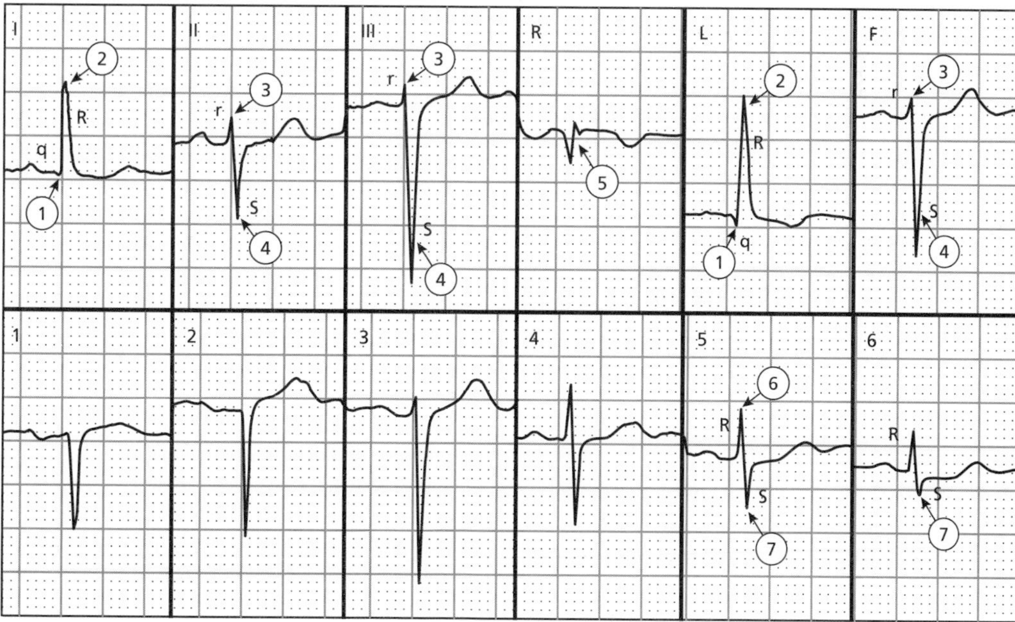

Figure 4.3 Left anterior fascicular block.

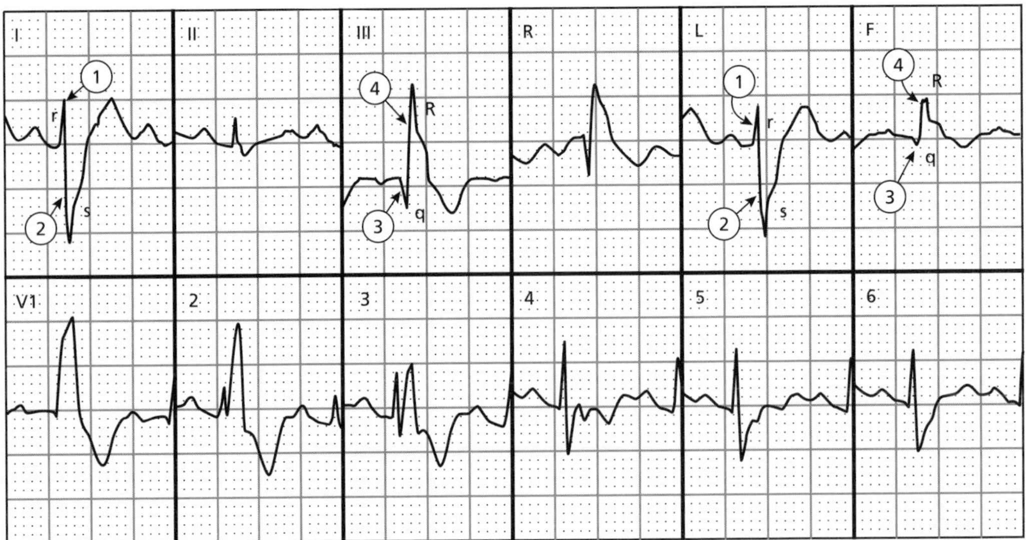

Figure 4.4 Left posterior fascicular block and right bundle branch block (bifascicular block).

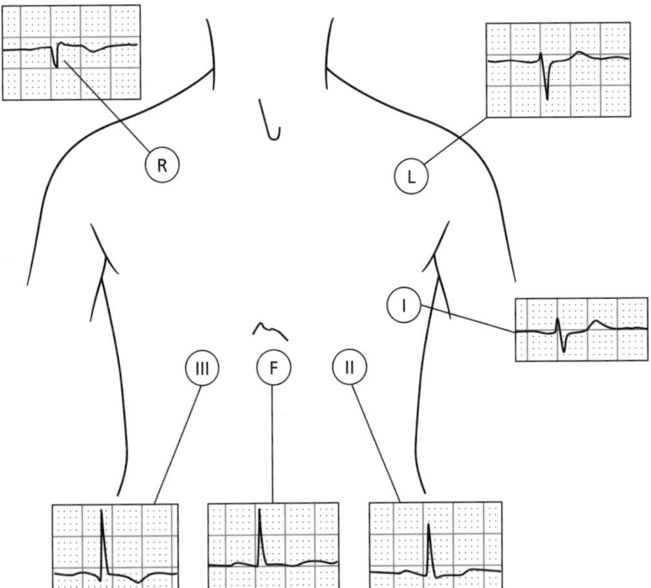

Figure 4.5 Isolated left posterior fascicular block.

lead V1 (Figure 4.6). The QRS axis may be normal, or be deviated to the left or right, particularly if accompanied by left anterior fascicular block (which is often the case) or by left posterior fascicular block.

In the case of RBBB, the QRS complex in V1 can exhibit a fairly wide range of morphologies, but it is always predominantly positive (Figure 4.7).

Increased *ventricular activation time* (VAT) in the right precordial leads is due to delayed or absent conduction in the right bundle branch. Ventricular activation time is reflected by the *QR interval*, measured from the beginning of the QRS complex to the lowest point of the S wave in lead V1 during normal intraventricular conduction, or from the beginning of the QRS complex to the peak of the R′

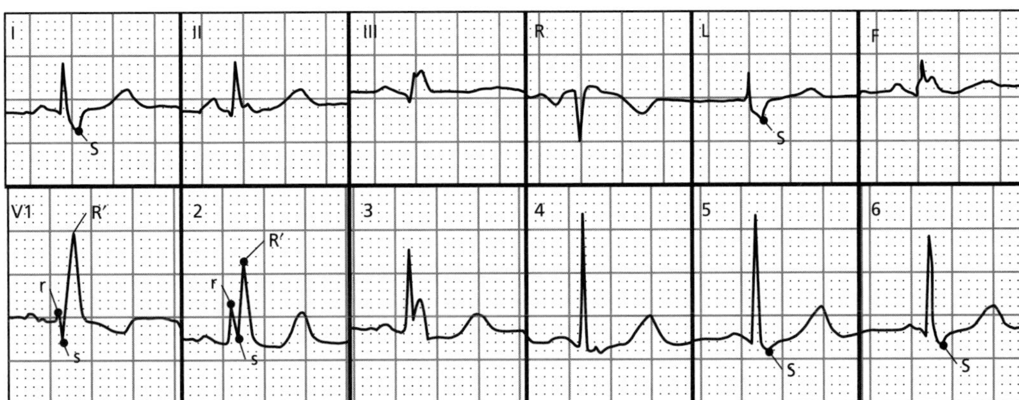

Figure 4.6 Right bundle branch block.

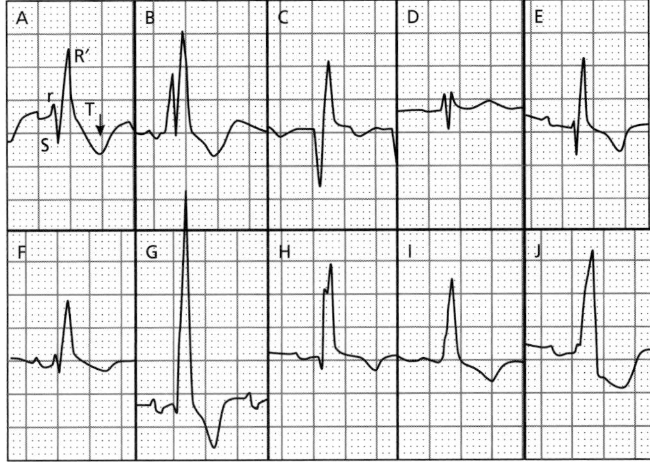

Figure 4.7 Right bundle branch block morphology in lead V1.

wave in the case of RBBB (Figure 4.8). The normal VAT does not exceed 35 msec (0.035 sec) in lead V1.

Ventricular activation in right bundle branch block

Because the integrity of the left bundle branch is undisturbed in RBBB, ventricular activation begins normally, starting from the surface of the left ventricular septum. The electrical forces generated by septal activation are directed anteriorly and rightward, producing a normal septal vector (*arrow 1* in Figure 4.9). The septal vector, responsible for the *small initial r wave* in lead V1, is lost in the event that RBBB is associated with septal infarction – which is often the case (compare C in Figure 4.7). As with normal intraventricular conduction, the septal vector produces a *small initial q wave* in the left lateral leads (I and V6).

Because there is no block in the left bundle branch, depolarization of the left ventricular muscle mass occurs next. The forces produced by the left ventricular vector (*arrow 2*, Figure 4.9) are directed leftward and posteriorly, producing an *S wave* in V1 and *tall R waves* in the left lateral leads (I, II and V6). The height of the R wave in the frontal plane leads reflects the net QRS axis in that plane, which is frequently abnormal owing to concomitant fascicular block.

Slow conduction through the septum eventually results in right ventricular septal activation, producing the right septal vector (*arrow 3*), which is directed rightward and anteriorly, producing the *upstroke of the R′ wave* in V1 and the beginning of

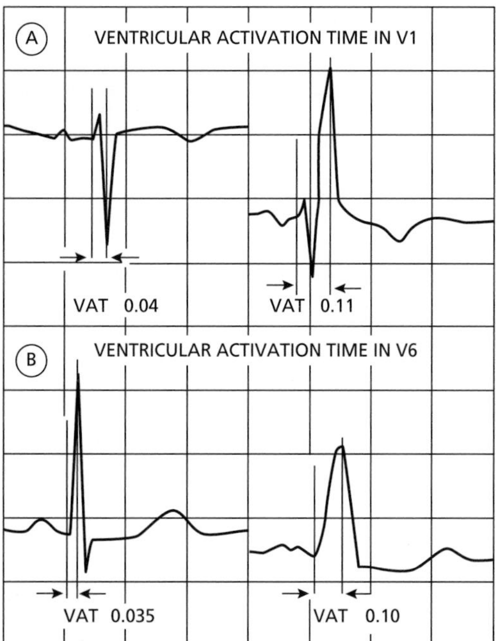

Figure 4.8 Ventricular activation time (VAT).

the *widened terminal S wave* in the left lateral leads (I, aVL, V5 and V6).

A fourth instantaneous vector (*arrow 4*) results from depolarization of the right ventricular free wall and outflow tract. Oriented rightward and anteriorly, these forces result in the inscription of the *peak of the R′ wave* in V1 and the *terminal portion of the S wave* in the left lateral leads. An electrode overlying the transition zone in the horizontal plane may record a polyphasic *transition complex*, like the one shown in lead V4 of Figure 4.9.

Left bundle branch block

Delay or loss of conduction in the left bundle branch results in *left bundle branch block* (*LBBB* in Figure 4.2) and the appearance of characteristic QRS deformities, which include: (1) *QRS complex prolongation* to 120 msec (0.12 sec) or more, (2) a *wide, slurred S wave* in the right precordial leads (V1 and V2), (3) a *wide R wave* that often displays notching and/or slurring in the left lateral leads (I, aVL, V5 and V6), (4) *prolonged ventricular activation time*, and (5) *ST segment and T wave displacement* in the direction opposite to the polarity of the QRS complex. Preserved right ventricular septal activation (which may be lost in the case of septal infarction) results in a *small initial r wave* in leads V1 and V2 (Figure 4.10).

Increased ventricular activation time in the left precordial leads V5 and V6 – a QR interval greater than 45 msec (0.045 sec) in Figure 4.8 – is due to delayed or absent conduction in the left bundle branch.

Ventricular activation in left bundle branch block

In left bundle branch block, ventricular depolarization begins on the right ventricular septal surface, producing an initial vector (*arrow 1*, Figure 4.11) that is directed anteriorly and leftward. This vector may result in a *small initial r wave* in the right precordial leads V1 and V2 and contributes to the upstroke of the R wave in the left lateral leads I, aVL, V5 and V6.

The second instantaneous vector (*arrow 2*), representing depolarization of the lower septum, is directed leftward and posteriorly, producing the *downstroke of the s wave* in the right precordial leads and the *ascending limb of the R wave* in the left lateral leads. As septal depolarization continues, a third vector (*arrow 3*) is generated. This vector is reflected by the *notching or slurring of the peak of the R wave* in the left lateral leads.

Depolarization of the left ventricular free wall and base of the left ventricular cone produces a fourth vector (*arrow 4*), directed leftward and posteriorly, that is responsible for the *descending limb of the R wave* in the left lateral leads and the *ascending limb of the S wave* in the right precordial leads. Occasionally this vector is directed extremely posteriorly in the horizontal plane with the result that leads I and aVL record the typical upright R wave morphology, but leads V5 and V6 record a biphasic RS (transition) complex or a deep S wave.

Multifascicular block

The most frequently encountered form of multifascicular block is a *bifascicular block*: right bundle branch block and left anterior fascicular block (*RBBB + LAFB*, Figure 4.2). The least common of the bifascicular blocks is right bundle branch block and left posterior fascicular block (*RBBB + LPFB*). Multifascicular block can also present as *bilateral bundle branch block* (BBBB), in which right bundle branch block alternates with left bundle branch

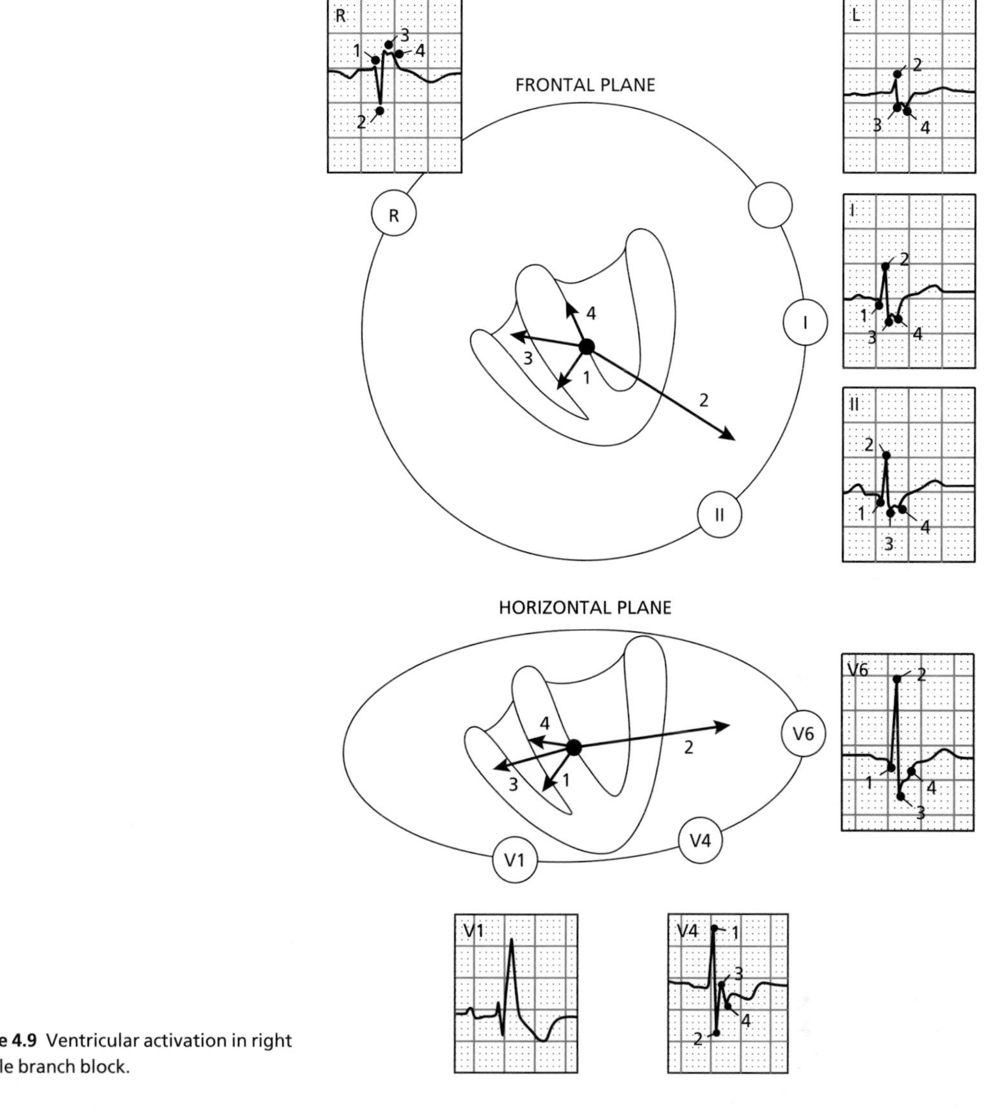

Figure 4.9 Ventricular activation in right bundle branch block.

Figure 4.10 Left bundle branch block.

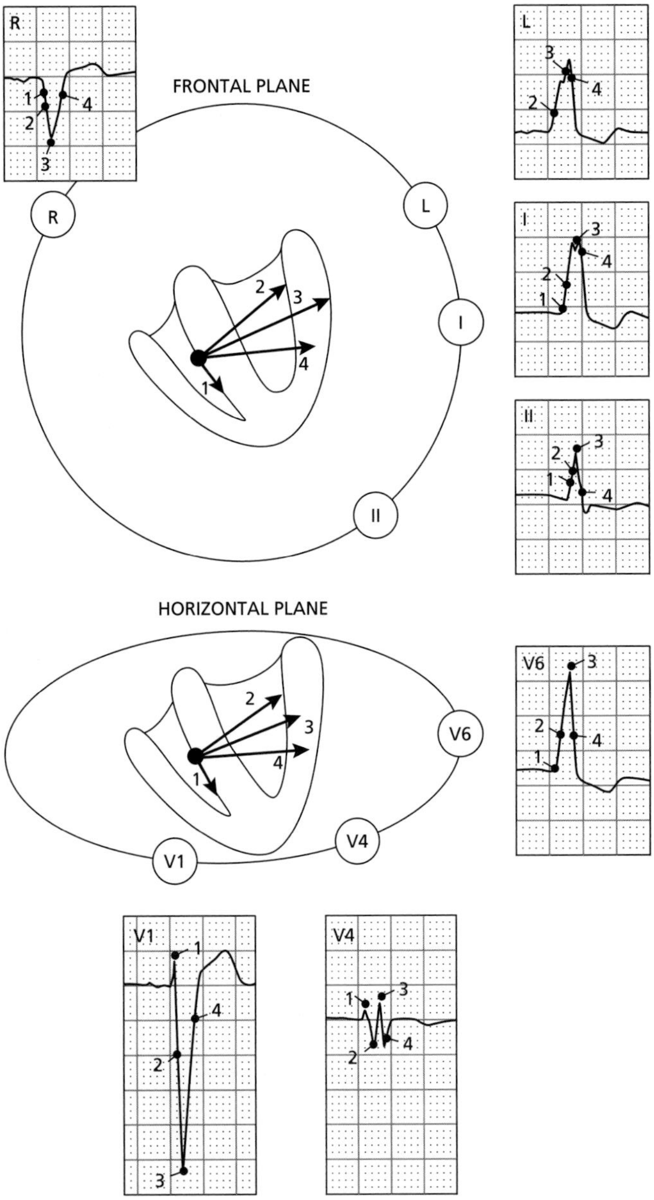

Figure 4.11 Ventricular activation in left bundle branch block.

block on tracings taken at different times or even on the same tracing. Second-degree, type II (Mobitz II) atrioventricular block with widened QRS complexes usually represents intermittent bilateral bundle branch block. Bundle branch block with first-degree atrioventricular block can represent conduction loss in one bundle branch with slow conduction through the other.

Three etiologies account for the majority of distal conduction disturbances in the industrialized world: ischemic heart disease, diffuse sclerodegenerative disease (Lenègre's disease), and calcification of the cardiac fibrous skeleton that impinges upon or invades the adjacent conduction structures (Lev's disease). However, the alert clinician should always suspect the presence of *Chagas' disease*

(American trypanosomiasis) in subjects from Central and South America who present with heart failure due to cardiomyopathy or with conduction deficits or arrhythmias. Indeed, identification of the fascicular blocks was first made by cardiologists treating patients with Chagas' disease.

Incomplete bundle branch block

Varying degrees of bundle branch block are recognized (Figure 4.12) and are frequently seen in clinical practice.

Aberrant ventricular conduction

A change in cycle length, particularly if abrupt, often precipitates functional bundle branch block, a phenomenon known as *aberrant ventricular conduction*. The most common form of aberrant conduction is *acceleration-dependent* bundle branch block (Figure 4.13). In most cases, this form of bundle branch block occurs when an impulse enters the distal conduction system prematurely, before the process of bundle branch repolarization is complete.

Ordinarily, *the time required for repolarization shortens incrementally as cycle length shortens incrementally*. Therefore when cycle length shortens abruptly, as in the case of premature atrial extrasystoles, for example, acceleration-dependent bundle branch block (aberrancy) may occur. Aberrant conduction following a long–short cycle sequence

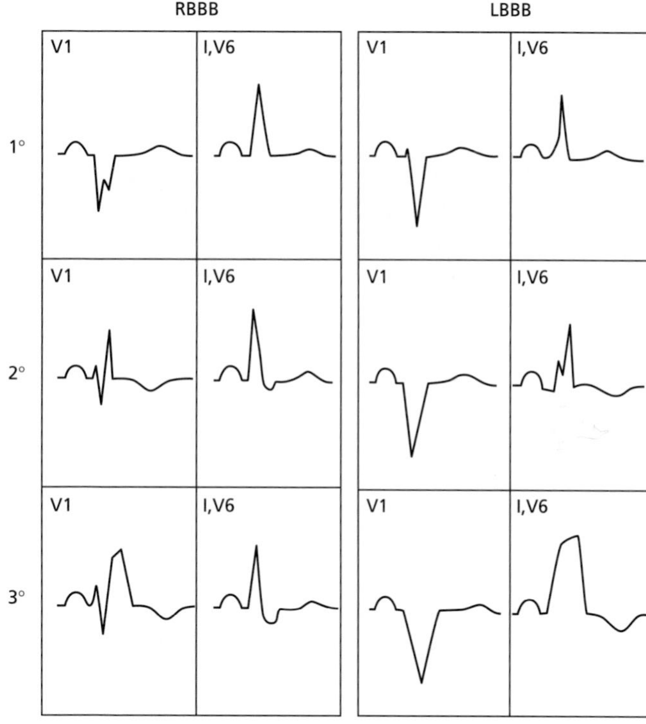

Figure 4.12 Degrees of bundle branch block.

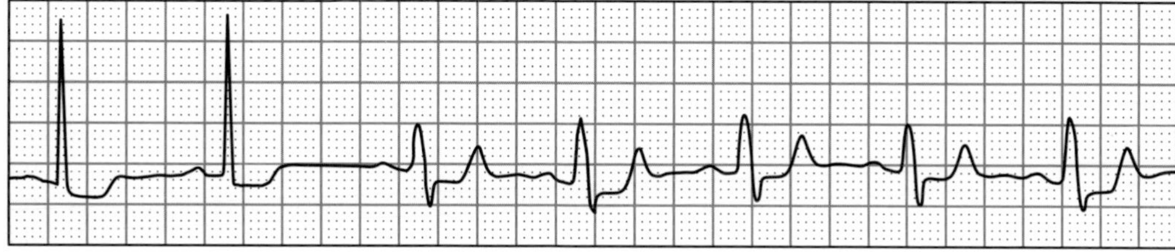

Figure 4.13 A slight acceleration in the rate precipitates left bundle branch block.

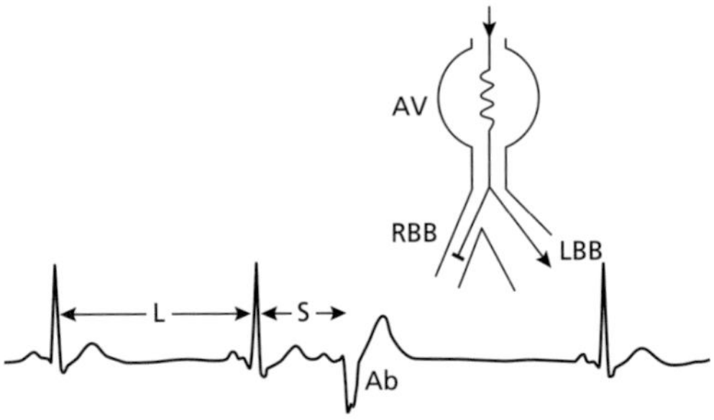

Figure 4.14 Ashman's phenomenon: a short cycle following a long cycle triggers acceleration-dependent bundle branch block.

is called *Ashman's phenomenon* (Figures 4.14 and 4.15).

Deceleration-dependent bundle branch block, a much less common form of aberrant conduction, occurs when cycle length *increases*. Spontaneous depolarization of fibers within one of the bundle branches is the most likely physiologic substrate of this form of aberrancy, the spontaneous automaticity of the affected segment creating a zone of defective conduction.

Nonspecific intraventricular conduction delay

Nonspecific intraventricular conduction delay (NSIVCD) is a term reserved for intraventricular conduction deficits that exhibit slow conduction (QRS >120 msec) but do not conform to the morphologic criteria for bundle branch block. The QRS morphology in these cases is often polyphasic and bizarre and occasionally manifests splintering of the QRS complex.

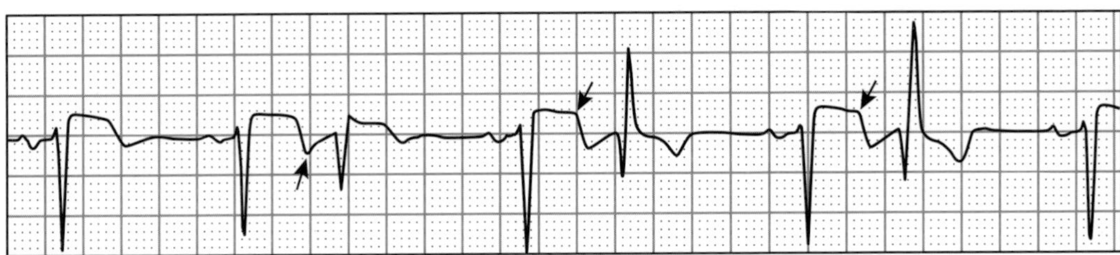

Figure 4.15 Ashman's phenomenon: atrial extrasystoles (*arrows*) ending long–short R–R intervals are conducted with varying degrees of right bundle branch block (V1).

5

CHAPTER 5

Myocardial ischemia and infarction

Coronary atherosclerosis, progressive obliteration of the arterial lumen, is the anatomic substrate of the *acute coronary syndromes.* Despite technological advances in the diagnosis of coronary artery disease (CAD), the patient interview and history remain a primary diagnostic tool, and the ECG an essential secondary tool for diagnosing and localizing ischemia in the evaluation of chest discomfort. Evidence of angina or an anginal equivalent, such as shortness of breath, must be diligently sought, bearing in mind that many individuals' perceptions have been colored by popular depictions of 'heart attack' as an instantly and dramatically catastrophic event and that many have a strong sense of denial. Diabetics may experience asymptomatic infarcts, and for others discomfort is unrelated to the chest, manifesting instead as referred sensations perceived as numbness, tingling, aching, or burning or as a sensation so poorly characterized that no term for it is offered. Misidentification of symptoms may prove more attractive if accompanied by nausea, clammy skin, or other manifestations of 'feeling sick' such as increased salivation.

Coronary artery anatomy

Two coronary arteries, the *right* and *left*, originate from the corresponding sinuses of Valsalva as the first branches of the aorta. Their points of origin, seen from within the aortic lumen, are called *ostia* (Figure 5.1).

The *left coronary artery* or *left main coronary artery* (1 in Figure 5.1) originates from the left aortic sinus of Valsalva, passes posterior to the trunk of the pulmonary artery, and emerges onto the sternocostal surface of the heart. Its distribution is illustrated in Figure 5.1. The left main coronary artery is a vessel of variable length, ranging from a very short trunk to a vessel of several centimeters.

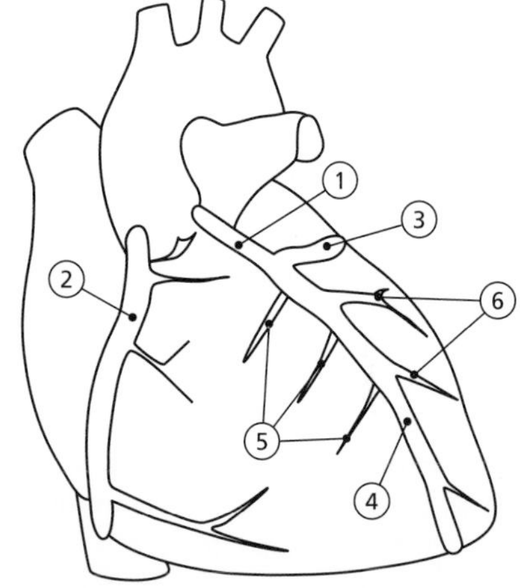

Figure 5.1 Coronary artery anatomy. 1: Left main, 2: Right coronary, 3: Circumflex, 4: Left anterior descending, 5: Septal perforators, 6: Diagonals.

Upon reaching the anterior interventricular sulcus, it divides into two constant branches: the left anterior descending artery, its more direct continuation, and the left circumflex artery.

The *left anterior descending artery* (4, Figure 5.1) and its branches are the principal blood supply of the anterior myocardial segment, which includes the left anterior free wall and anterior ventricular septum (Figure 5.5). Two important sets of secondary branches arise from the left anterior descending artery (LAD), the *septal perforating arteries* (5) and the *diagonal arteries* (6). The one to three diagonal branches supply the anterolateral free wall of the left ventricle and the three to five septal perforating branches supply the anterior two-thirds of the interventricular septum and the associated conduction structures, the right bundle branch and the anterior radiations of the left bundle branch.

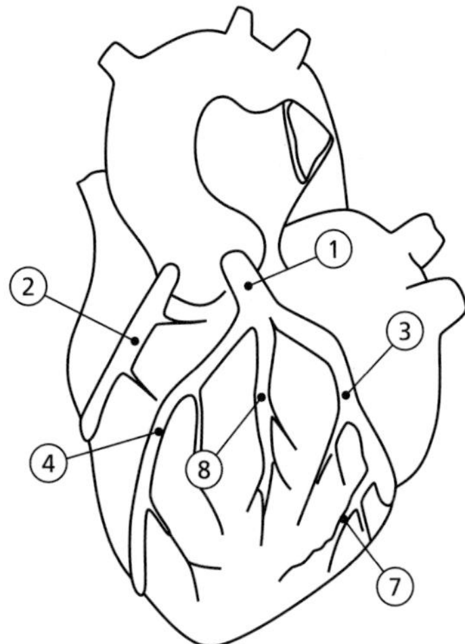

Figure 5.2 Coronary artery anatomy. 7: Obtuse marginals, 8: Ramus intermedius.

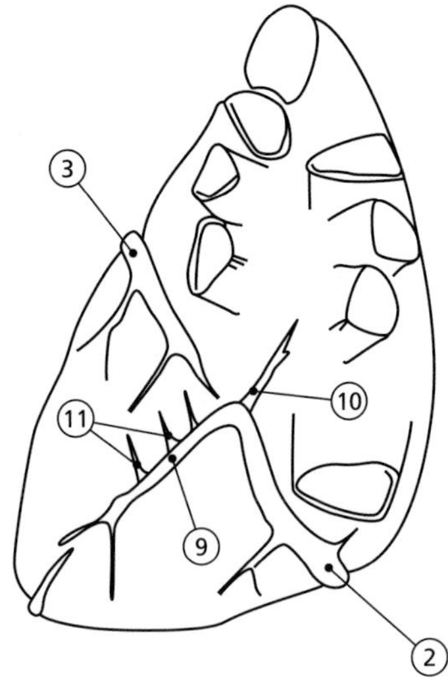

Figure 5.3 Coronary artery anatomy. 9: Posterior descending, 10: AV nodal, 11: Septal perforators.

The *left circumflex artery* (3, Figure 5.1 and Figure 5.2), the less direct continuation of the left coronary artery, originates from it at an angle and curves inferiorly in the atrioventricular sulcus toward the inferior (diaphragmatic) surface of the heart. It supplies the lateral wall of the left ventricle and the dorsal section of the left ventricular cone (compare Figure 5.11). As many as three *obtuse marginal arteries* (7, Figure 5.2) originate from the circumflex. In the majority of subjects the circumflex ends in a variable number of small muscular branches, but in 10% the circumflex reaches the *crux* (the intersection of the atrioventricular and posterior interventricular sulci) and continues in the posterior interventricular sulcus as the *posterior descending artery* (PDA). If the posterior descending artery is supplied by the left circumflex artery, the subject is said to be 'left coronary artery dominant.'

Sometimes the left main coronary artery does not end in a true bifurcation but terminates in three or more branches. If a trifurcation is present, with three vessels originating from the terminus of the left main coronary artery, the anterior is the left anterior descending artery (LAD), the posterior is the circumflex artery, and the remaining intermediate vessel is the *ramus intermedius* (8, Figure 5.2).

The *right coronary artery* (2 in Figures 5.1 to 5.3) originates from the right aortic sinus of Valsalva, passes between the pulmonary artery and the right atrial appendage, and turns downward in the atrioventricular sulcus toward the inferior surface of the right ventricle. In 55% of the population the sinoatrial node (2 in Figure 5.4) is supplied by a relatively large branch of the right coronary artery, the sinus node artery (1, Figure 5.4). As it circles the heart toward the inferior surface, the right coronary artery (RCA) supplies branches to the right atrium and ventricle, and at the crux the important *atrioventricular nodal artery* (7, Figure 5.4).

At the crux the RCA turns sharply downward, forming the 'shepherd's crook,' to continue as the *posterior descending artery* (9, Figure 5.3 and 10, Figure 5.4). The posterior descending artery (PDA) is the parallel counterpart of the left anterior descending artery and like the LAD supplies septal perforating branches (11, Figure 5.3) to the posterior one-third of the septum and associated conduction structures, the posterior and septal radiations of the left bundle branch (6 and 9, Figure 5.4). The septal perforating branches of the right and left coronary arteries form anastomoses, establishing an important source of collateral circulation. When the posterior descending artery is supplied by the right coronary artery, as in the majority of cases, the subject is said to be 'right coronary dominant.'

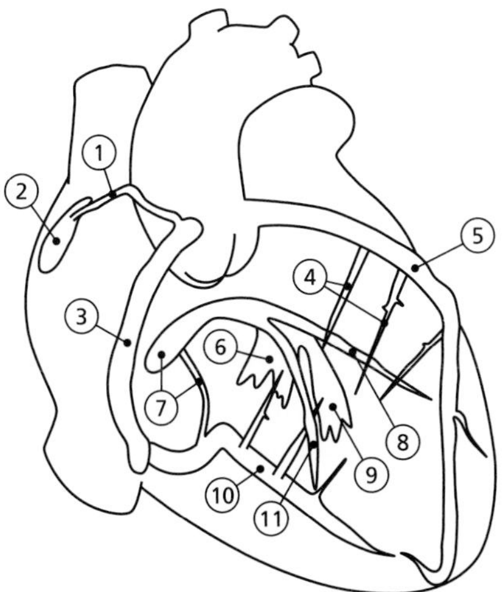

Figure 5.4 The distal conduction system. 1: Sinus node artery, 2: Sinus node, 3: Right coronary artery, 4: Septal perforators, 5: Left anterior descending artery, 6: Left posterior fascicle, 7: AV node & artery, 8: Left anterior fascicle, 9: Left septal fascicle, 10: Posterior descending artery, 11: Right bundle branch.

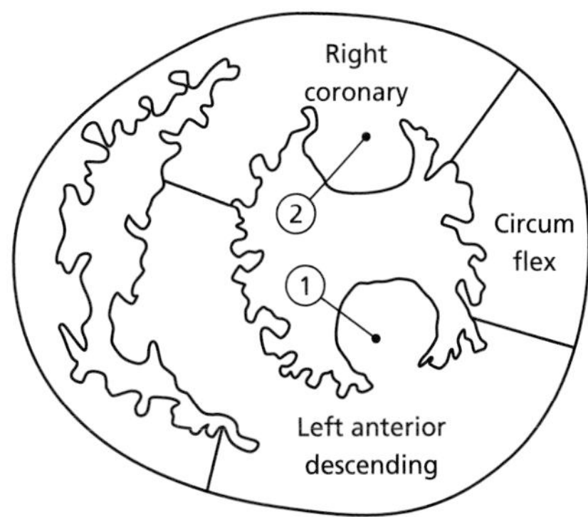

Figure 5.5 The major myocardial segments and their arterial supply. 1: Anterior papillary muscle, 2: Posterior papillary muscle.

The electrocardiogram of myocardial ischemia

The ECG findings indicative of myocardial ischemia may be, and often are, totally absent from a tracing taken with the subject comfortable and at rest. In fact, *it may be flatly asserted that a normal ECG obtained under such conditions is meaningless as far as the detection of ischemia is concerned.*

Some of the ECG findings suggestive of ischemia are shown in Figure 5.6. These markers involve changes in the ST segment and T wave. It should be recalled that the upslope of the normal ST segment is gradual, merging imperceptibly with the proximal limb of the T wave *without abrupt angles* or changes in polarity. *A normal ST segment is not flat and it is not normally elevated or depressed.*

Ischemia often causes *ST segment depression* with a sharp angle at the junction of the ST segment and T wave (2 and 3 in Figure 5.6). The classic ST segment depression that usually indicates ischemia is in sharp contrast to the ST segment change that occurs during *variant* or *Prinzmetal's angina*. During these attacks, provoked by transient coronary vasospasm, ST segment elevation is seen (5 in Figure 5.6); after vasospasm subsides, the ST segment returns to baseline. Although not specific, *flattening of the ST segment* is a suspicious finding (Figure 5.7) that often reflects ischemia.

Another commonly seen indication of ischemia is *T wave inversion* (4, Figure 5.6). Inverted T waves due to ischemia are typically narrow and relatively symmetrical ('arrowhead T waves'). Bundle branch

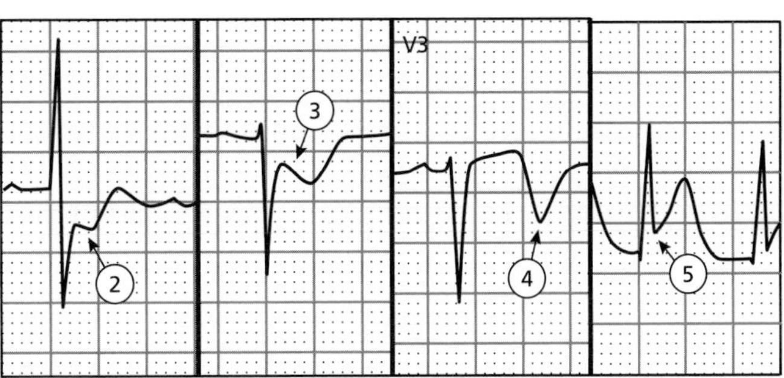

Figure 5.6 Ischemic changes.

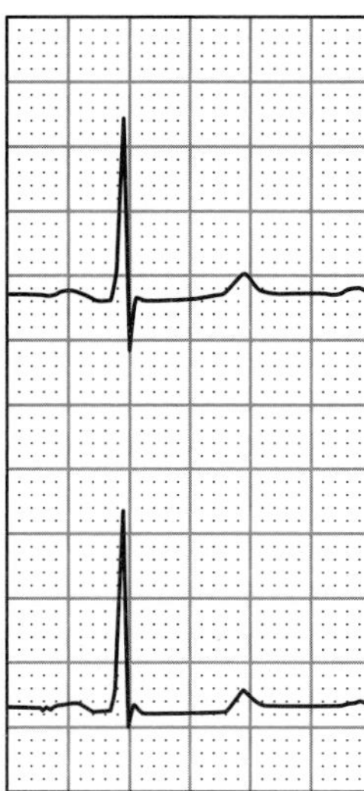

Figure 5.7 Flattening of the ST segment (leads V5 and V6).

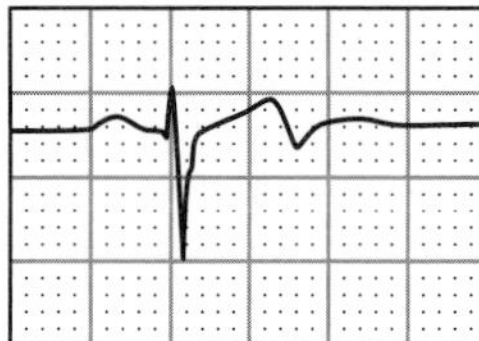

Figure 5.8 The T wave deformity of Wellen's syndrome (lead V2).

block, fully evolved pericarditis and ventricular hypertrophy are also common causes of T wave inversion.

Wellen's syndrome refers to *T wave inversion or biphasic T waves* usually noted in precordial leads V1–V3 (Figure 5.8). Patients presenting with these findings may be experiencing chest discomfort or may be asymptomatic at the time the ECG is recorded. Cardiac enzymes are usually within normal limits, but because this ECG presentation often correlates with critical stenosis in the proximal left anterior descending (LAD) artery and impending anterior wall infarction, exercise testing is contraindicated and angiography should be performed at the earliest opportunity.

Myocardial infarction

According to classic ECG theory, three markers are used to diagnose *acute myocardial infarction* (AMI): (1) T wave inversion; (2) ST segment elevation; and (3) abnormal Q waves. In the classic paradigm, T wave inversion is thought to reflect myocardial ischemia, ST segment changes represent myocardial injury and pathologic Q waves indicate necrosis. Infarction Q waves are by definition 40 msec (0.04 sec) or more in duration. Changes that appear in leads facing the ischemic segment are called *indicative changes* whereas changes that occur in leads facing away from the ischemic areas are known as *reciprocal changes.*

Using these criteria, the incidence of myocardial infarction would be grossly underestimated and many infarctions missed; the majority of infarctions presenting in emergency departments result *only in T wave inversion and ST segment depression.* These infarctions, formerly known as 'subendocardial' infarctions, are better called *non-Q wave* infarctions. A more subtle but equally important indication of infarction is *loss of R wave amplitude*, which can be confirmed when serial ECG tracings are examined.

Other conditions, including the cardiomyopathies, left ventricular hypertrophy, and the Wolff–Parkinson–White syndrome, can produce spurious infarct patterns.

The ECG pattern of infarction typically evolves in stages. The *hyperacute stage*, the very earliest stage, represents the first ECG manifestation of infarction; the *acute phase* is observed in the first day to week; the *recent phase* reflects an infarct less than a month old; and the term *old infarction* refers to those healing infarcts generally over three months old.

The *hyperacute phase* is characterized by abnormally tall, symmetrical T waves with or without ST segment elevation (Figure 5.9). Prompt recognition of this phase is necessary for timely intervention.

As the infarction progresses to the *acute phase*, ST segment elevation occurs in those leads facing the ischemic area and persists as a feature of subsequent stages. Early in the evolution of the infarct pattern, T waves begin to invert. Finally, Q waves, the classic *sine qua non* of infarction, appear in the leads facing the infarcted area (indicative leads). Elevation of the ST segment and inversion of the T wave combine to produce a gracefully arched ST–T complex ('coving'), while the distal limb of the T wave straightens ('planes'), producing the typical *cove-plane T wave.* An infarction Q wave

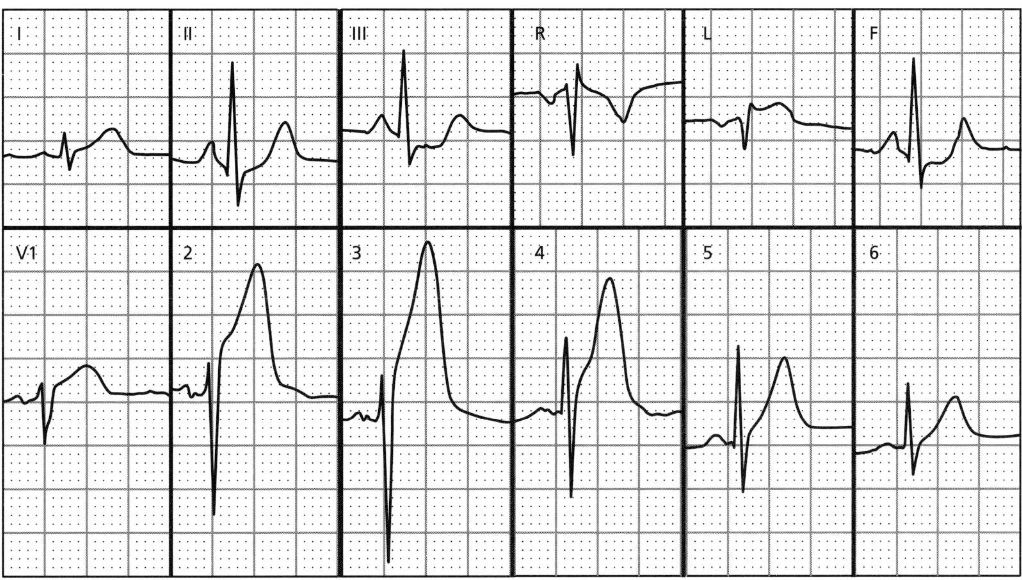

Figure 5.9 The hyperacute phase of myocardial infarction. Tall, symmetrical T waves appear in the ischemic segment (V2–V5).

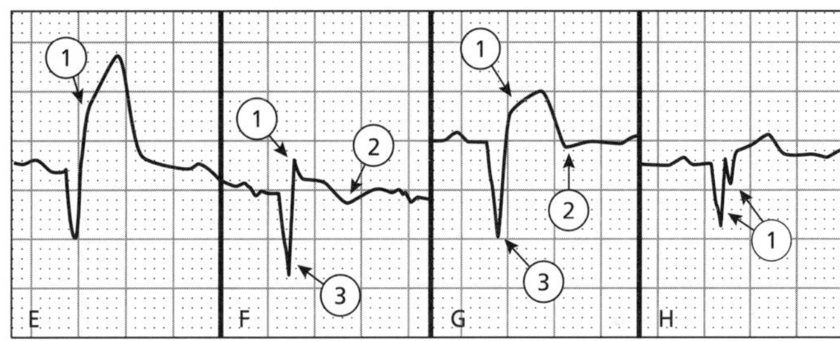

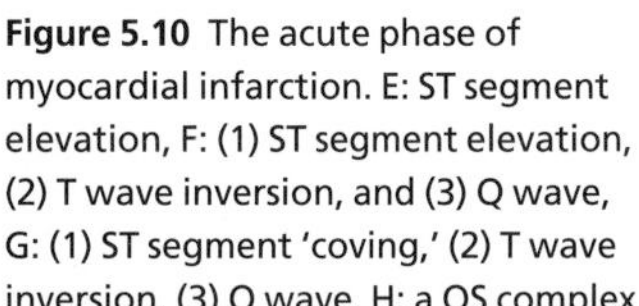

Figure 5.10 The acute phase of myocardial infarction. E: ST segment elevation, F: (1) ST segment elevation, (2) T wave inversion, and (3) Q wave, G: (1) ST segment 'coving,' (2) T wave inversion, (3) Q wave, H: a QS complex.

may result in two successive negative waves written below the baseline so that a *QS complex* results (Figure 5.10).

The following myocardial segments can be distinguished electrocardiographically: *anterior* (leads V3 and V4), *septal* (V1 and V2), *anteroseptal* (V1–V4), *lateral* (I, aVL, V5 and V6), *anterolateral* (I, aVL and V3–V6), *inferior* (II, III and aVF), and *posterior* (reciprocal changes V1–V3).

Anterior wall myocardial infarction (AWMI) is diagnosed when ST segment elevation, T wave inversion and Q waves appear in the precordial leads. The infarction may remain localized (septal), or involve all or part of the left ventricular free wall. Anterior wall infarction results from occlusion of the left coronary artery or its anterior descending branch. An evolving anterior wall infarction is shown in Figure 5.11, in which coving of the ST segments, T wave inversion, and abnormally wide Q waves are noted in leads V1–V4. The loss of R wave amplitude in V5 and V6 reflects loss of voltage due to necrosis of the myocardium underlying those leads. Anterior wall infarctions are associated with serious atrioventricular and intraventricular conduction defects preceded by fascicular and/or bundle branch blocks, a higher incidence of cardiogenic shock, and an overall higher mortality than infarctions of other segments.

Lateral wall myocardial infarction (LWMI) is diagnosed when ST segment elevation, T wave inversion and Q waves appear in the lateral leads. Lateral wall infarcts generally result from occlusion of the circumflex branch of the left coronary artery. An example of remote lateral wall infarction shows that ST segment displacement and T wave inversion resolve over time as the infarction heals

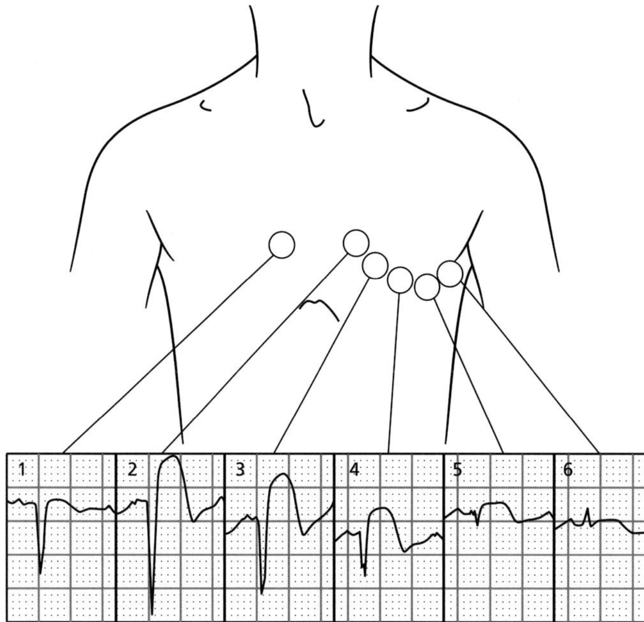

Figure 5.11 Anterior wall myocardial infarction.

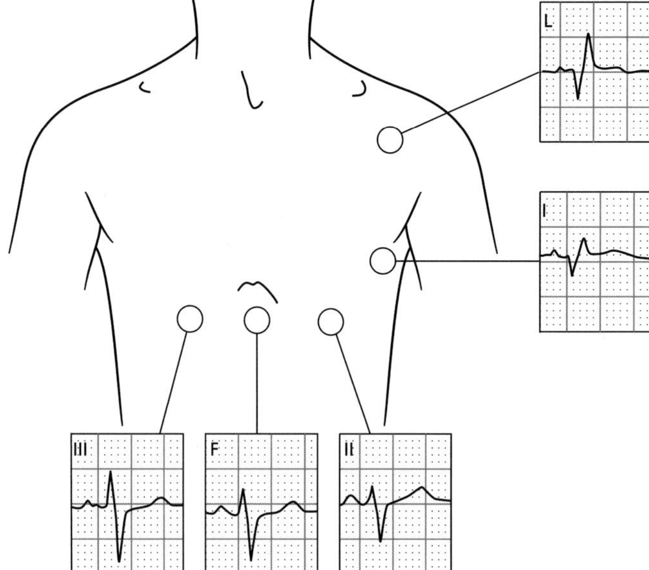

Figure 5.12 Lateral wall myocardial infarction.

(Figure 5.12). Conduction deficits rarely accompany lateral wall infarcts.

Inferior wall myocardial infarction (IWMI) is diagnosed when ST segment elevation, T wave inversion and Q waves appear in the inferior leads. Figure 5.13 illustrates the acute stage of an inferior wall infarct. The leads facing the infarction record the classic *indicative changes*, which at this stage consist of marked ST segment (J point) elevation and pointed, symmetrical T waves. The leads facing away from the infarcting segment record a mirror image of the ST–T wave abnormalities, the *reciprocal changes*. Inferior wall infarctions are due to occlusion of the right coronary artery and are often

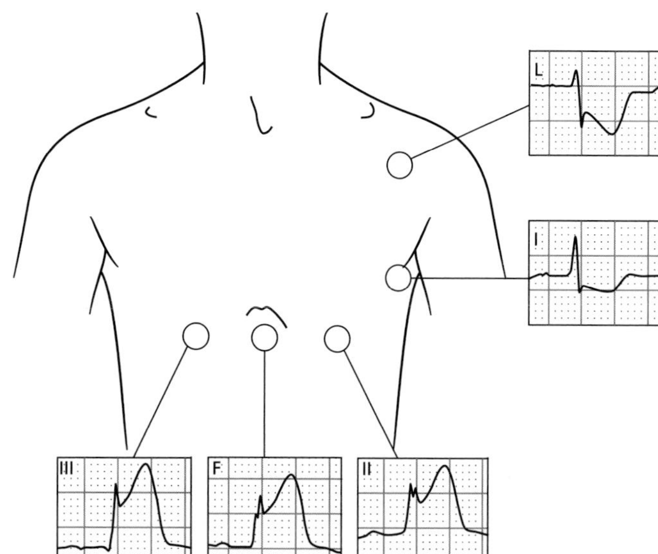

Figure 5.13 Inferior wall myocardial infarction.

accompanied by bradyarrhythmias, particularly sinus bradycardia and accelerated idioventricular rhythm (AIVR), and all degrees of atrioventricular block. Right ventricular infarction commonly complicates right coronary artery occlusion.

Because no conventional ECG leads face the posterior wall (Figure 5.14), the diagnosis of *posterior wall myocardial infarction* (PWMI) is made from reciprocal changes that appear in the anterior leads (V1–V3). Figure 5.15 shows the characteristic triad of (1) tall R waves, (2) depressed ST segments, and (3) tall, symmetrical T waves in leads V2 and V3. Coexisting inferior or lateral wall infarctions are commonly noted, with many posterior infarcts representing territorial extension of an inferior wall infarction. *Voltage drop-off*, a marked loss of R wave amplitude in the left precordial leads, is common.

Traditional teaching long held that the abnormal Q wave is the essential marker of a transmural ('full-thickness') infarction. Less than full-thickness infarcts were known as *subendocardial infarcts*, but subsequent study demonstrated that the distinctions were untenable. Current terminology favors the term *non-Q wave infarction* for this common subset. It would appear that infarctions that initially exhibit Q waves carry a higher *initial* mortality rate, but non-Q wave infarcts, which are prone to subsequent extension, were frequently noted to 'complete' to Q wave infarcts with high risk to patients.

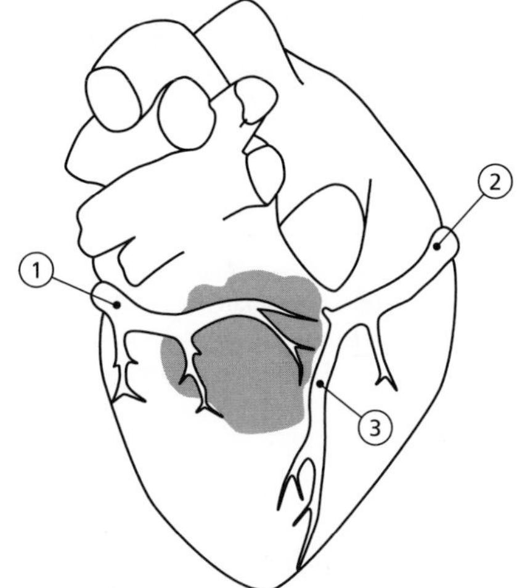

Figure 5.14 The posterior myocardial segment and its blood supply. 1: circumflex coronary artery, 2: right coronary artery, 3: posterior descending coronary artery.

The electrocardiogram of subarachnoid hemorrhage

For reasons that are not entirely clear, *subarachnoid hemorrhage* (SAH) is well known to produce acute

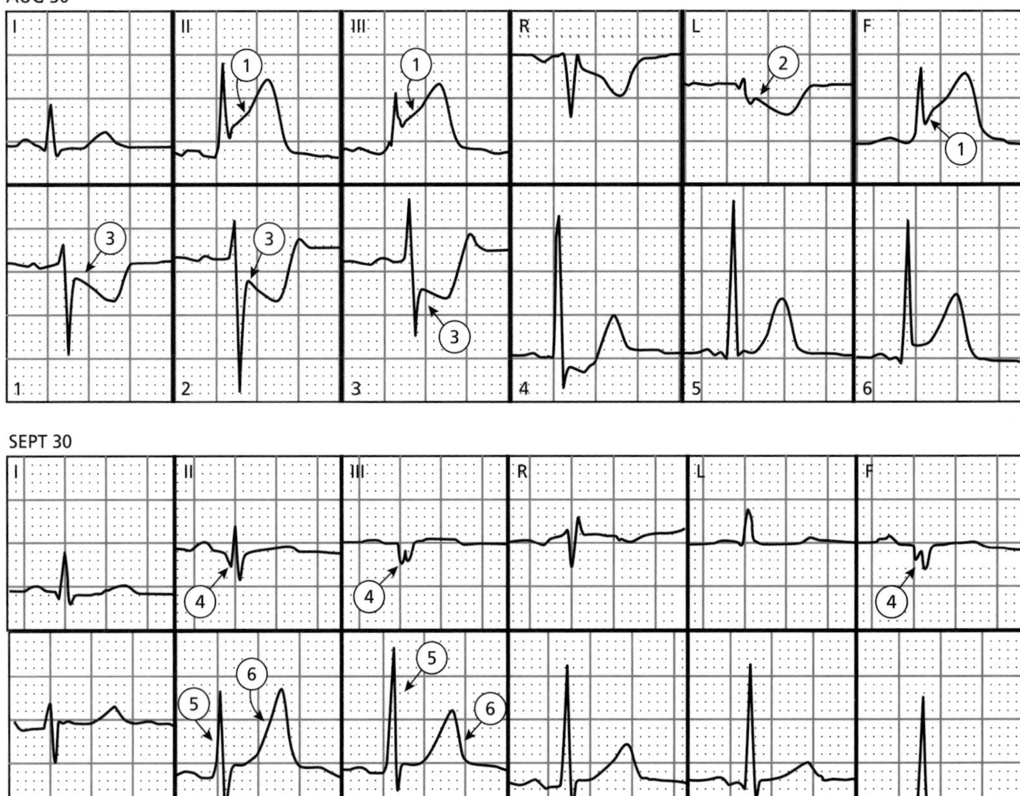

Figure 5.15 Posterior wall myocardial infarction complicating an inferior wall infarct: precordial ST segment depression (V1–V3) represents the hyperacute phase of the posterior infarction (3, Aug 30 tracing). Concomitant infarction of the inferior wall resulting in QS complexes (4) are noted on the Sept 30 tracing as well as prominent R waves (5) and tall T waves (6) that signal posterior wall extension.

ECG changes that closely mimic those of myocardial ischemia. Ventricular wall motion abnormalities and even acute pulmonary edema have also been documented. Marked T wave inversion, in which the depth of the T wave may occasionally equal or surpass the amplitude of the QRS complex, is occasionally seen (Figure 5.16). Sometimes called 'cerebral T waves' or 'giant T waves,' these are probably the largest T waves seen in clinical practice.

More commonly, widespread T wave inversion and QT prolongation are noted, particularly in the lateral and precordial leads (Figure 5.17). Unlike typical ischemic changes, which are usually limited to affected myocardial segments, the T wave

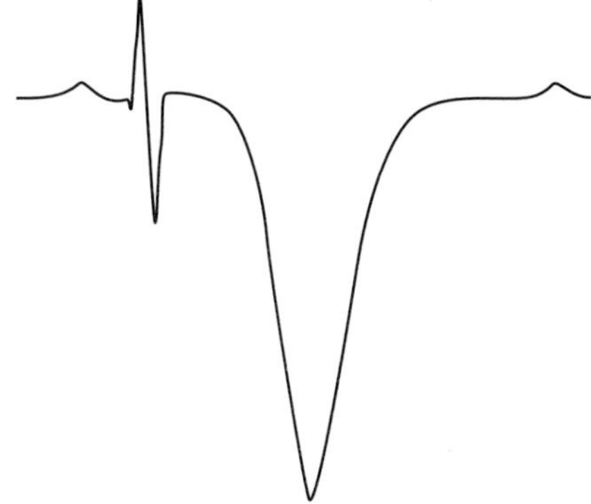

Figure 5.16 The giant inverted T wave of subarachnoid hemorrhage.

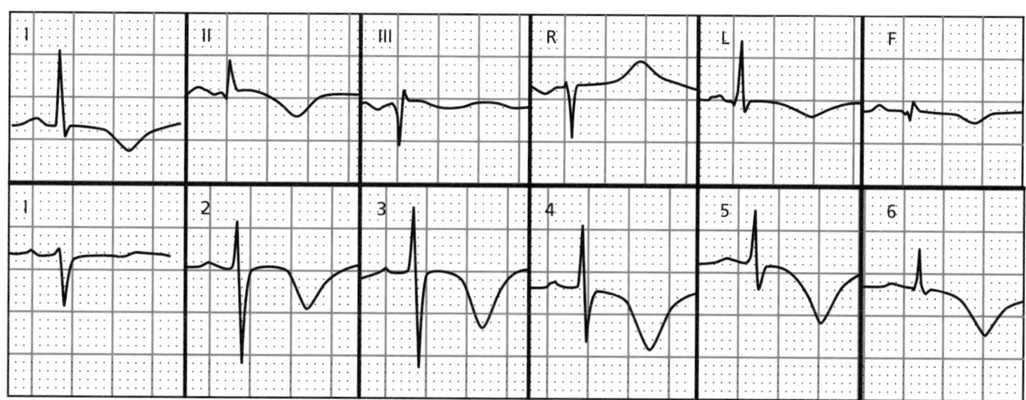

Figure 5.17 The ECG of a patient with subarachnoid hemorrhage: widespread T wave inversion and prolongation of the QT interval.

inversion of SAH tends to occur across the usual segmental boundaries, giving the appearance of 'global ischemia.' Atrial and ventricular arrhythmias, including torsade de pointes, are well documented in this setting. Increased sympathetic tone appears to be the trigger event leading to polymorphic ventricular tachycardia, and β-blockers may suppress arrhythmias in this setting.

Self-Assessment Test Two

Identify the abnormalities in the following three tracings.

2.1.

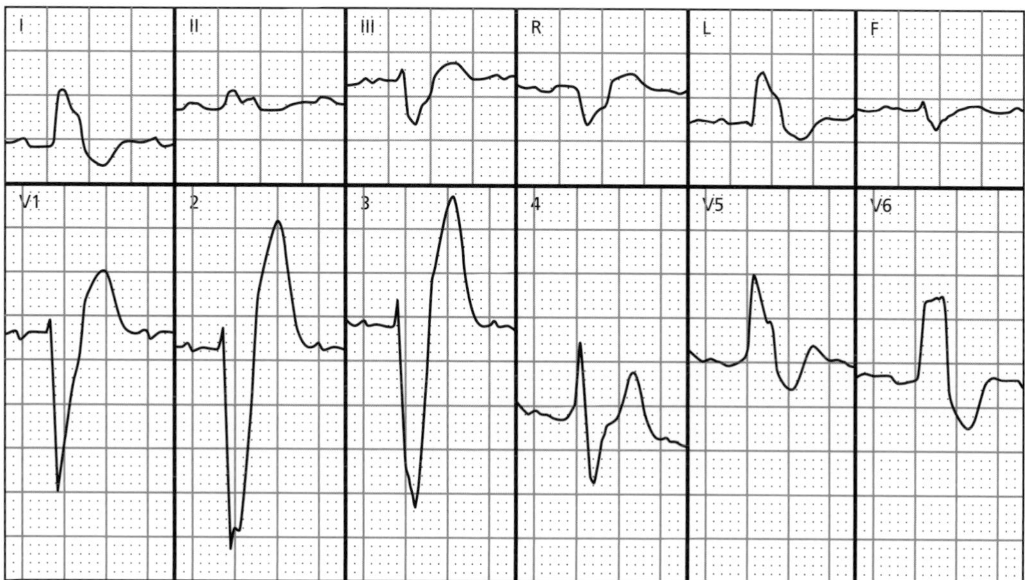

2.2.

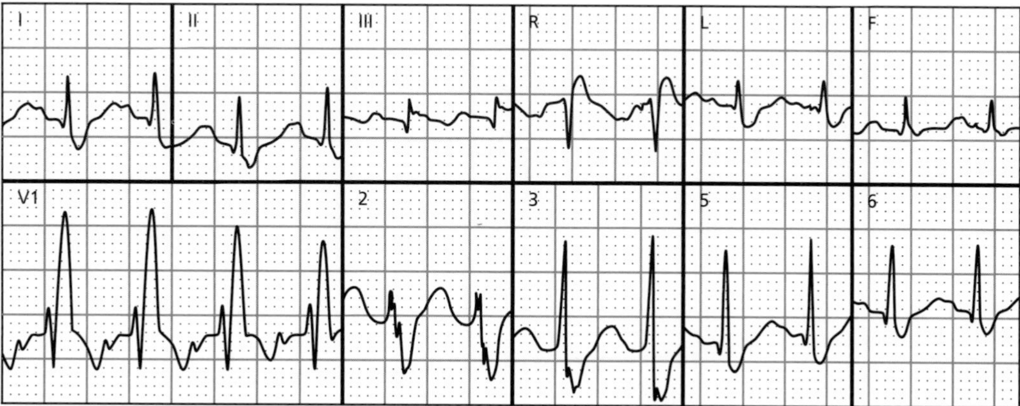

2.3.

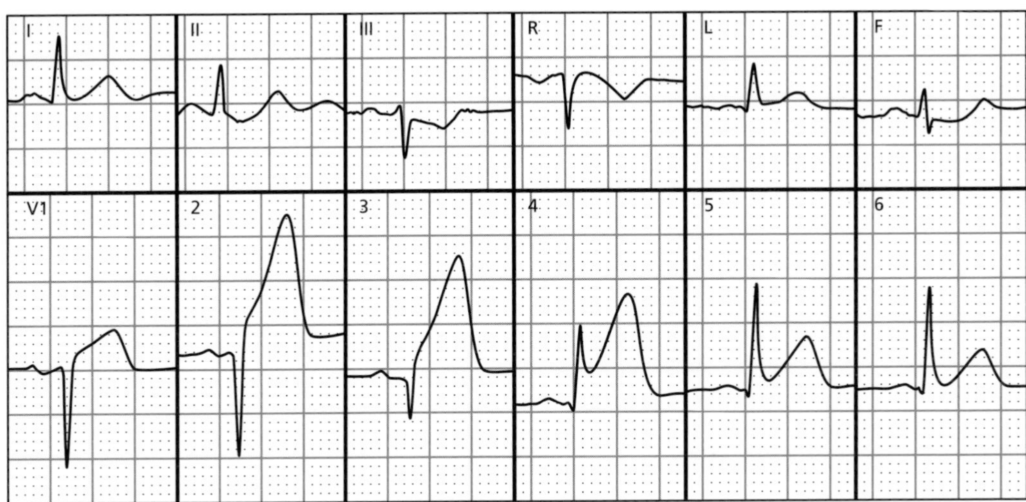

2.4. The acute phase of myocardial infarction is diagnosed primarily by the observation of . . .
   a. diagnostic Q waves in leads facing the infarcted area
   b. marked T wave inversion in the leads facing the infarcted area
   c. tall, symmetrical T waves with or without ST segment elevation

2.5. Variant or Prinzmetal's angina is associated with . . .
   a. widespread ST segment depression and T wave inversion
   b. transient ST segment elevation that persists during the bout of angina
   c. no diagnostically significant ST segment or T wave changes

2.6. Inferior wall myocardial infarction is diagnosed from ST–T wave changes and/or Q waves in . . .
   a. leads II, III and aVF
   b. leads V1–V6
   c. leads I and aVL

Identify the abnormalities in the following three tracings.

2.7.

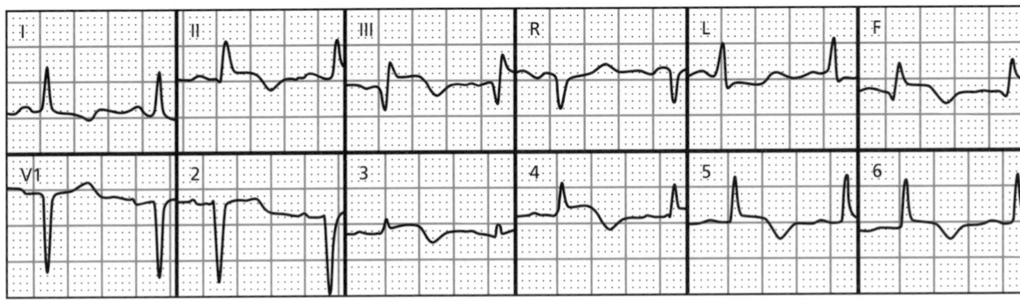

2.8.

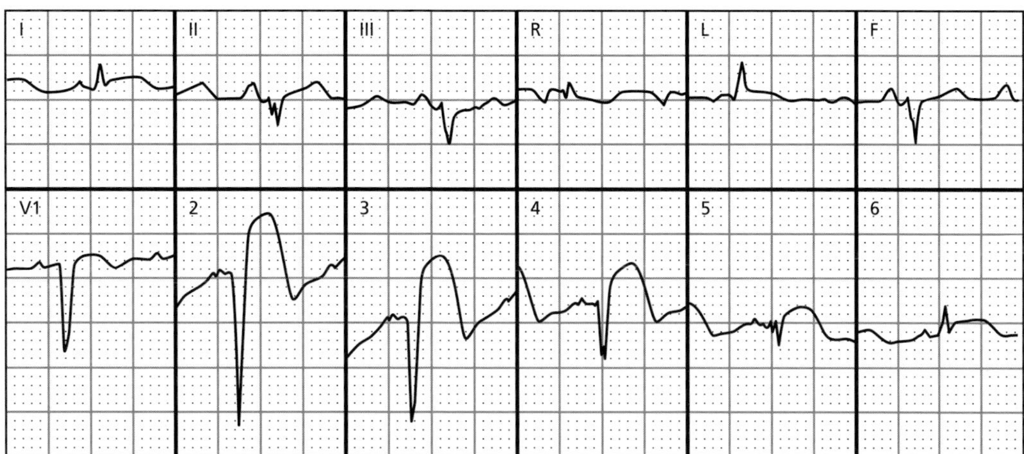

2.9.

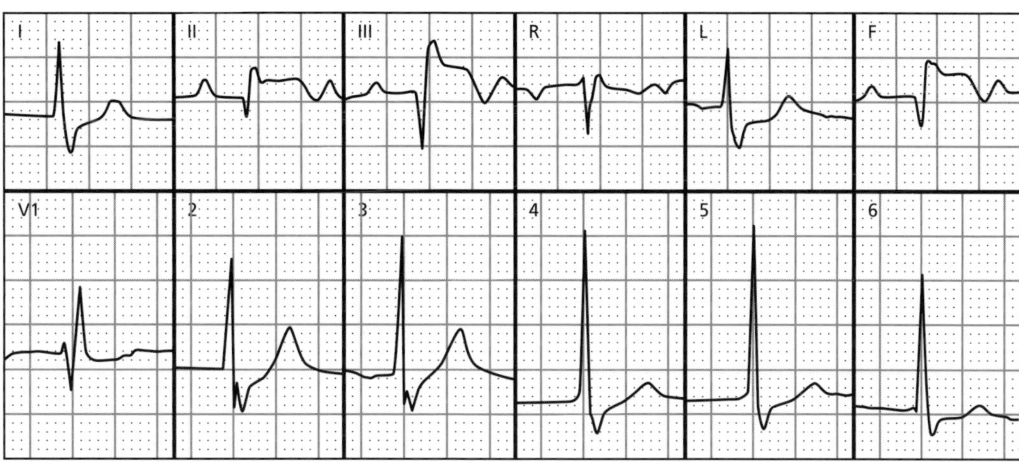

2.10. Ventricular activation time is reflected by the . . . interval, which normally does not exceed . . . second in lead V6.

a. QT, 0.12
b. QR, 0.035
c. QR, 0.45

2.11. T wave inversion across segmental boundaries tends to occur in connection with . . .

a. Wellen's syndrome
b. subarachnoid hemorrhage
c. vasospastic (Prinzmetal's) angina

2.12. Identify the abnormality in the following tracings.

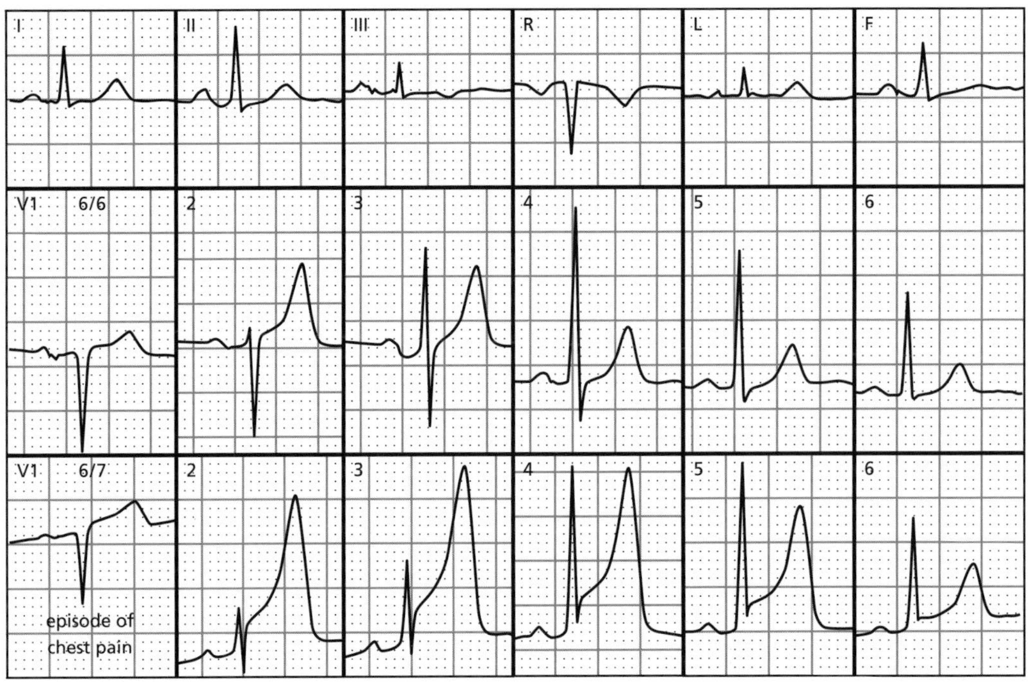

2.13. Left anterior fascicular block results in left axis deviation, . . . complexes in the lateral leads and . . . complexes in leads III and aVF.

a. qR, RS
b. rS, qR
c. qR, rS

Identify the abnormalities in the following twelve tracings.

2.14.

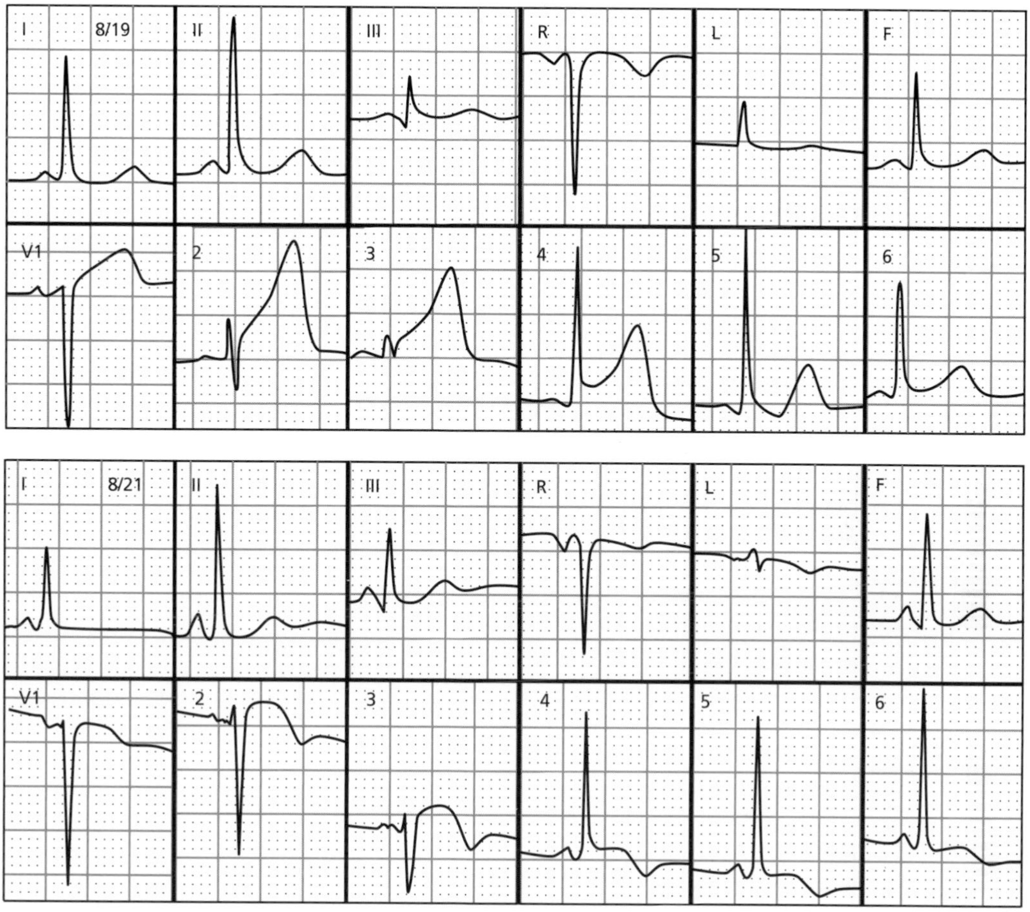

2.15.

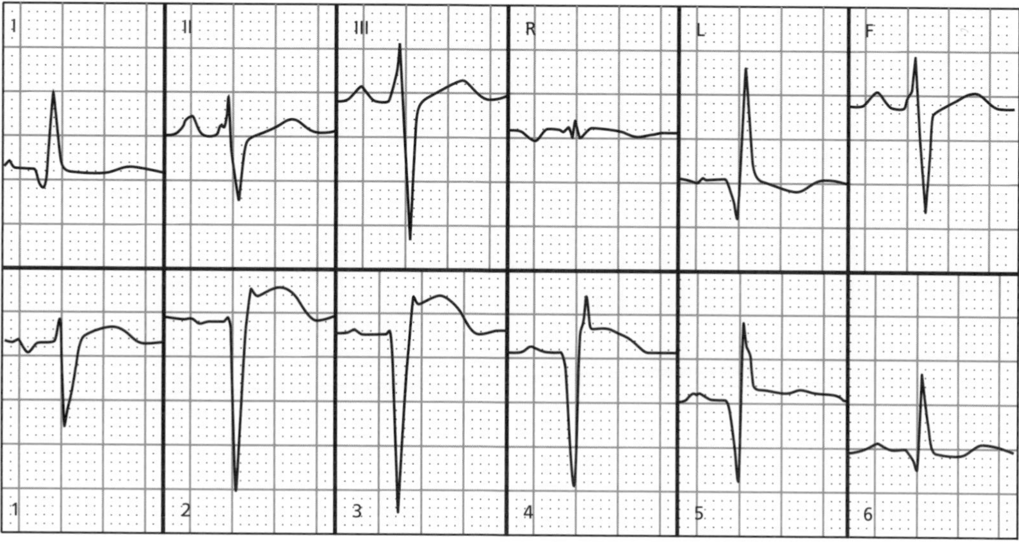

2.16.

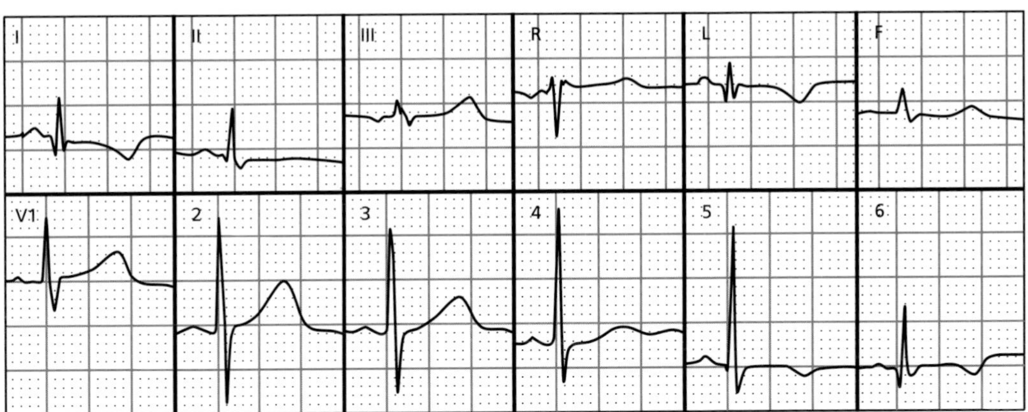
I
II
III
R
L
F
V1
2
3
4
5
6

2.17.

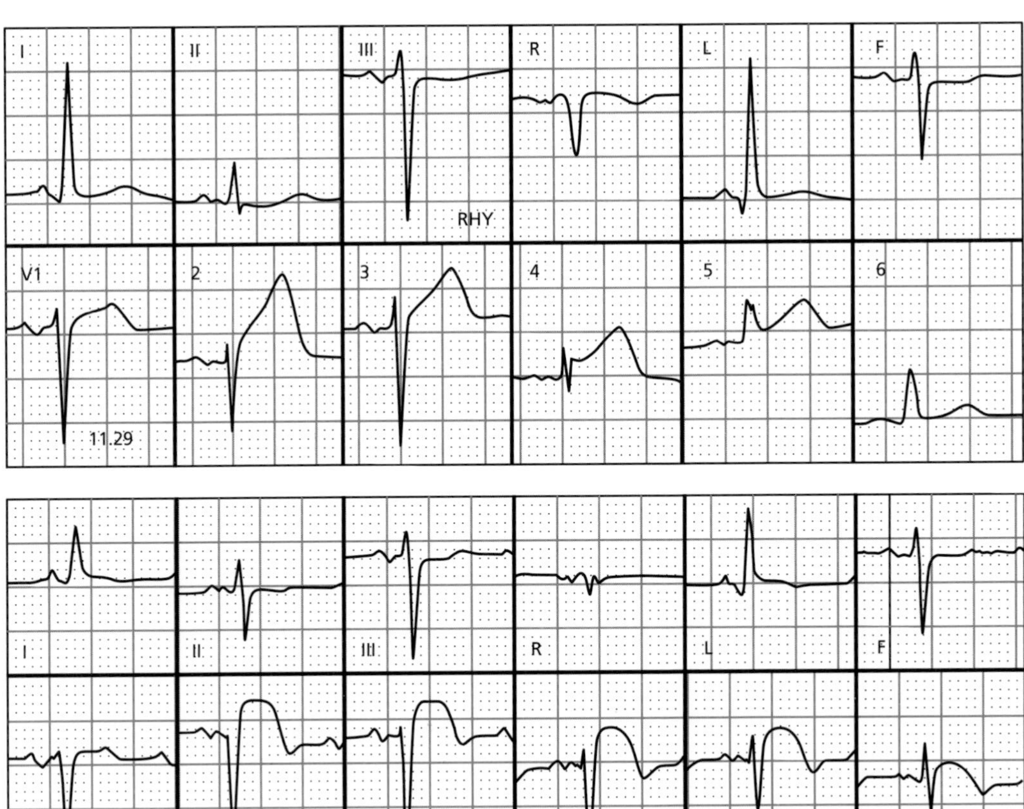
I
II
III
RHY
R
L
F
V1
11.29
2
3
4
5
6
I
II
III
R
L
F
V1
11.30
2
3
4
5
6

2.18.

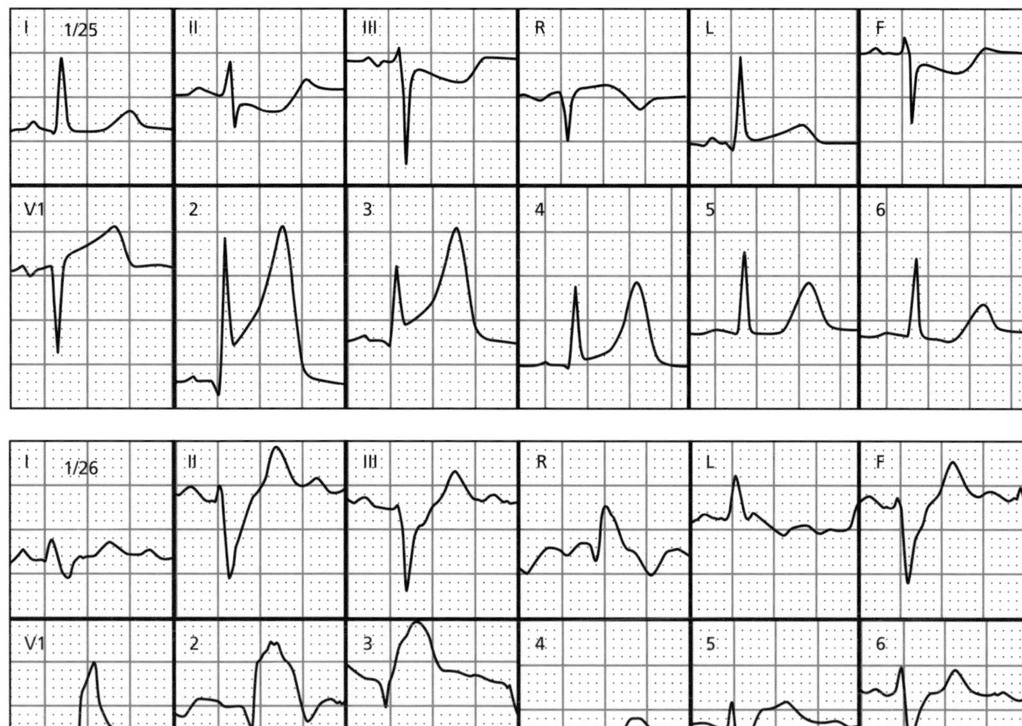
I
1/25
II
III
R
L
F
V1
2
3
4
5
6
I
1/26
II
III
R
L
F
V1
2
3
4
5
6

2.19.

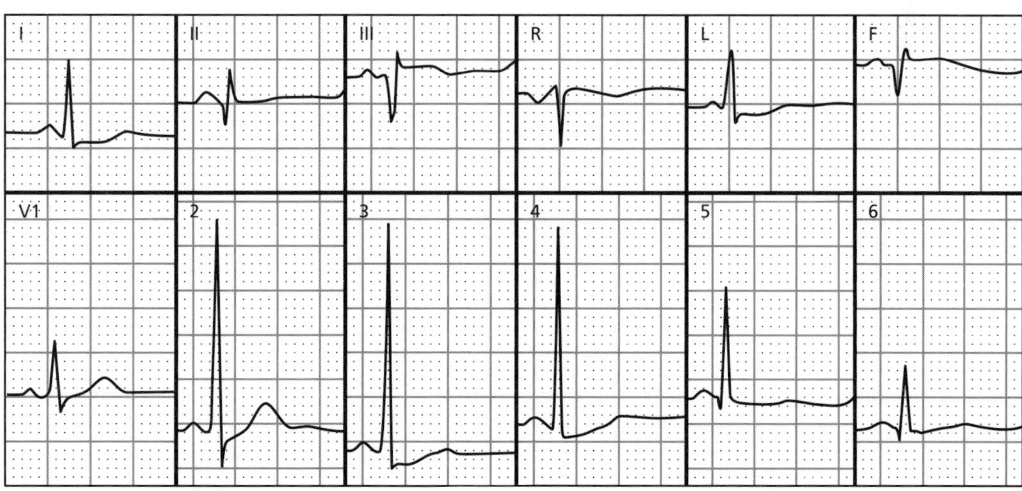
I
II
III
R
L
F
V1
2
3
4
5
6

2.20.

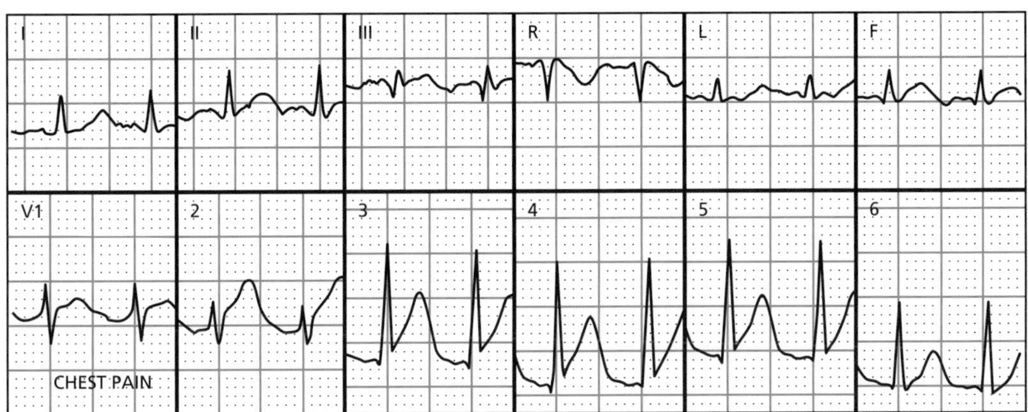
I
II
III
R
L
F
V1
2
3
4
5
6
CHEST PAIN

2.21.

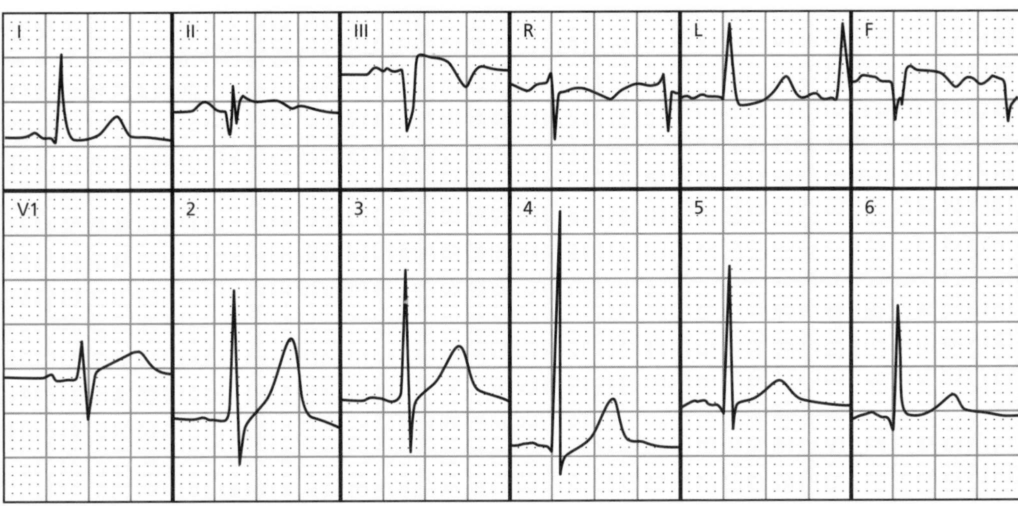
I
II
III
R
L
F
V1
2
3
4
5
6

2.22.

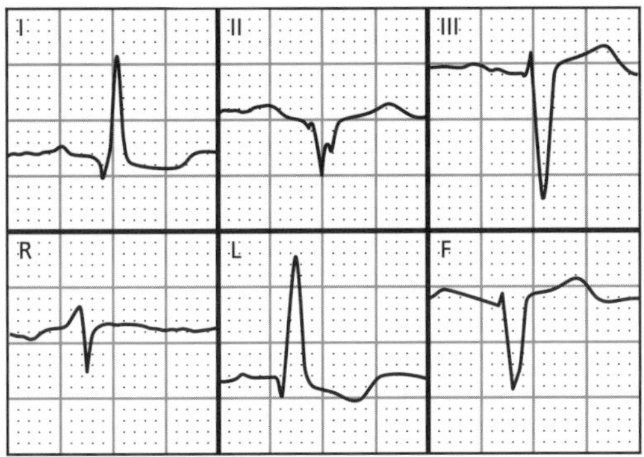
I
II
III
R
L
F

2.23.

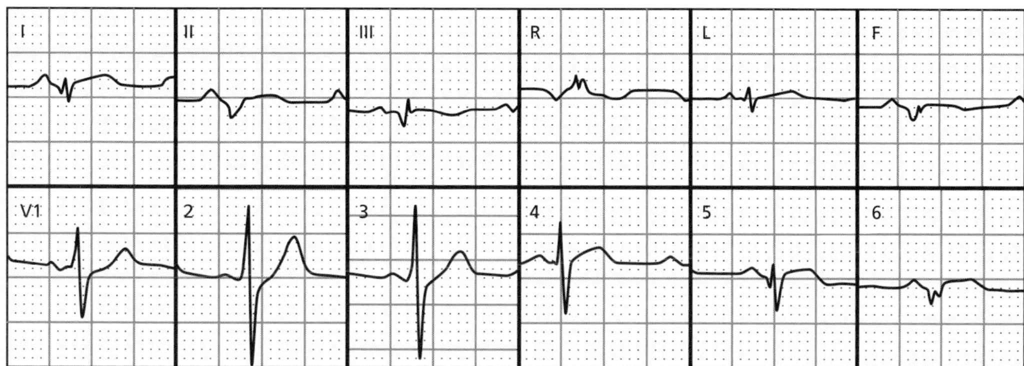
I
II
III
R
L
F
V1
2
3
4
5
6

2.24.

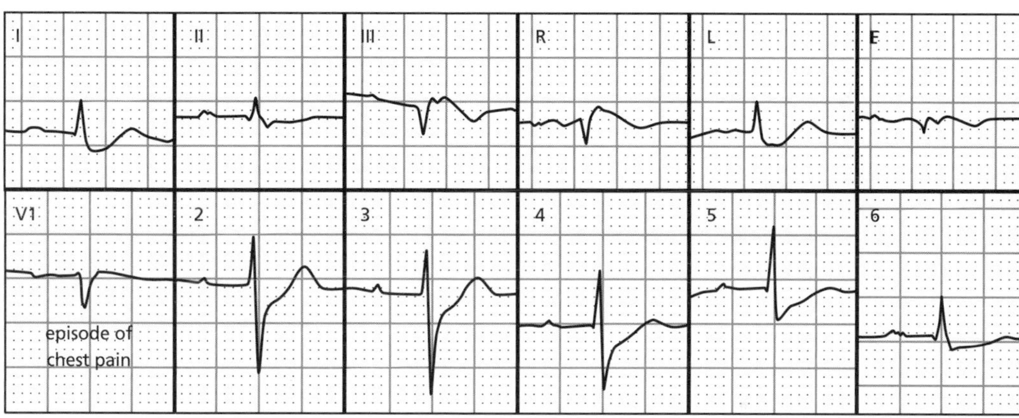
I
II
III
R
L
F
V1
episode of
chest pain
2
3
4
5
6

2.25.

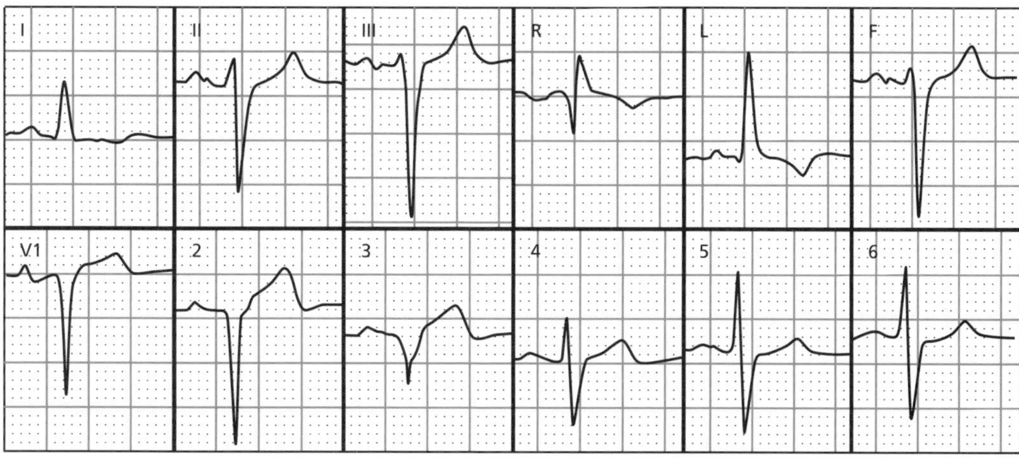
I
II
III
R
L
F
V1
2
3
4
5
6

CHAPTER 6

Chamber enlargement and hypertrophy

The forces that produce the ECG originate primarily from the left ventricle and therefore reflect its normal preponderance. However, factors other than simple muscle mass influence the QRS complex, among them the conductivity of body tissue, the distance of the surface electrodes from the heart, and intraventricular pressure and volume. Because air and fat are poor conductors, subjects with emphysema or obesity are more likely to produce tracings with low voltage. On the other hand, larger than average QRS complexes are commonly recorded from young, asthenic subjects with thin chest walls, producing high-amplitude tracings lacking in diagnostic significance.

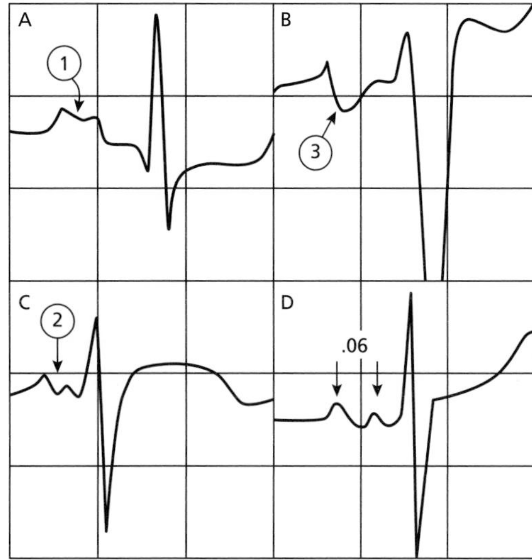

Figure 6.1 Left atrial abnormality showing wide, notched P waves.

Atrial abnormalities

The normal sinus P wave, representing the sequential depolarization of the atria, assumes the shape of a truncated pyramid with rounded contours. Normal P wave height does not exceed 2.5 mm, and the duration does not exceed 110 msec (0.11 sec). The normal P wave axis is +15 to +75 degrees, making it tallest in lead II, and positive in leads I, II and aVF and precordial leads V4–V6.

Because the left atrium is depolarized slightly later than the right, its electrical potentials account for the inscription of the last half of the P wave. Conduction delay through the left atrium (usually due to dilatation) results in changes that are labeled *left atrial abnormality* (LAA). The criteria for left atrial abnormality include: increased P wave duration (> 120 msec); notching of the P wave with a 'peak to peak' interval of 40 msec or more (1–2 in Figure 6.1); and increased *P terminal force*, a terminal negative deflection in V1 greater than 40 msec (3, Figure 6.1).

The term *P mitrale* is sometimes used to describe P waves that are both notched and abnormally wide, since P waves of this type were frequently noted on tracings taken from subjects with mitral stenosis, but an equally important correlation points to left *ventricular* dysfunction due to hypertension and/or coronary artery disease.

Because the right atrium is depolarized first, its electrical potentials determine the formation of the first half of the P wave, increasing the height of the P wave but not its duration. *Right atrial abnormality* is diagnosed if the P waves in lead II, III or aVF are 2.5 mm or more in height, or when the initial positive portion of the P wave in lead V1 is 1.5 mm or more in height. Since such P waves are observed most often in subjects with severe lung disease, they have acquired the name *P pulmonale* (Figure 6.2).

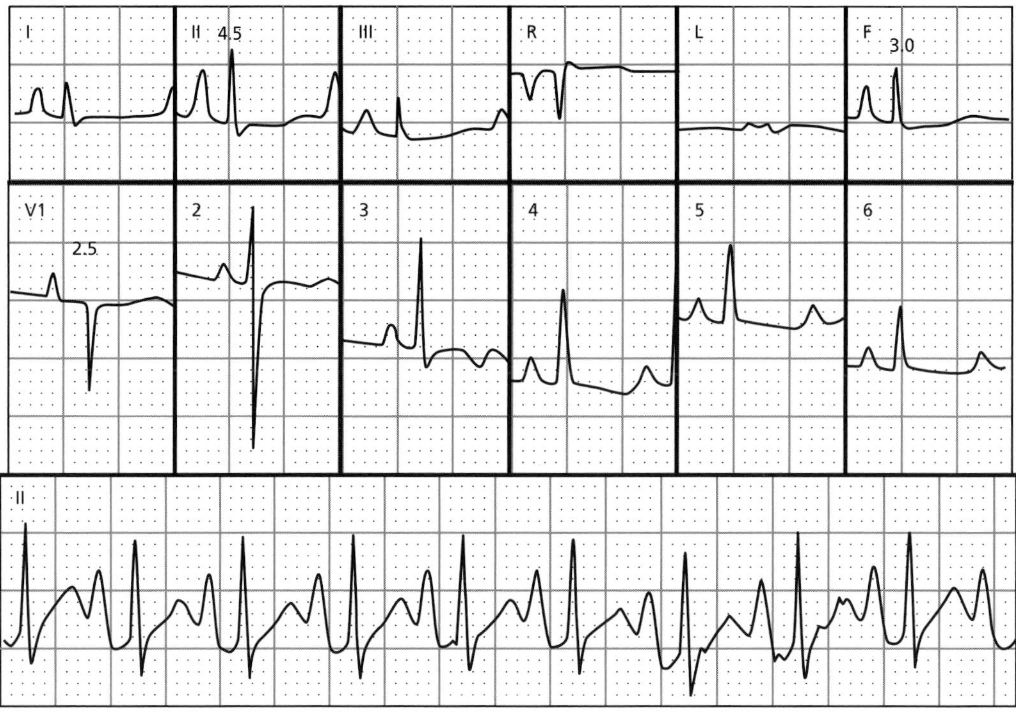

Figure 6.2 Right atrial abnormality – tall, narrow P waves.

In actual practice, *P pulmonale* likely represents an extreme of increasing P wave amplitude, and the observation of right atrial abnormality and right ventricular hypertrophy is therefore a poor prognostic sign in patients with lung disease and/or pulmonary hypertension.

Left ventricular hypertrophy

The diagnosis of *left ventricular hypertrophy* (LVH) is made primarily on the basis of *increased QRS amplitude* and is supported by the finding of *secondary ST segment and T wave changes* and *prolonged ventricular activation time* (VAT). Unfortunately for diagnostic accuracy, none of the ECG criteria taken individually is very sensitive, nor does LVH alone produce marked axis deviation or distinctive deformities of the QRS complex.

Many ECG criteria as well as more or less complex scoring systems for diagnosing LVH have been proposed. Some of the more widely recognized criteria are listed below.

Frontal plane leads:

- R wave in I + S wave in III = 25 mm
- R wave in aVL = 11 mm
- R wave in aVF = 20 mm.

Horizontal plane leads:

- S wave in V1 + R wave in V5 or V6 = 26 mm
- R wave in V5 or V6 = 26 mm
- Largest S wave + largest R wave = 45 mm
- Secondary ST segment and T wave abnormalities
- Prolonged QR interval in V6.

It should be noted that computerized ECG machines routinely scale the precordial leads to *half size* when high-amplitude QRS complexes are encountered. This reduction in scale is indicated on the tracing and must be taken into account if the amplitude of the precordial complexes is to be interpreted accurately. High voltage in the precordial leads is far more commonly noted than in the limb (frontal plane) leads, although high voltage in the limb leads is more specific for diagnosing LVH (Figure 6.3).

Frequently subjects with LVH manifest changes in the ST segment and T wave that occur secondarily to ventricular hypertrophy. The ST segments typically exhibit *upward concavity* in the right precordial leads (1 in Figure 6.3) and *upward convexity* in the left precordial leads (2, Figure 6.3). The T

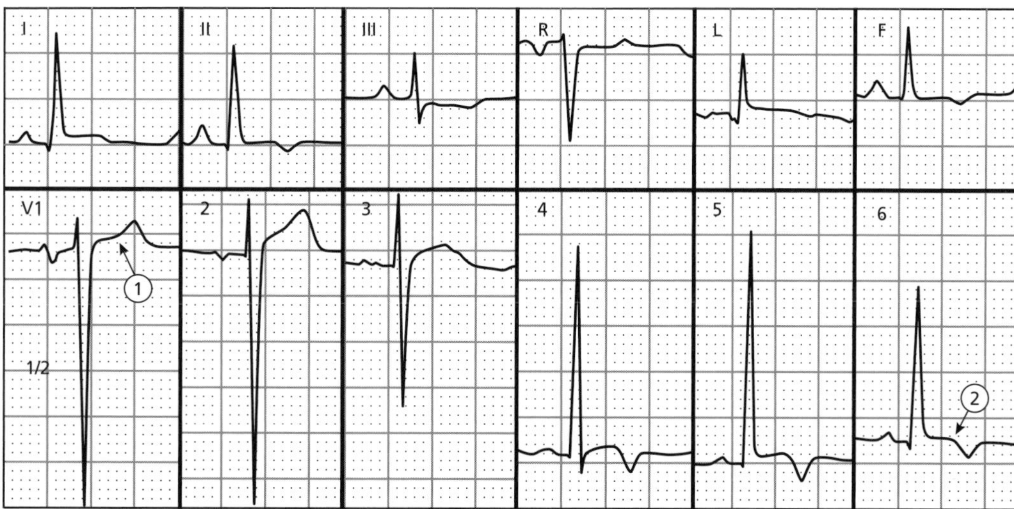

Figure 6.3 Left ventricular hypertrophy.

waves are usually opposite in polarity to the QRS complexes. Taken together, these ST–T wave changes are called the *strain pattern*, a term firmly embedded in ECG terminology despite the fact that 'strain' characterizes a physical, not electrical, event. In many subjects the ECG pattern of LVH will eventually progress to, or even alternate with, the pattern of left bundle branch block.

Ventricular activation time (VAT) is related to the speed of impulse conduction through the bundle branches or the ventricular muscle itself. Delayed conduction through a bundle branch or through the ventricular myocardium (owing to increased thickness) will prolong the VAT, making it an expected finding in both conditions. The VAT is determined by measuring the *QR interval* from the beginning of the QRS complex to the peak of the R wave. The end of the VAT is marked by the inscription of the *intrinsicoid deflection* (*ID* in Figure 6.4), the descending limb of the R wave. The normal QR duration is 35 msec (0.035 sec) in lead V1 and 45 msec (0.045 sec) in lead V6.

Despite the shortcomings of the electrocardiographic markers compared to more accurate means of detection such as echocardiography, LVH by ECG has proven to be a reliable indicator of cardiovascular pathology in general. In addition to having an expectedly higher incidence of hypertension, subjects with LVH–ECG have a higher incidence of left ventricular dysfunction and an increased risk of sudden death, congestive failure, infarction and stroke.

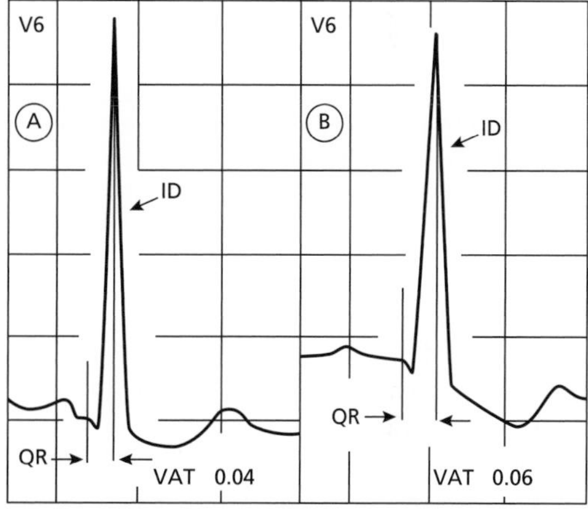

Figure 6.4 Ventricular activation time in LVH.

Right ventricular hypertrophy

If the reliability of the criteria for left ventricular hypertrophy is suspect, the dependability of the individual criteria for *right ventricular hypertrophy* (RVH) can only be considered worse. This is largely owing to the fact that the normally predominant left ventricular forces must be overshadowed by right ventricular forces before RVH becomes apparent on the ECG. Such a dramatic shift in the balance of electrical forces may take place suddenly, as in the case of massive pulmonary embolism, but the manifestation of RVH–ECG more commonly represents long-standing and severe pulmonary or cardiac disease.

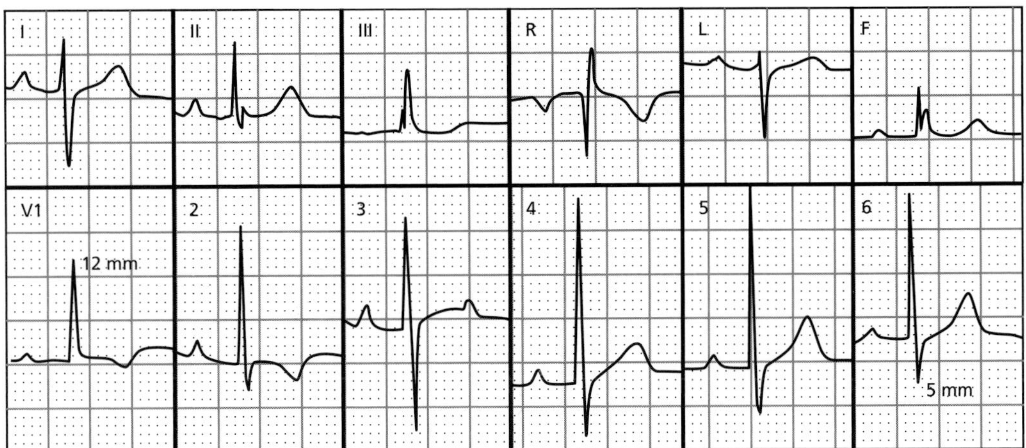

Figure 6.5 Right ventricular hypertrophy.

Some of the generally accepted diagnostic criteria for RVH are shown below.

Frontal plane leads:

- Right axis deviation of at least +110 degrees.

Horizontal plane leads:

- R:S ratio in V1 greater than 1.0
- R wave in V1 = 7 mm
- S wave in V1 is less than 2 mm
- qR or qRS pattern in V1
- S wave in V5 or V6 = 7 mm
- rSR′ in V1 with R′ wave greater than 10 mm
- R in V1 + S in V5 or V6 greater than 10.5 mm.

Because lead V1 most directly faces the right ventricular muscle mass, any increase in right ventricular forces will be most clearly reflected in that lead. Some authorities distinguish between as many as three types of RVH based on the QRS morphology in V1. *Type A* consists of a single large R wave, *Type B* is represented by an equiphasic RS complex, and *Type C* consists of an rSr′ or rSR pattern essentially identical to the QRS pattern of right bundle branch block. Type A RVH, shown in Figure 6.5, probably represents right ventricular pressure overloading like that seen in subjects with pulmonic stenosis. Type C RVH may represent volume overloading like that seen in subjects with atrial septal defect.

In severe cases – such as those found among children and young adults with congenital cardiac anomalies – a strain pattern like that described in connection with LVH may appear, accompanied by peaked P waves that have accordingly been christened *P congenitale*.

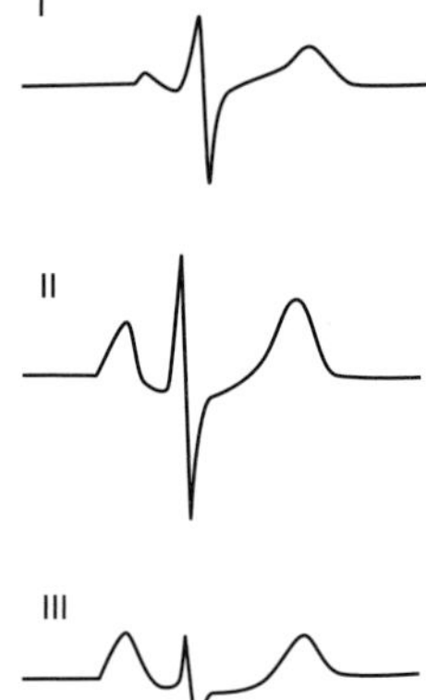

Figure 6.6 The S1,S2,S3 sign.

Three conditions in particular are likely to produce RVH–ECG: severe mitral stenosis with pulmonary hypertension, chronic cor pulmonale, and congenital heart disease. Patients with pulmonary hypertension or massive pulmonary embolus may exhibit S waves in all three standard leads – the *S1,S2,S3 sign* – an indicator of a poor prognosis in subjects with cor pulmonale (Figure 6.6).

Right axis deviation, an expected finding in subjects with RVH, is a normal feature in tracings recorded from infants and young children, and in the adult population some persons with a tall, slender body habitus tend to have rightwardly directed QRS axis. Extensive lateral wall infarction can shift the axis to the right owing to loss of countervailing left ventricular muscle mass, and right axis deviation is the *sine qua non* of left posterior fascicular block.

CHAPTER 7
Acute pericarditis

Pericarditis is an important differential diagnosis that must be made in cases of both *de novo* and recurrent chest pain. Acute pericarditis, usually a transitory affliction, is a frequent complication of both open heart surgery and myocardial infarction and poses a clinical problem for two reasons: it is often the cause of intense physical discomfort, and it predisposes the patient to atrial tachyarrhythmias, particularly atrial fibrillation and flutter. The pain of pericarditis can mimic angina, and like angina, can radiate, particularly to the interscapular area and base of the neck. Pericardial pain is often aggravated by deep inspiration and rotation of the trunk and relieved by sitting up or leaning forward. The pain may have a sharp, stabbing quality that generates intense anxiety.

The ECG findings in *acute pericarditis* include widespread ST segment elevation (1 in Figure 7.1), notching at the J point (2), reciprocal ST segment depression (3), PR segment depression (4), and *late* T wave inversion noted as pericarditis resolves and atrial arrhythmias.

Elevation of the ST segment in acute pericarditis differs significantly from ST elevation due to ischemia in that *it is not isolated to discrete segments*, and the ST segment exhibits *upward concavity* as opposed to upward convexity ('coving') typical of ischemia.

Inversion of T waves does occur in pericarditis, but ordinarily not until the acute phase has passed and the ST segment elevation has returned to baseline. This is in marked contrast to T wave behavior in cases of ischemia, in which T wave inversion occurs early while the ST segment is still elevated. In pericarditis uncomplicated by infarction, Q waves never appear. Depression of the PR segment, the interval between the end of the P wave and the beginning of the QRS complex, is a common but subtle sign most often noted in lead II (4, Figure 7.1) and the precordial leads. PR segment depression is quickly detected by laying a straight edge along the isoelectric line between P–QRS–T sequences. In some cases, PR segment depression may be the only ECG sign of acute pericarditis.

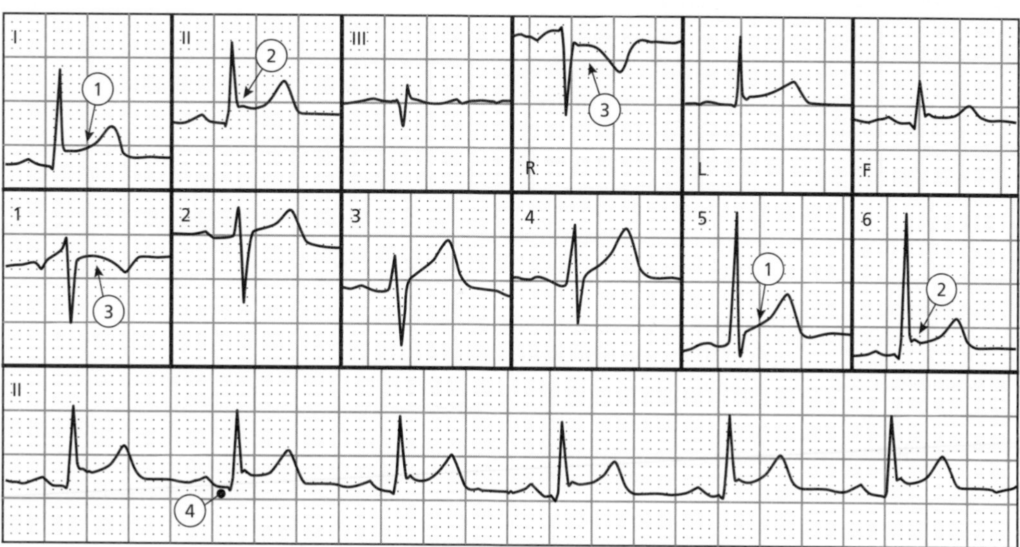

Figure 7.1 Acute pericarditis.

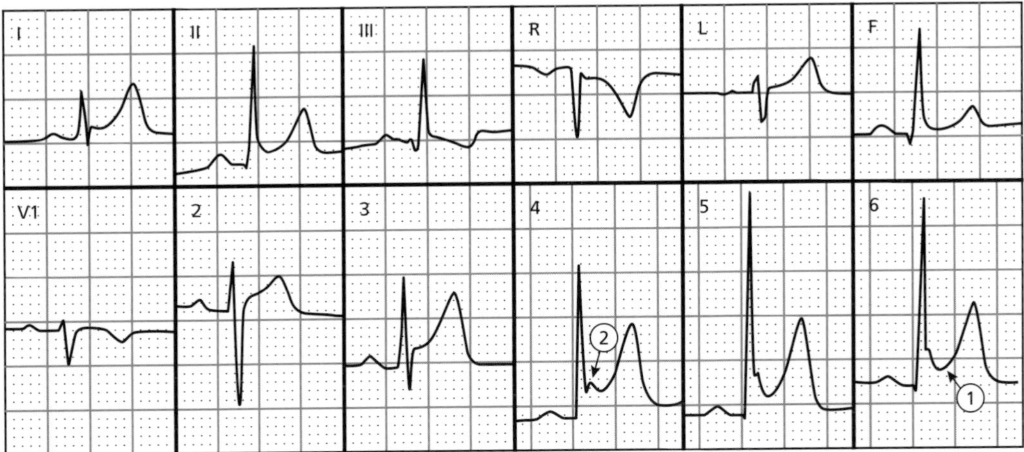

Figure 7.2 Early repolarization.

Early repolarization

Early repolarization is a normal ECG variant of striking appearance that closely resembles both acute pericarditis and the hyperacute phase of myocardial infarction. The pattern is most often seen in young, thin-chested adults, particularly black men. There is almost never any clinical or laboratory evidence of heart disease.

The features of early repolarization, shown in Figure 7.2, include ST segment elevation (1), particularly noticeable in the lateral precordial leads, concave upward ST segments identical to those seen during the acute phase of pericarditis, notching of the J point (2) which is also reminiscent of pericarditis, and tall, symmetrical T waves that closely mimic the vaulting T waves of the hyperacute phase of infarction. In marked contrast to the evolution of the acute pericarditis and infarction patterns, *the ECG findings of early repolarization are stable over long periods of time.*

The Osborne wave

The *Osborne wave* or *J wave* refers to a hump-like deflection inscribed at the J point (Figure 7.3) that is seen in cases of severe hypothermia and hypercalcemia. The prominence of the Osborne wave varies inversely with body core temperature and is most clearly seen in the inferior and lateral precordial leads. As rewarming occurs, Osborne waves shrink and disappear.

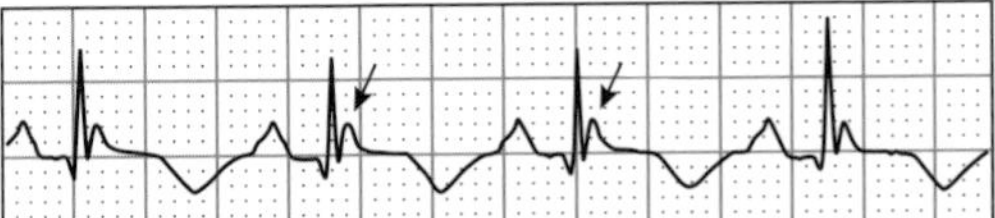

Figure 7.3 The Osborne wave of hypothermia (lead II) in a subject with a core temperature of 32°C.

Hyperkalemia

Tall, symmetrical T waves, particularly noticeable in the precordial leads, are a relatively early sign of *hyperkalemia* (Figure 7.4). The T waves of hyperkalemia are sometimes described as 'pinched at the base.' As hyperkalemia progresses, the P waves flatten and then disappear and the QRS complex widens, eventually assuming a wide sine wave shape as hyperkalemia progresses to lethal levels.

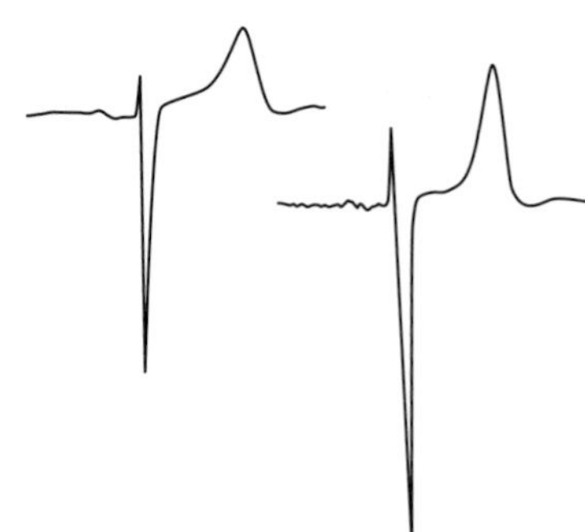

Figure 7.4 Hyperkalemia: the complex on the left recorded with normal serum potassium, the complex on the right with a serum potassium level of 7.1 mmol/l (both from V2). Hyperkalemia causes the T wave to become tall, narrow, and symmetrical.

8

CHAPTER 8

Sinus rhythm and its discontents

Normally the driving impulse of the heart arises in the P cells of the sinoatrial (SA) node, a spindle-shaped cluster of about 5000 specialized myocardial cells located at the junction of the superior vena cava and the lateral wall of the right atrium. Although this aggregate of spontaneously depolarizing cells functions as the primary cardiac pacemaker, other natural pacemaking foci, sometimes known as 'the line of fire' or 'atrial pacemaking complex,' extend along the crista terminalis. The most superior of these sites are the fastest, and the inherent rates of subsidiary sites decrease as one moves caudally toward the inferior vena cava.

A significant percentage of the right atrial surface consists of electrically silent holes: the openings of the superior and inferior venae cavae, the fossa ovalis, and the ostium of the coronary sinus. Atrial myocardial fibers are deployed around these openings in thicker strands that conduct the sinus impulse more efficiently. The irregular geometry of the right atrium therefore tends to channel the spreading wave of excitation through certain areas of myocardium called *preferential pathways*, three of which are recognized: the *anterior*, *middle* and *posterior*. Another preferential pathway, *Bachmann's bundle*, connects the right and left atria. These pathways, determined by the anatomical arrangement of the atrial muscle fibers, are myocardial strands, i.e. not specialized conduction tissue.

Sinus rhythm

Sinus rhythm is determined by P wave morphology and P wave axis. Normal P waves are rounded, 80–110 milliseconds (0.08–0.11 sec) in duration, with an axis of +15 to +75, making them positive in leads I and II, negative in lead aVR, and variable in leads III, aVL and aVF. Sinus P waves are frequently biphasic in leads V1 and V2, but the initial deflection should be positive in those leads. Initial *P wave negativity in leads V1 and V2* is an indication of ectopic origin (Figure 8.1).

The rate of normal sinus rhythm is conventionally given as 60–100 beats per minute, although a rate of 50–90 is probably normal in the majority of subjects (A in Figure 8.2). The *intrinsic sinus rate* can be determined by giving atropine and propranolol intravenously, temporarily disconnecting the sinus node from autonomic modulation. The normal intrinsic rate is usually greater than 100 beats per minute, implying that parasympathetic influence predominates in most subjects. Elderly subjects frequently exhibit some degree of *chronotropic incompetence*: compared to younger subjects, the

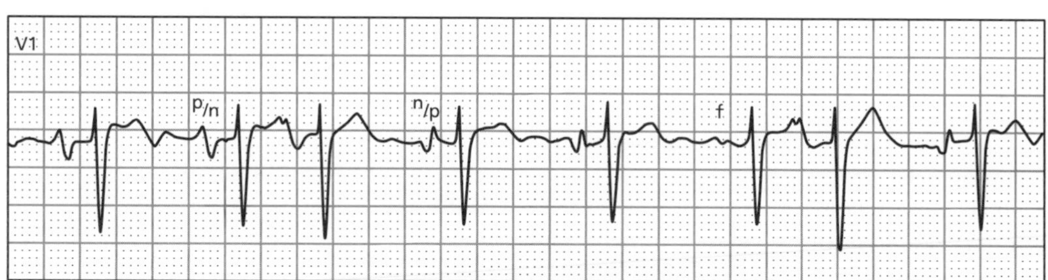

Figure 8.1 Sinus beats are positive/negative (p/n) in lead V1, low atrial beats are negative/positive, and 'f' is an atrial fusion beat.

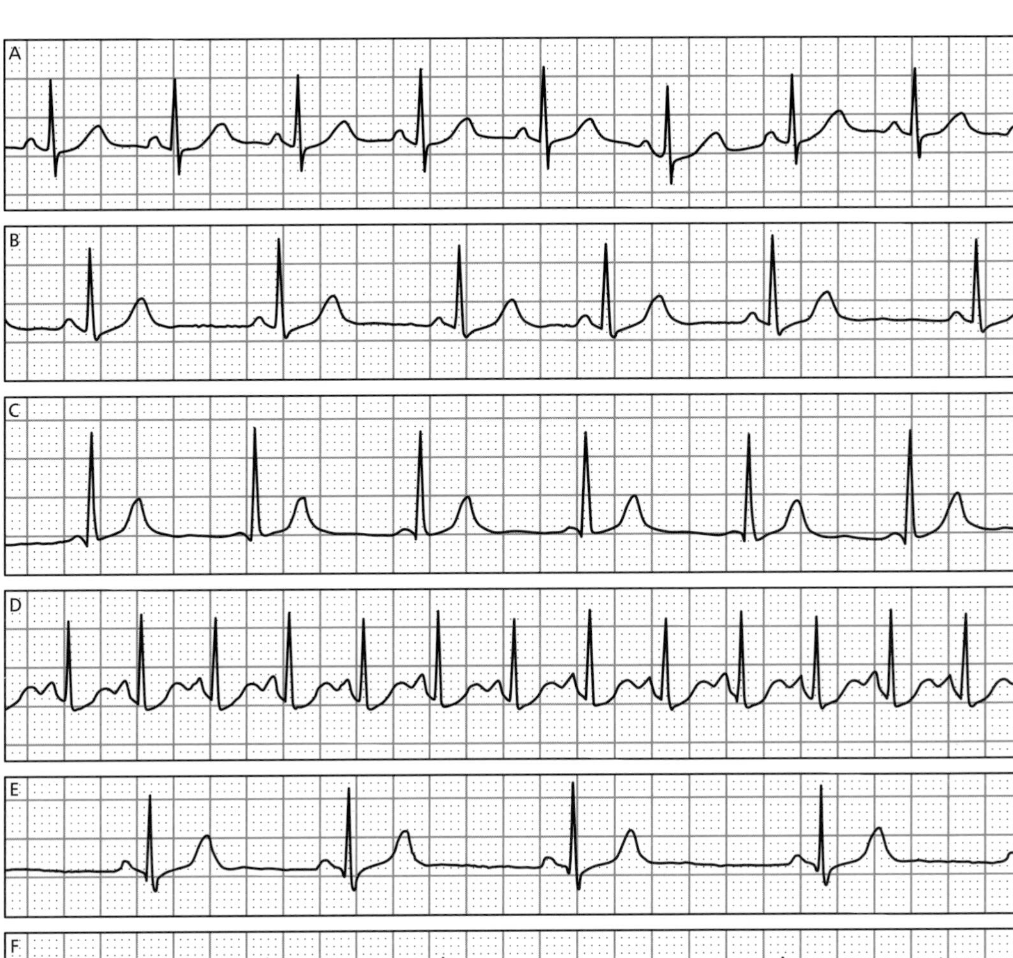

Figure 8.2 The sinus rhythms.

heart rate does not increase appropriately in response to metabolic demands – elderly patients may not mount an appropriate sinus tachycardia in response to fever or low cardiac output.

If P wave to P wave (P–P) variability exceeds 160 milliseconds (0.16 sec) in duration and all other criteria for sinus rhythm are met, *sinus arrhythmia* is present (B, Figure 8.2). In this common variant of sinus rhythm, cyclical waxing and waning of the rate of P wave formation is typically entrained to the respiratory cycle. Sinus arrhythmia is particularly common in younger subjects and is usually noted when the sinus rate is relatively slow, since P–P intervals tend to regularize at faster rates.

A small percentage of normal subjects exhibit sinus P waves with short PR intervals (<120 msec). In the majority, *accelerated atrioventricular conduction* represents a normal variant (C, Figure 8.2). Unless accompanied by supraventricular tachyarrhythmias or other signs of abnormal atrioventricular connections, the presence of a short PR interval should be regarded as benign.

If the sinus rate exceeds 100 per minute, *sinus tachycardia* is diagnosed (D, Figure 8.2). A sinus rate above 100 in adults always raises the question of causation, and a reason should always be sought (e.g. fever, anxiety, pain, hypoxia, low cardiac output, thyrotoxicosis). Although the rate of sinus tachycardia rarely exceeds 140 beats per minute, it can rise above 200 in healthy young subjects. In cases in which P waves are not clearly visible owing to rapid rate, sinus tachycardia may mimic other supraventricular tachycardias.

If other criteria for sinus rhythm are met and the rate is less than 60 per minute, *sinus bradycardia* is diagnosed (E, Figure 8.2). The upper limit of 60 beats per minute is widely recognized as an unrealistic figure; sinus bradycardia is not usually clinically significant unless the rate falls below 50 per minute, and many subjects, particularly young athletic individuals, regularly tolerate rates of 40 or less at rest without adverse effects. Inappropriate sinus bradycardia, particularly in the elderly, is a frequent manifestation of sinoatrial nodal disease and this is especially likely if other indications of conduction system disease (atrioventricular block, fascicular or bundle branch block) are observed.

Wandering atrial pacemaker (F, Figure 8.2) is distinguished from sinus rhythm by changing P wave morphology that is often accompanied by changes in P wave axis, PR interval and heart rate. Atrial fusion beats are also commonly produced as the site of impulse formation moves from the sinus node to lower subsidiary pacemaking sites along the line of fire and then back again to the sinus node. Like sinus arrhythmia, wandering pacemaker usually exhibits a waxing and waning effect and is nearly always observed at slower heart rates. Wandering pacemaker is harmless.

Disorders of sinus rhythm

Disorders of sinus rhythm can be divided into two broad categories: pacemaker failure and sinoatrial exit block.

Pacemaker failure most commonly presents as inappropriate sinus bradycardia, a reflection of chronotropic incompetence, and more rarely by *sinus arrest*, the failure of sinus impulses to form. Sinus arrest may be episodic or permanent, and if intermittent it may last for seconds to hours.

Sinoatrial (SA) exit block occurs when the SA node forms impulses that are blocked in the transitional zone separating the electrical syncytium of the SA node from the contiguous atrial myocardium. Broadly speaking, *exit block* exists whenever impulses are formed but fail to conduct ('exit') out of the pacemaking focus. Sinoatrial exit block, considered to be analogous to atrioventricular block for descriptive purposes, can be classified as first, second or third degree (complete). First-degree SA block cannot be diagnosed from the scalar ECG because the proximal point of reference, the firing of the SA node, leaves no deflection on surface tracings. For the same reason, third-degree SA block is impossible to distinguish from sinus arrest on the scalar ECG.

Like its atrioventricular counterpart, *second-degree sinoatrial block* is divided into two subtypes: Mobitz type I (Wenckebach) and Mobitz type II. All variants of the *Wenckebach phenomenon* require a proximal impulse source (1 in Figure 8.3), separated by a zone of defective conduction (2) from distal myocardium (3). During each *Wenckebach cycle*, conduction exhibits *progressive delay* that culminates in the block of an impulse. After each blocked impulse the cycle repeats.

In the case of sinoatrial Wenckebach, the impulse source is the sinoatrial node, and the distal myocardium is the atrial muscle. Discharge of the sinus node is silent on the surface ECG, so no proximal point of reference is visible. Atrial depolarization, signaled by the P wave, marks the distal point of reference.

Classic *type I (Wenckebach) sinoatrial block* is characterized by (1) progressive shortening of the P–P intervals followed by (2) a pause in sinus rhythm that is less than the sum of any two preceding P–P intervals (sinus cycles). The progressive shortening of the P–P intervals in classic type I SA block conforms to the principle that in textbook Wenckebach cycles the rate of the chamber distal to the block steadily accelerates before each pause in rhythm.

Unfortunately, atypical Wenckebach cycles are as common in sinoatrial block as in atrioventricular

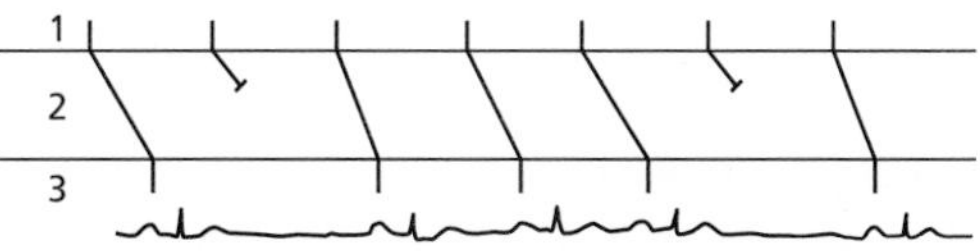

Figure 8.3 Type I (Wenckebach) sinoatrial block with a 4:3 conduction ratio: P–P intervals shorten and the pause in sinus rhythm is less than the sum of two sinus cycles. Progressive conduction delay (decremental conduction) ends in block, after which the cycle repeats. 1: SA node, 2: zone of conduction delay, 3: atrial muscle.

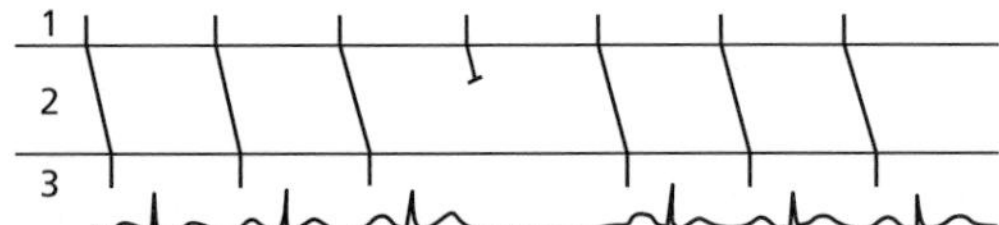

Figure 8.4 Type II (Mobitz II) sinoatrial block: P–P intervals are the same and the pause is twice the cycle length. Conduction is all-or-none. 1: SA node, 2: zone of conduction delay, 3: atrial muscle.

block. Therefore the diagnosis of type I sinoatrial block should be entertained whenever clusters of P waves separated by pauses are observed. In actual practice, some cases of sinus arrhythmia are difficult to distinguish from atypical sinoatrial Wenckebach cycles.

Mobitz type II sinoatrial block, like its atrioventricular counterpart, is characterized by sudden conduction loss, i.e. there is little to no antecedent or subsequent change in the P–P intervals before an expected P wave suddenly fails to appear (Figure 8.4). As a result, the pause in sinus rhythm equals two sinus cycles (two P–P intervals). Just as type II atrioventricular block may progress to higher grades, type II SA block can result in multiple dropped beats. The pause illustrated in Figure 8.5 is equal to three sinus cycles – in high-grade SA block, the length of the pause will be a multiple of the basic sinus cycle length. *High-grade* or *advanced block* occurs if three or more consecutive impulses are blocked.

Sinus arrest refers to a pause in sinus rhythm that is *not a multiple* of the basic sinus cycle. If sinus arrest is prolonged, single or repetitive escape beats may appear, but depression of subsidiary pacemakers is common in the setting of SA nodal disease, so that escape rhythms, if present, are often very slow.

Sick sinus syndrome refers to a constellation of disorders of sinus rhythm that includes (1) inappropriate sinus bradycardia, (2) sinoatrial block, (3) sinus arrest, (4) tachycardia–bradycardia syndrome ('tachy–brady' syndrome), (5) suppression of sinus rhythm by ectopic beats and (6) sinoatrial re-entry. Florid and rapidly changing manifestations of sick sinus syndrome are common and may present one after another within moments to hours. Sinoatrial block accompanied by atrioventricular block has been called '*dual* or *double nodal disease*' (Figure 8.6).

The *tachycardia–bradycardia* or '*tachy–brady*' syndrome is a frequently seen and quite dramatic

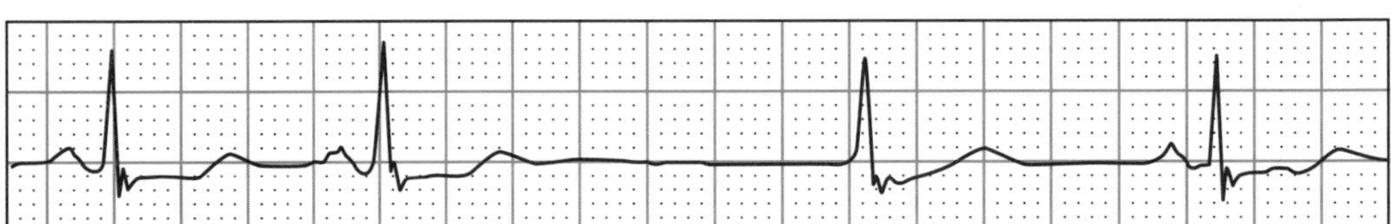

Figure 8.5 Sinoatrial block (3:1): there are two missing P waves, so the pause is equal to three sinus cycles. The third QRS complex is a junctional escape beat.

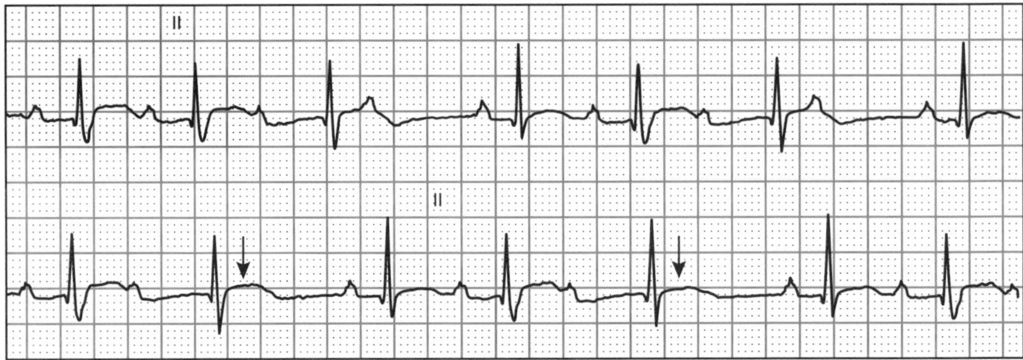

Figure 8.6 Double nodal disease: type II sinoatrial block (*arrows* mark the expected location of missing P waves), type I atrioventricular block (top strip), and rate-dependent right bundle branch block.

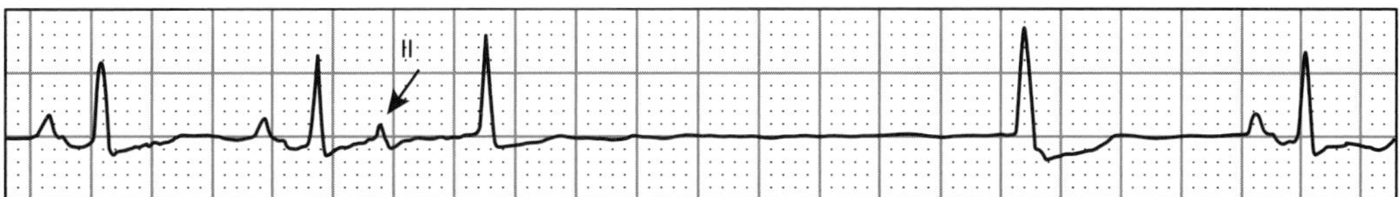

Figure 8.7 Sinus node suppression following an atrial extrasystole (*arrow*): a sinus pause of 2.8 seconds is interrupted by a single junctional escape beat.

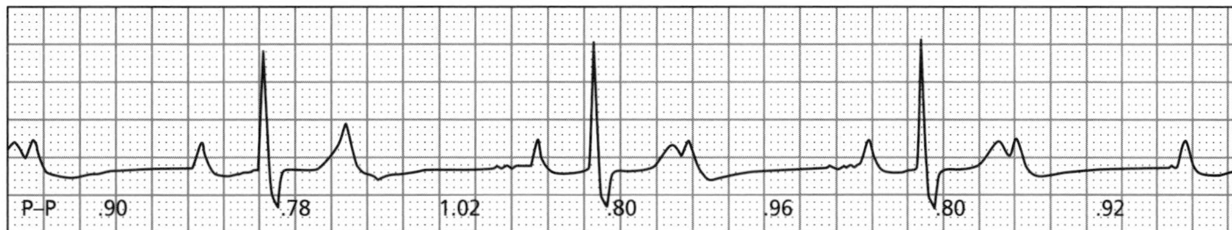

Figure 8.8 Ventriculophasic sinus arrhythmia.

manifestation of sick sinus syndrome. Typically atrial fibrillation or atrial flutter is abruptly replaced by asystole or extreme sinus bradycardia. Concomitant atrioventricular block and/or intraventricular block is a common finding.

Suppression of sinus impulse formation following ectopic beats, generally premature atrial systoles (Figure 8.7), is a reflection of prolonged *sinus node recovery time* (SNRT). Transient depression of impulse formation following early or repetitive depolarization, known as *overdrive suppression*, is a normal response to passive discharge of any pacemaking site, including the sinoatrial node. As a rule, sinoatrial nodal recovery time following depolarization by an ectopic pacemaker is equal to the basic sinus cycle length plus 600 milliseconds (0.60 sec). Values in excess of 125% of the baseline sinus cycle length imply impaired sinus node function.

Sinoatrial nodal re-entrant tachycardia is discussed in a subsequent chapter.

Ventriculophasic sinus arrhythmia

In some cases of third-degree atrioventricular block the P–P intervals containing a QRS complex are noted to be shorter in duration than P–P intervals in which no QRS falls, a phenomenon known as *ventriculophasic sinus arrhythmia* (Figure 8.8). Rarely, P–P intervals containing paced beats or premature ventricular complexes may exhibit ventriculophasic sinus arrhythmia. Various explanations for this finding have been advanced: (1) the sinus node accelerates because of the mechanical pull of ventricular contraction; (2) the ventricular beat transiently improves perfusion of the sinus node; or (3) ventricular contraction causes vagal inhibition due to atrial distension.

Self-Assessment Test Three

3.1. Identify the abnormality in the following tracing.

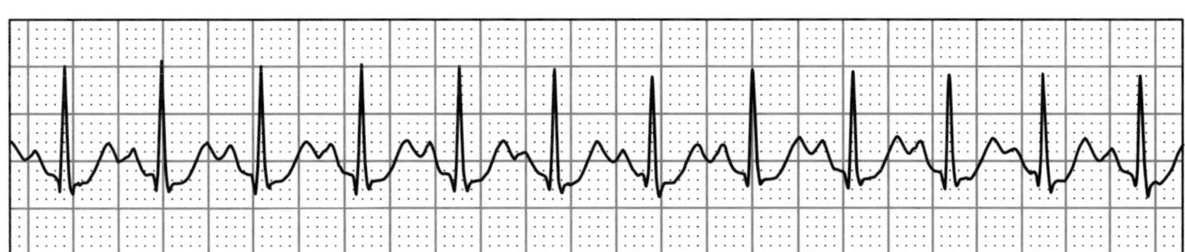

3.2. The Osborne wave is associated with . . .
   a. early repolarization
   b. hypothermia and hypercalcemia
   c. acute pericarditis

Identify the abnormalities in the following seven tracings.

3.3.

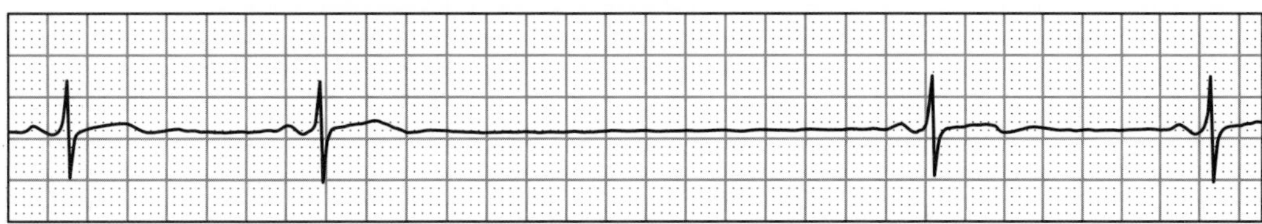

3.4.

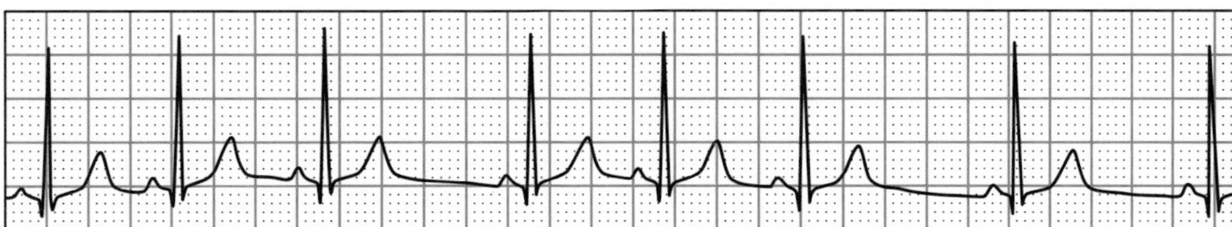

3.5. Set A

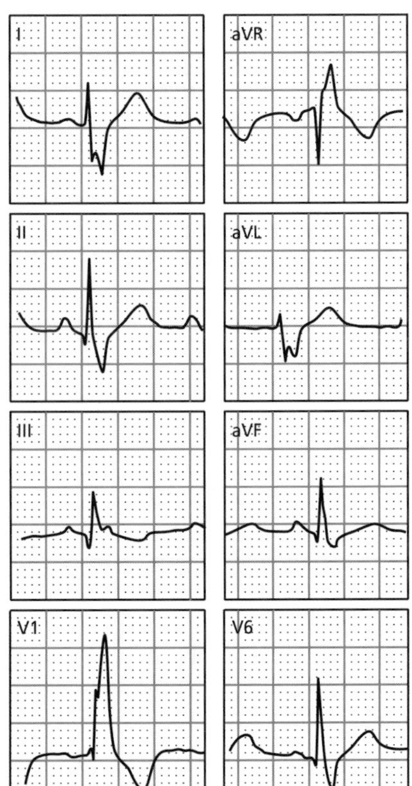

Set B

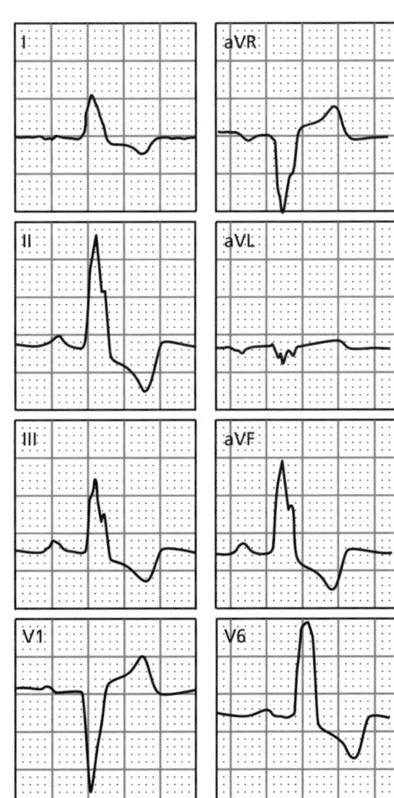

3.6.

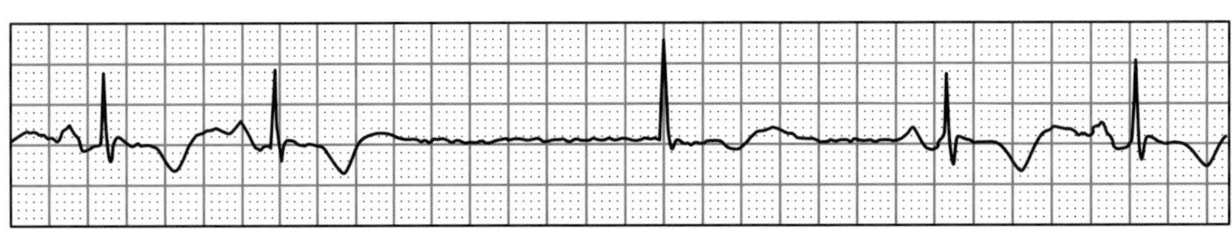

3.7.

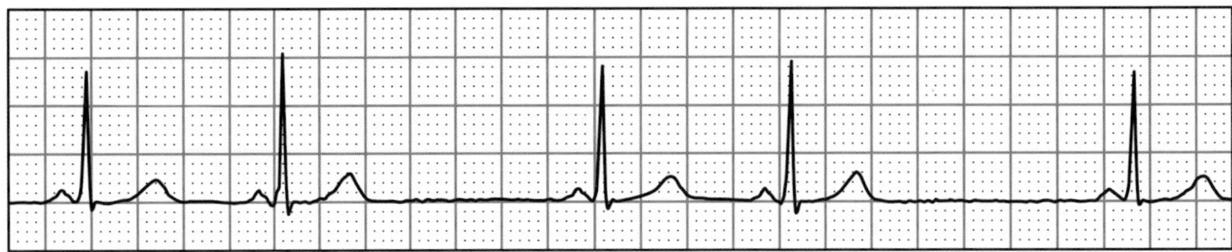

3.8.

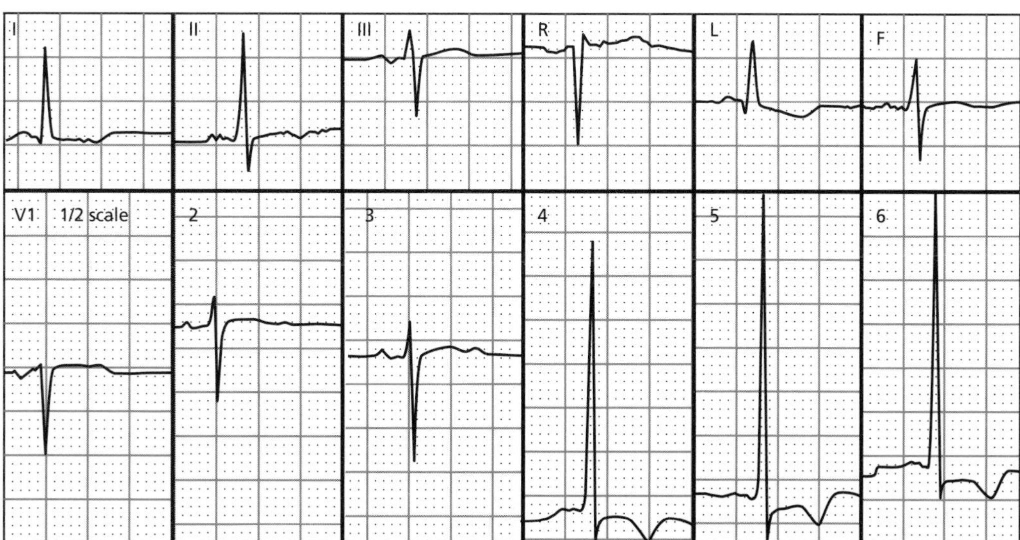

3.9.

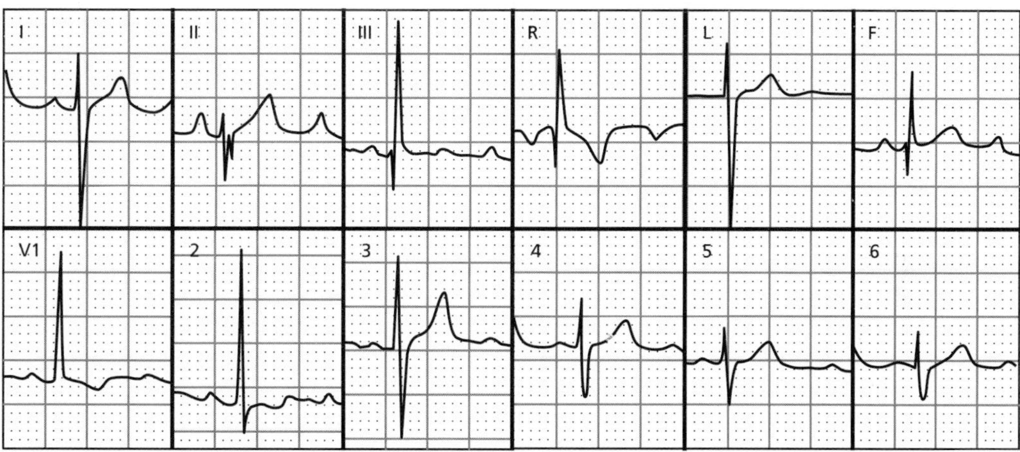

3.10. In early repolarization syndrome the ST segment . . . and . . .
   a. is upwardly concave . . . stable over time
   b. is upwardly convex . . . descends to the base-line over time
   c. begins at the baseline . . . elevates during ischemia

3.11. Type I (Wenckebach) sinoatrial block is characterized by . . .
   a. P–P intervals that shorten and a pause less than twice the P–P interval
   b. constant P–P intervals and a pause twice the P–P interval
   c. pauses that are multiples of the P–P interval

3.12. Identify the abnormality in the following tracings.

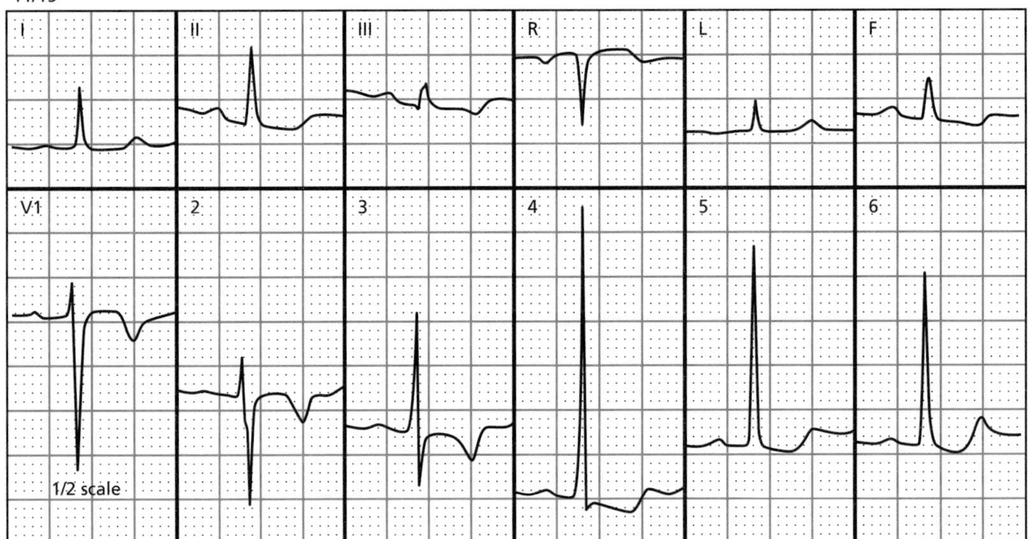

11/16

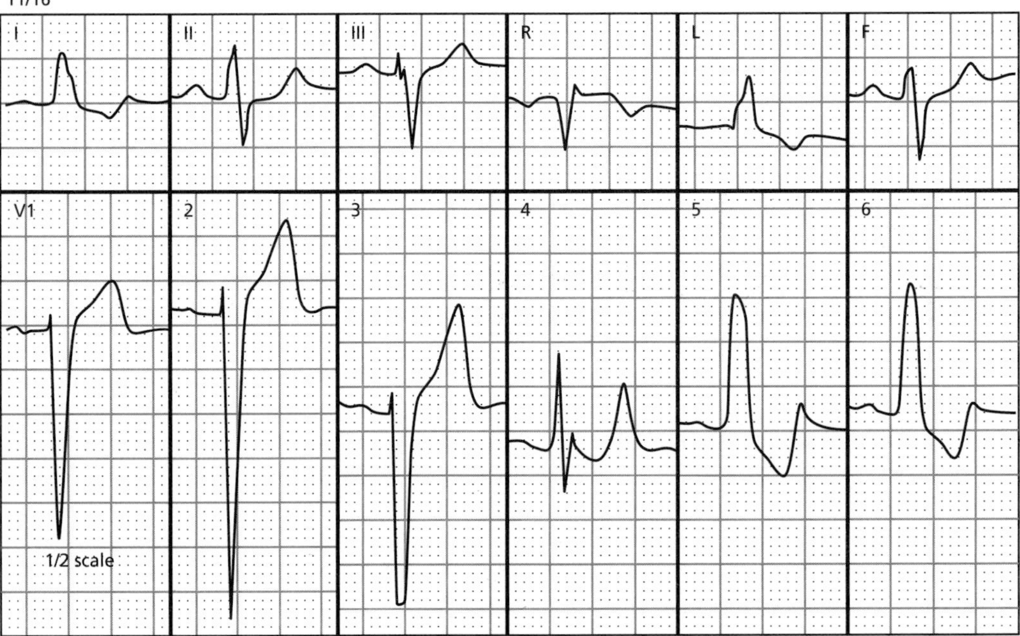

3.13. Identify the abnormality in the following tracing.

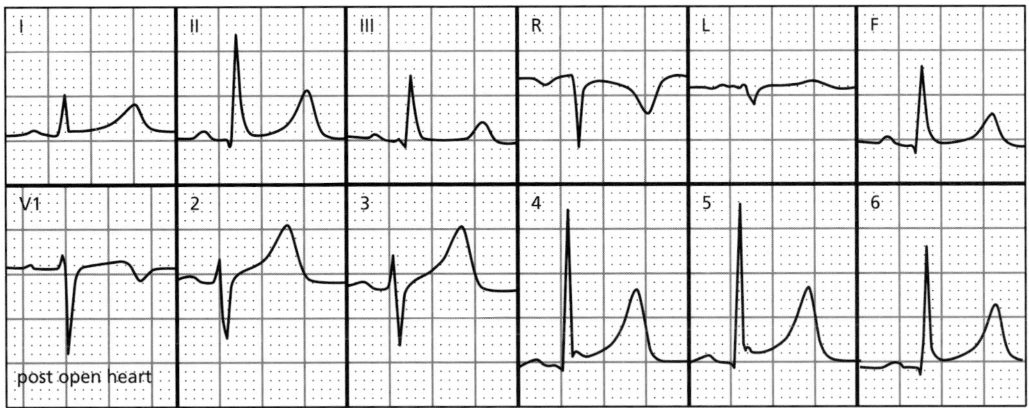

3.14. Sinoatrial block accompanied by atrioventricular block is called . . .

a. Mobitz II sinoatrial block
b. Ashman's phenomenon
c. double nodal disease

3.15. Identify the abnormality in the following tracing.

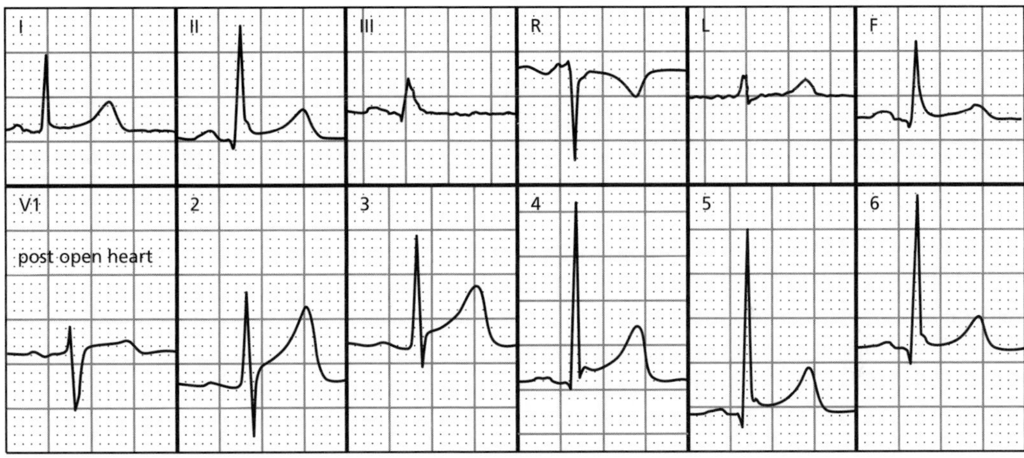

3.16. Identify the abnormality in the following tracing.

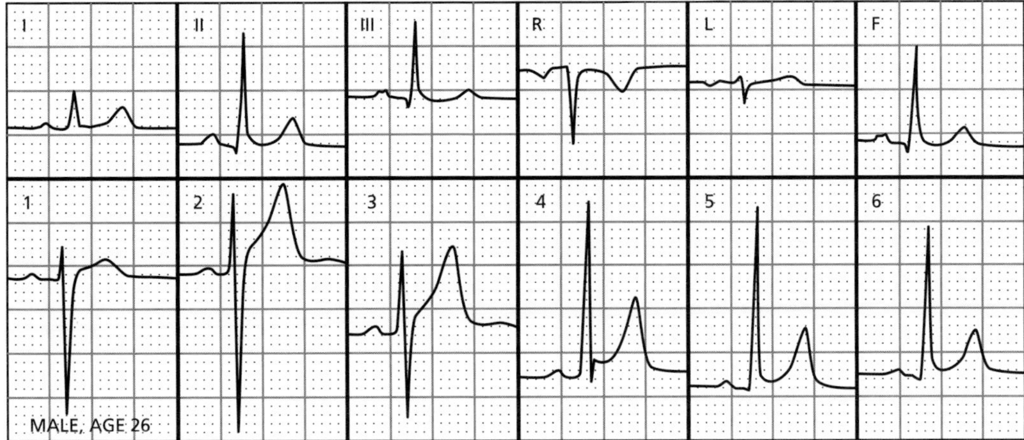

3.17. Right atrial abnormality is diagnosed when P waves are greater than . . . in the . . . leads.
  a. 2.5 mm . . . inferior
  b. 2.5 mm . . . lateral
  c. 2.0 mm . . . precordial

3.18. Identify the abnormality in the following tracings.

12/19

I
II
III
R
L
F
V1
2
3
4
5
6

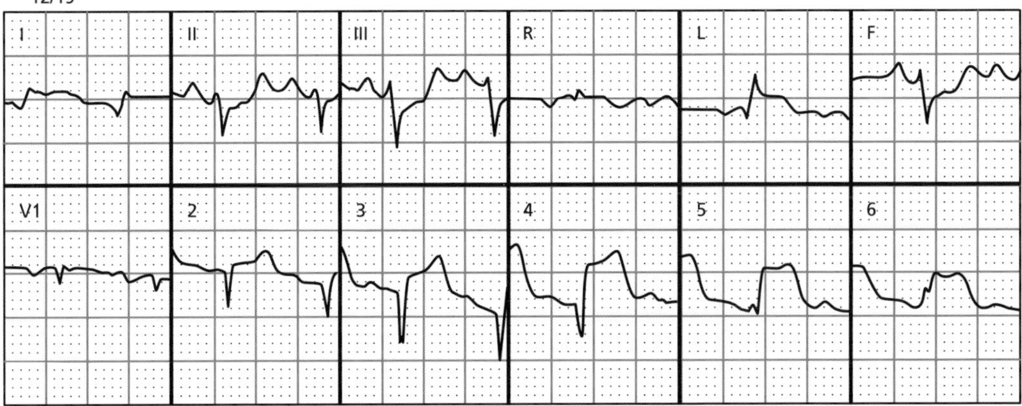

12/21

I
II
III
R
L
F
V1
2
3
4
5
6
II
1
2
3

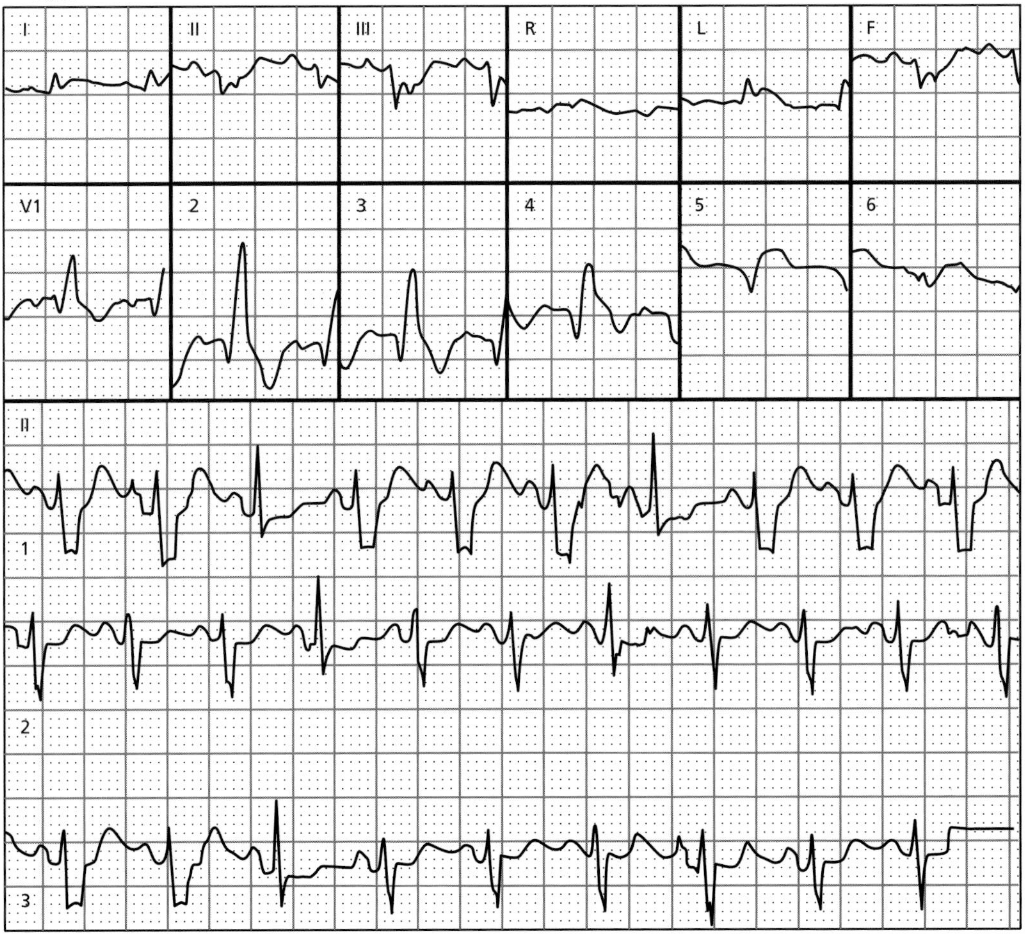

3.19. The two fascicles most likely to block are . . .
   a. the right bundle branch and left posterior fascicle
   b. the right bundle branch and left anterior fascicle
   c. the bundle of His and left anterior fascicle

3.20. Which is a feature of acute pericarditis?
   a. Depression of the ST segment
   b. Inversion of the T wave
   c. Depression of the PR interval

3.21. Wellen's syndrome is characterized by . . .
   a. negative or biphasic T waves in leads V1–V3
   b. a hump-like deformity at the J point with ST segment elevation
   c. tall, symmetrical T waves

3.22. Hyperkalemia is characterized by . . .
   a. flattened T waves in the precordial leads
   b. tall, symmetrical T waves in the precordial leads
   c. biphasic T waves in the inferior leads

Identify the abnormalities in the following 18 tracings.

3.23.

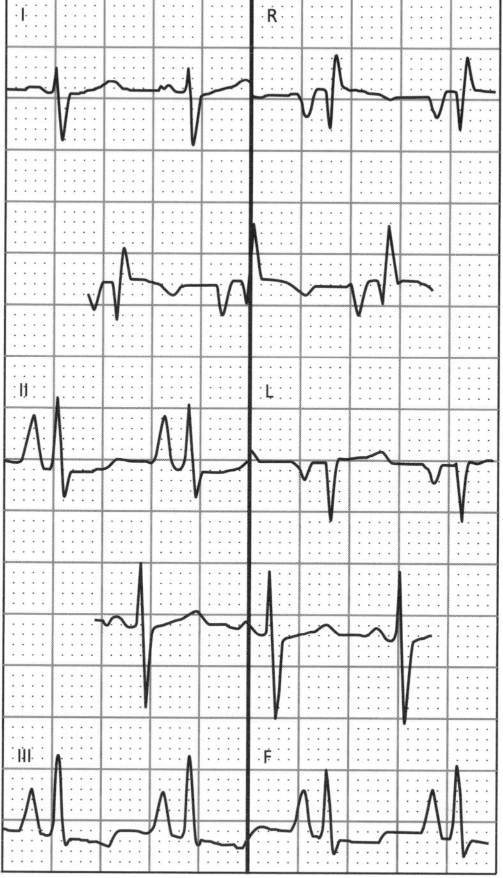

3.24.

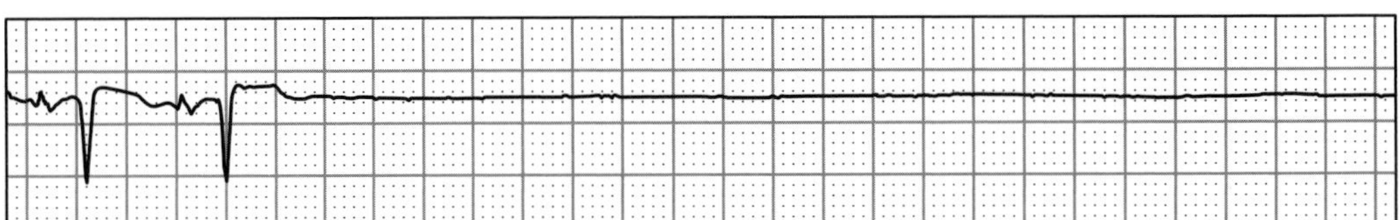

3.25.

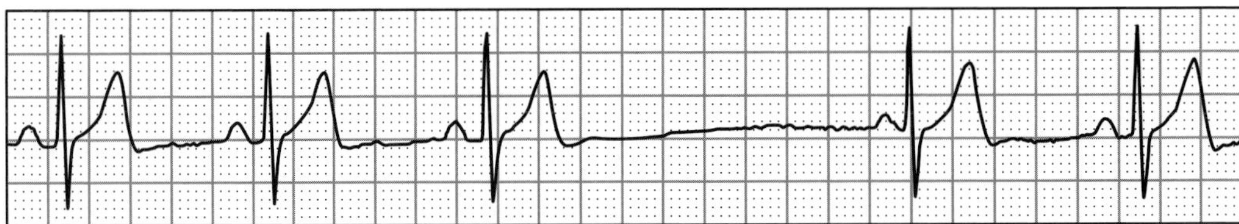

3.26.

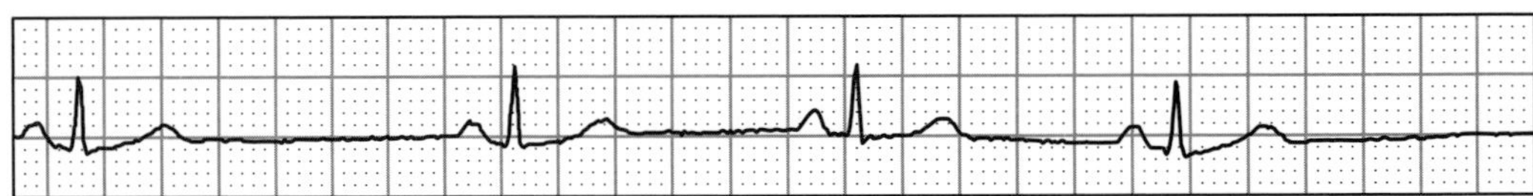

3.27.

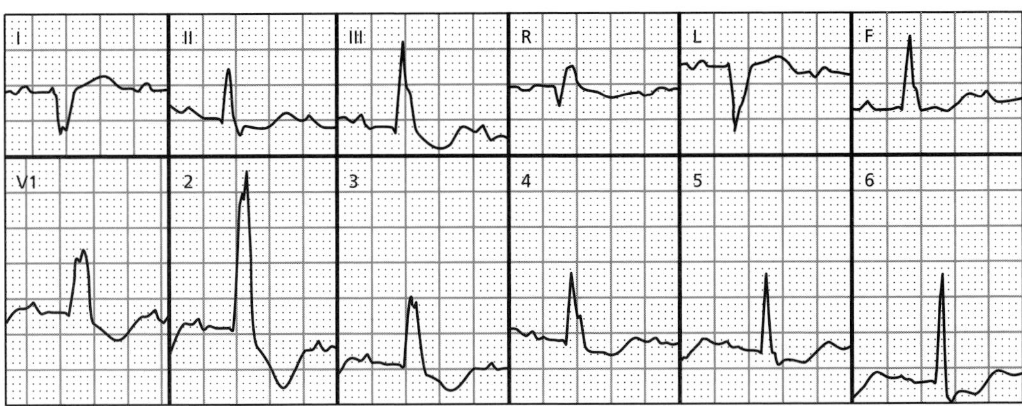

3.28.

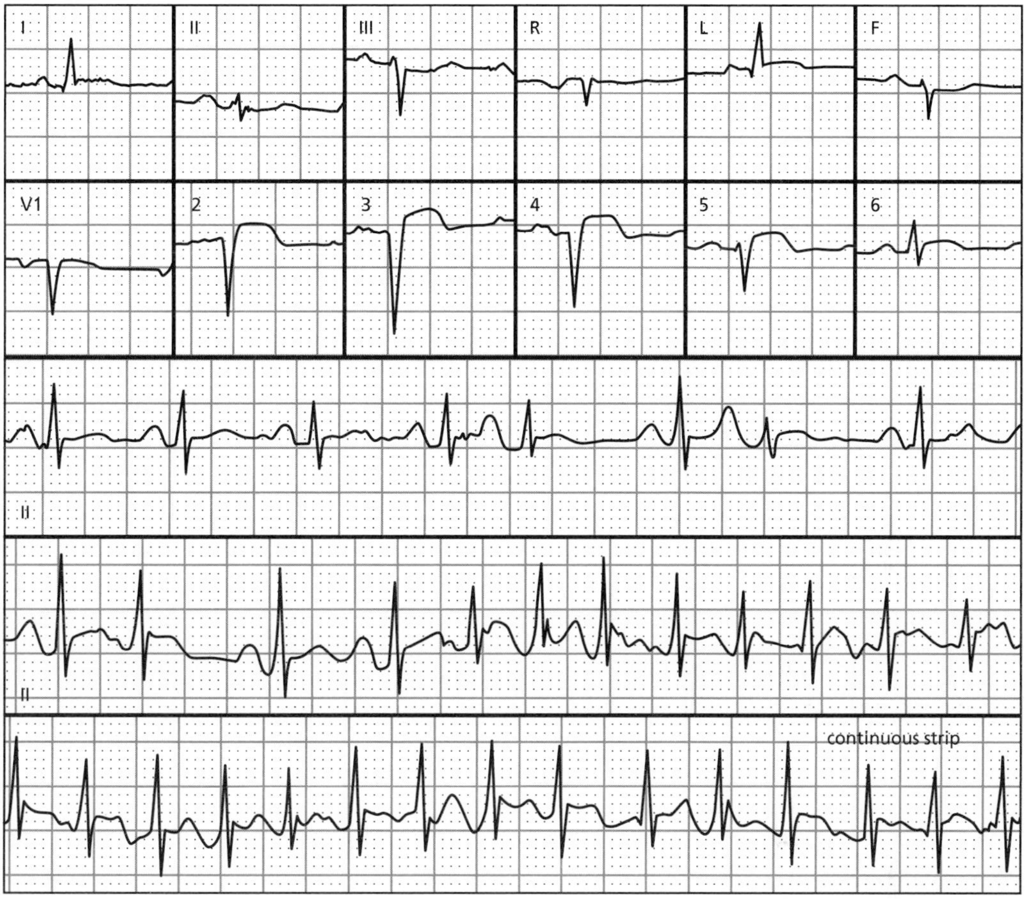

3.29.

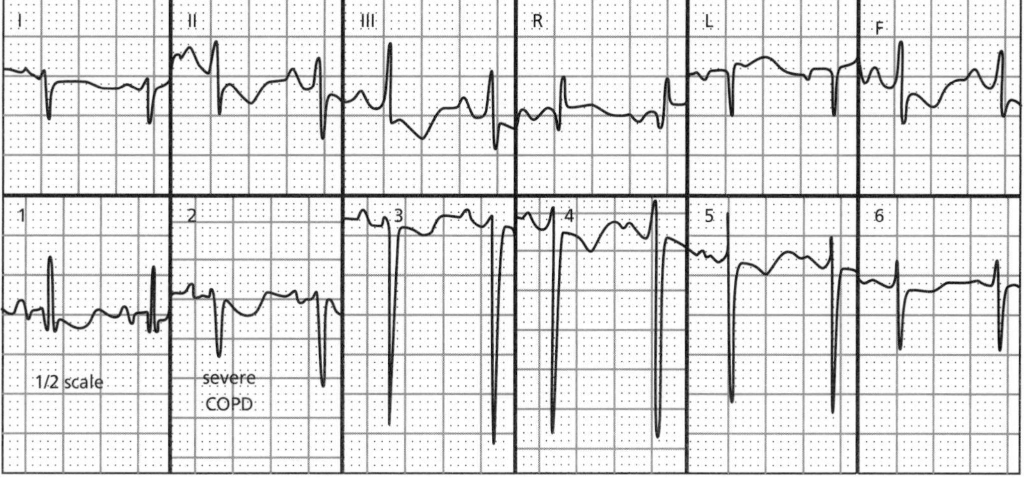

3.30.

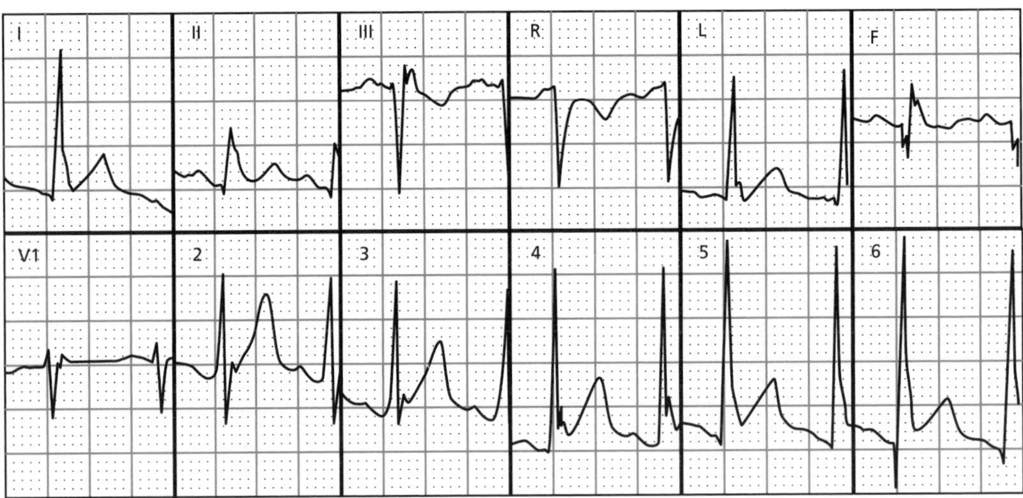

3.31.

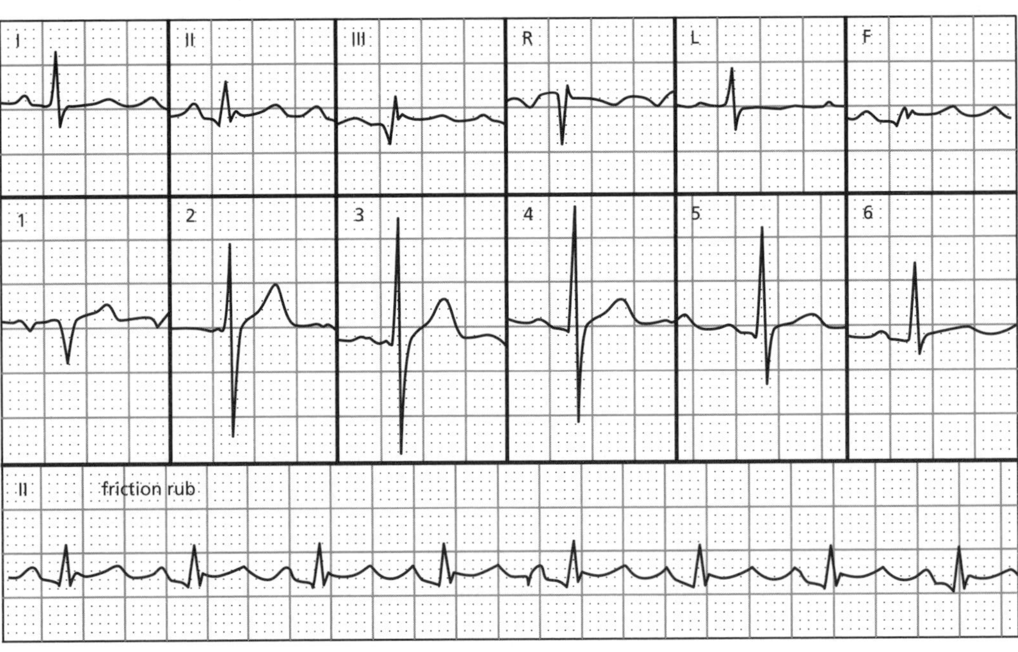

3.32.

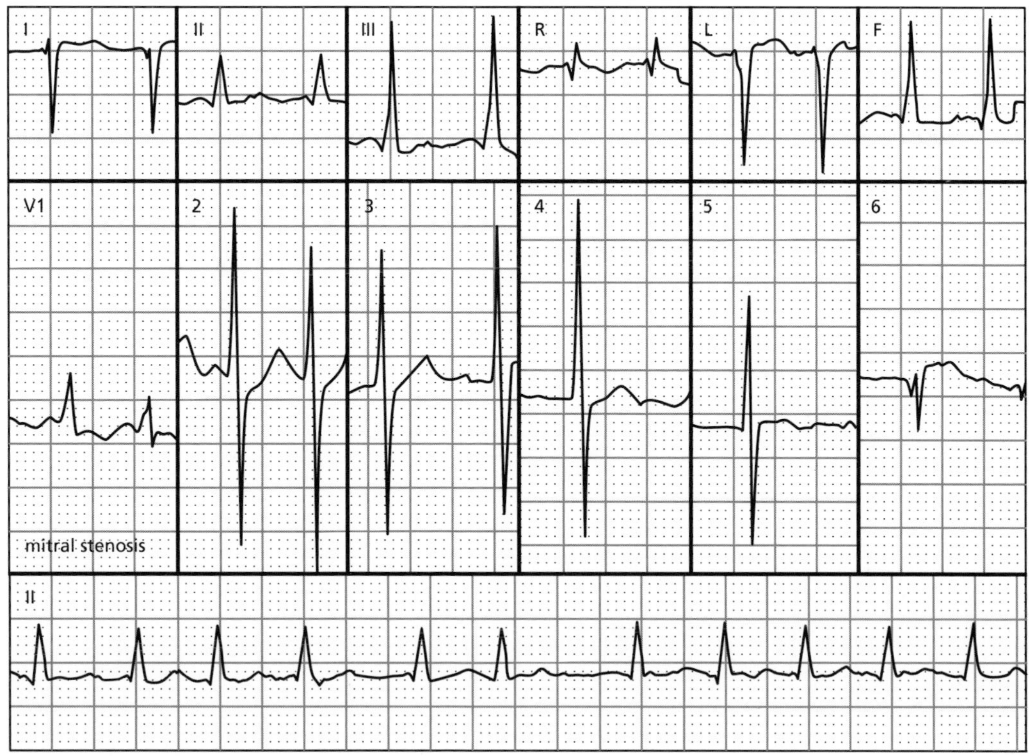
I
II
III
R
L
F
V1
2
3
4
5
6
mitral stenosis
II

3.33.

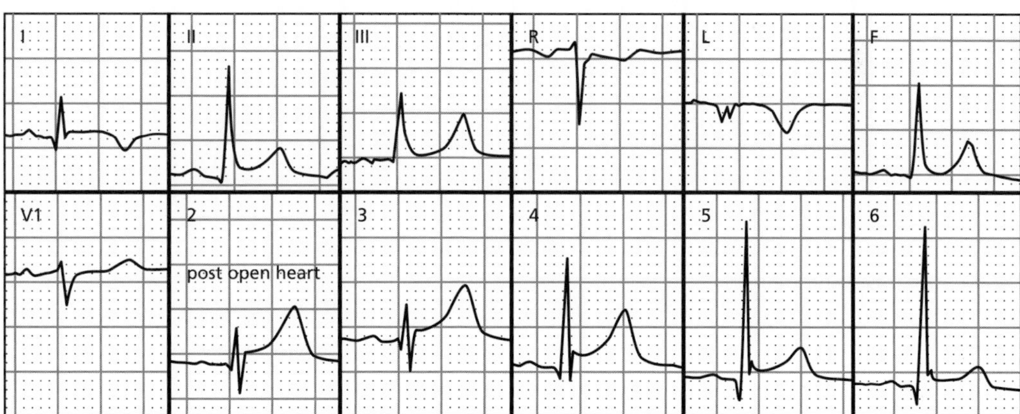
I
II
III
R
L
F
V1
2
post open heart
3
4
5
6

3.34.

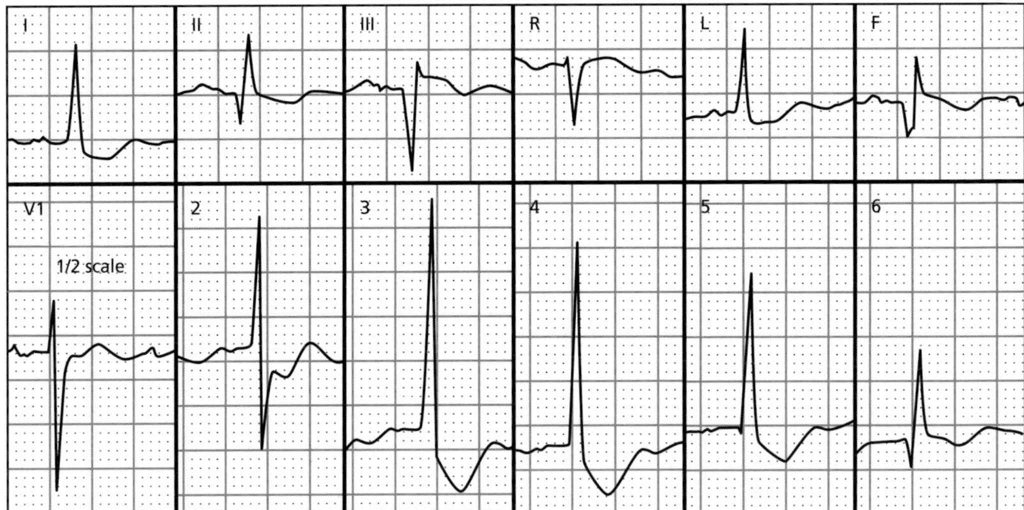
I
II
III
R
L
F
V1
1/2 scale
2
3
4
5
6

3.35.

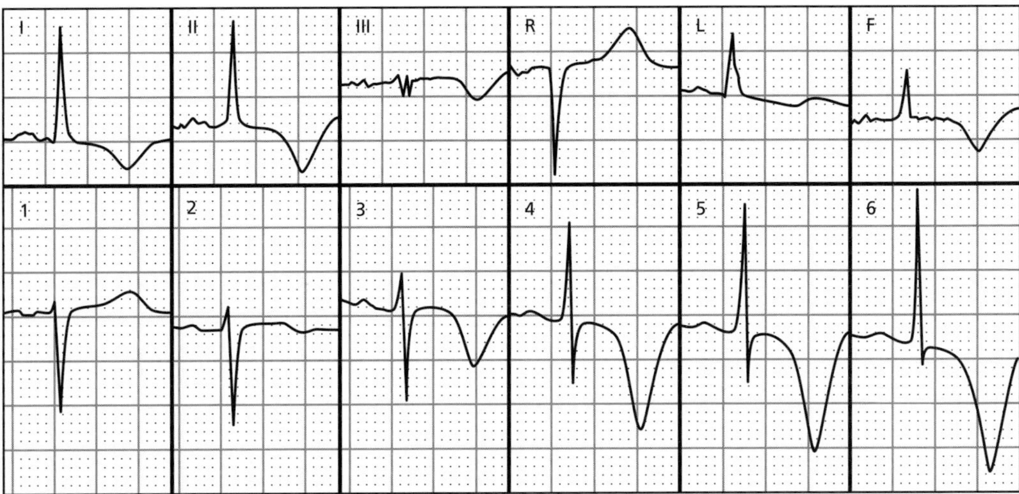
I
II
III
R
L
F
1
2
3
4
5
6

3.36.

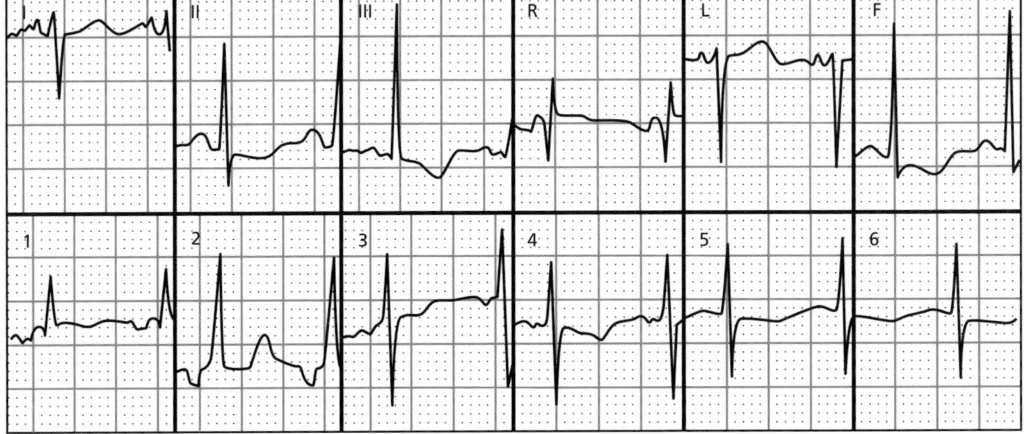
I
II
III
R
L
F
1
2
3
4
5
6

3.37.

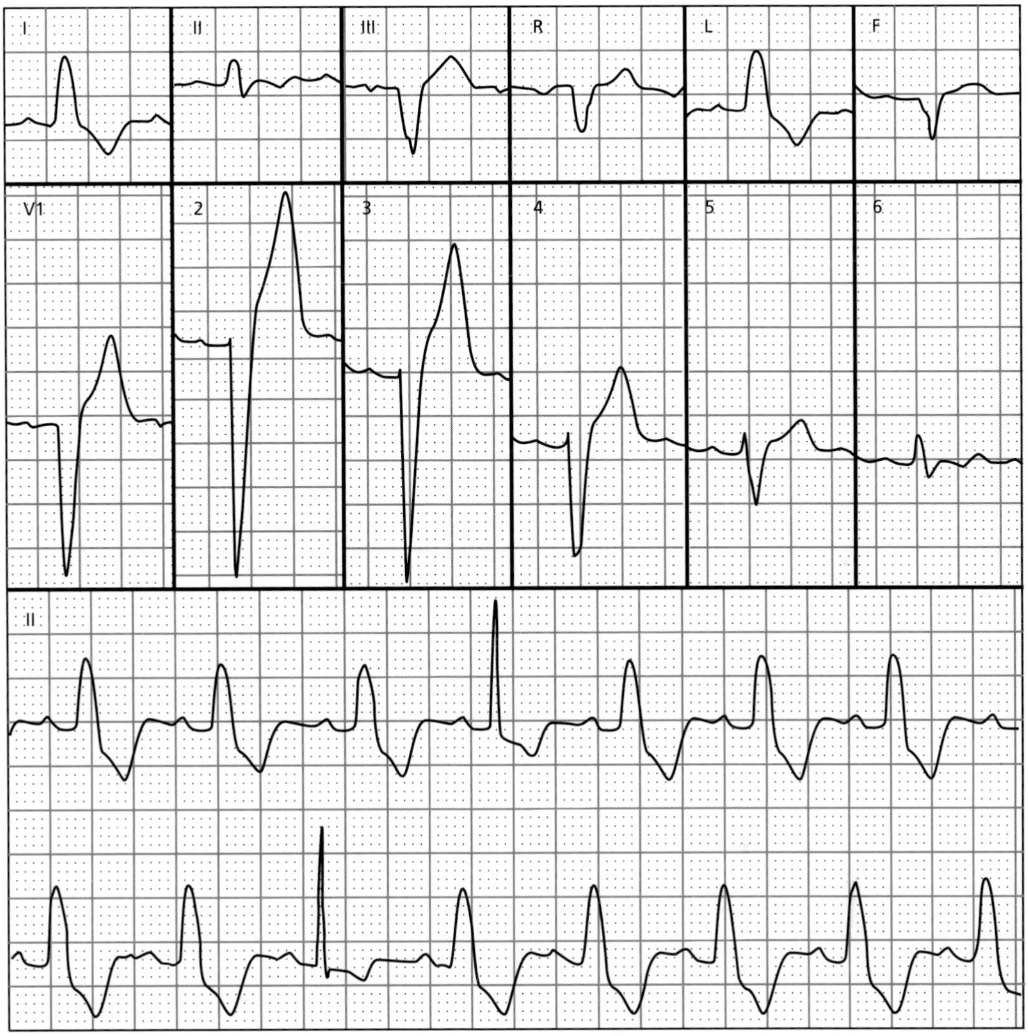

3.38.

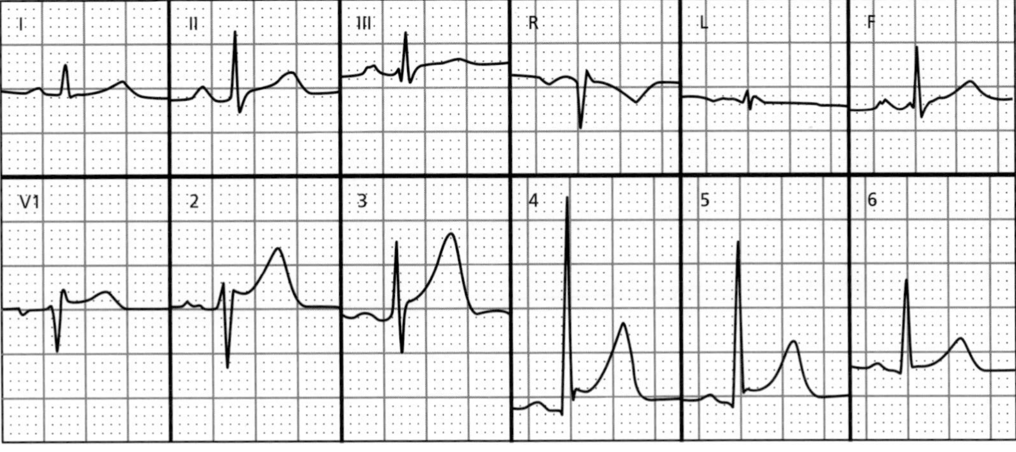

3.39.

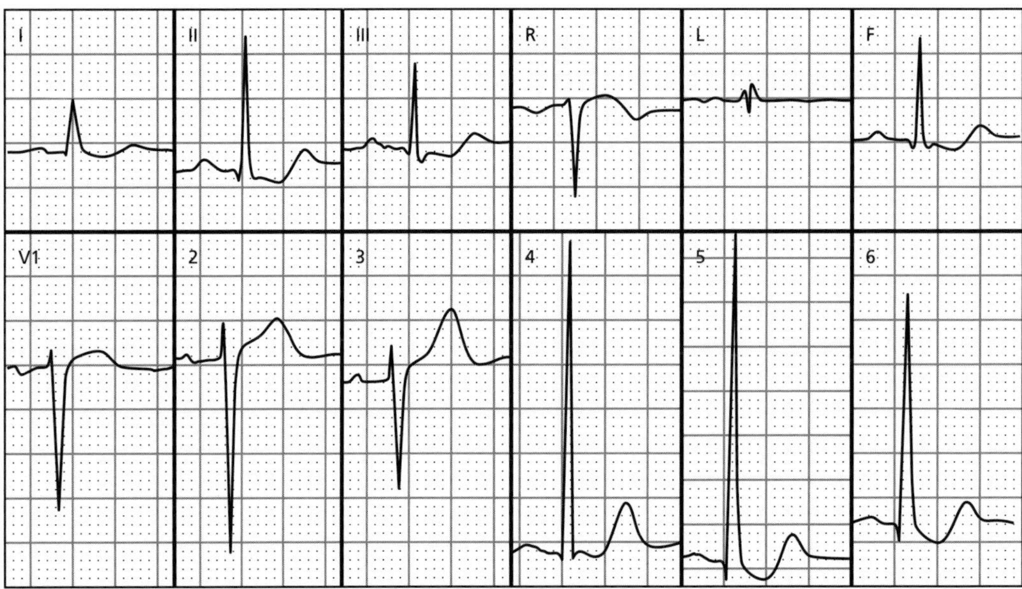

3.40.

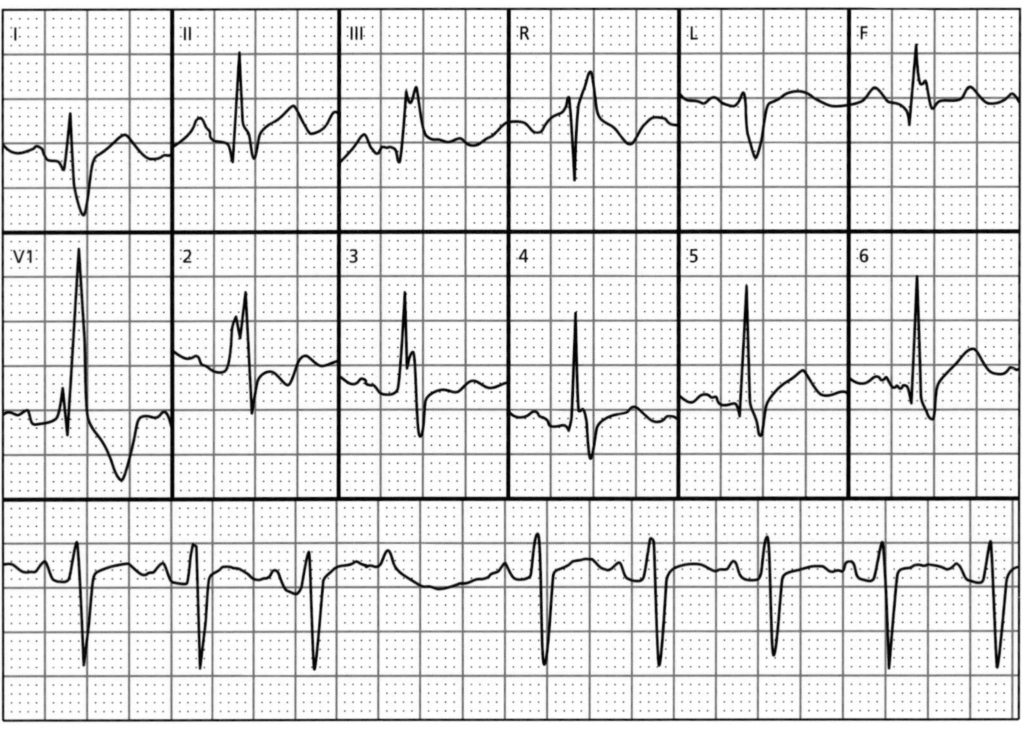

CHAPTER 9

Atrioventricular block

Atrioventricular block refers to slowing of conduction or loss of conduction between the atria and ventricles due to pathology of the conduction structures.

First-degree atrioventricular block

The normal PR interval ranges from 120 to 200 milliseconds (0.12 to 0.20 sec) in adults. Any interval longer than 200 msec is regarded as *first-degree atrioventricular* (AV) *block* (Figure 9.1). Harmless prolongation of the PR interval is occasionally noted in children, aerobically trained athletes, and the elderly. If 'block' is understood as the opposite of 'conduction,' then first-degree AV block is a complete misnomer, since the conduction ratio between the atria and ventricles remains 1:1. However illogical the term may be on analysis, it is firmly entrenched and universally used.

In young subjects changes in vagal tone may cause the PR interval to intermittently lengthen before returning to its baseline value, a finding known as *floating PR interval*. Other, more exotic, causes of variable PR intervals are discussed later in this chapter.

Second-degree atrioventricular block

Intermittent loss of conduction between the atria and ventricles results in *second-degree atrioventricular block*, which may take a number of forms.

Mobitz type I (Wenckebach) second-degree atrioventricular block is a common form of AV block characterized by *decremental conduction*: cycles of progressive conduction delay end with failure of impulse transmission (Figure 9.2). The typical ECG presentation consists of *clusters of QRS complexes separated by pauses*. The interval from the first conducted beat of one group to the first conducted beat of the next constitutes a *Wenckebach cycle* or *period*.

The conduction ratio of a Wenckebach cycle is determined by the number of P waves to the number of QRS complexes (P:QRS) (Figure 9.3).

In M*obitz type II second-degree atrioventricular block* progressive lengthening of the PR interval is absent. Consecutively conducted P waves are followed by constant PR intervals that may be of normal duration or prolonged but *do not lengthen* before a P wave fails to conduct (Figure 9.4). In Mobitz II block, atrioventricular conduction is often referred to as 'all or none.'

It must be emphasized that separation of type I from type II second-degree block is based on an examination of **consecutive PR intervals.** Many textbooks erroneously classify 2:1 atrioventricular conduction ratios as examples of type II AV block, a practice that has resulted in widespread misinformation and confusion. *Atrioventricular block with persistent 2:1 conduction ratios may be a variant of either type I or type II, but the type is impossible to specify unless* **consecutive** *PR intervals are available for examination.* The two types of second-degree

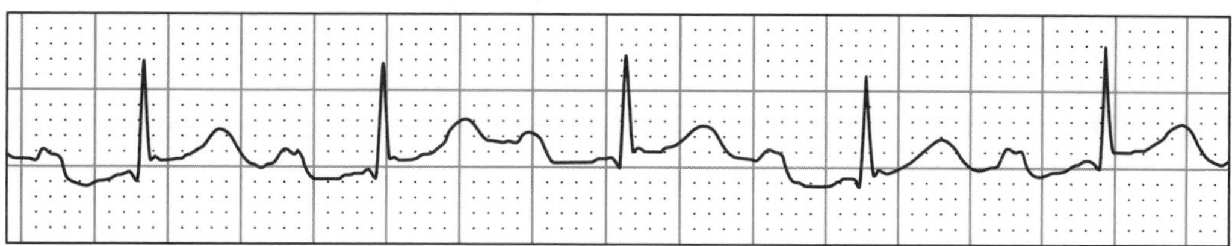

Figure 9.1 First-degree atrioventricular block: prolonged PR interval (280 msec).

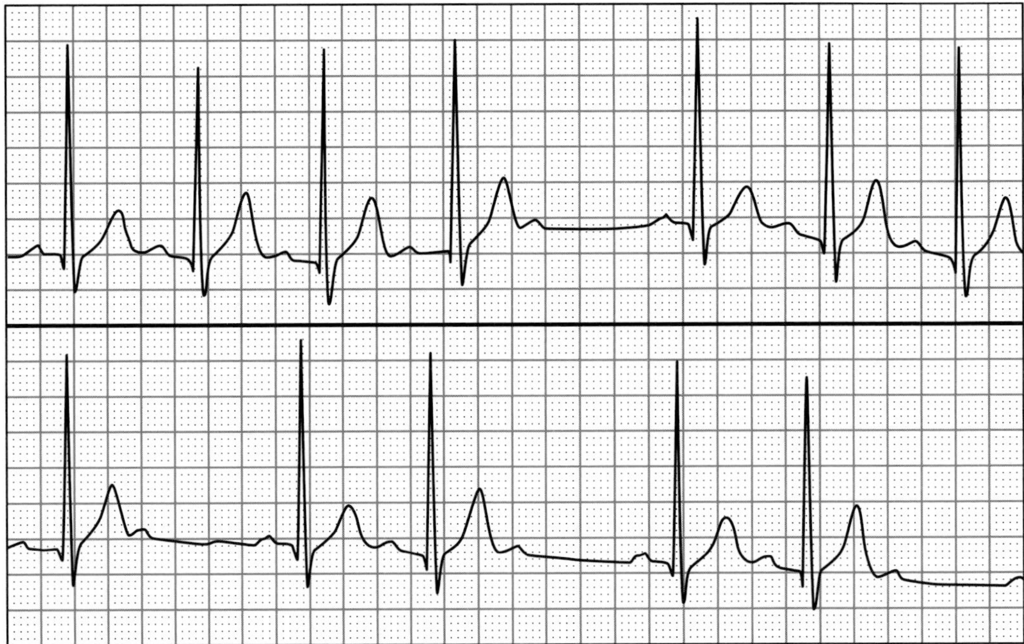

Figure 9.2 Second-degree atrioventricular block, type I (Wenckebach). Consecutive PR intervals lengthen before conduction fails.

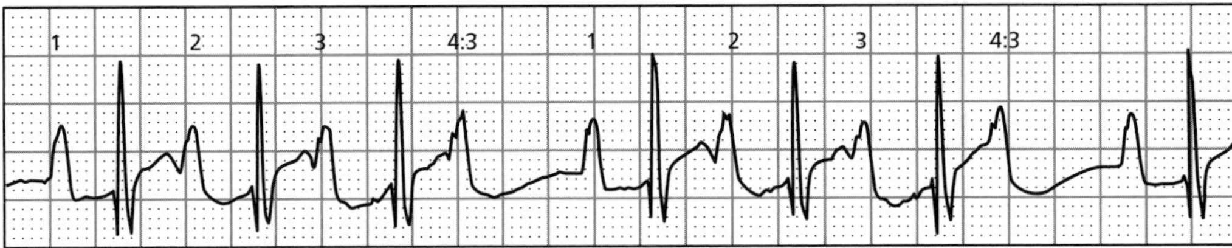

Figure 9.3 Atrioventricular Wenckebach cycles with 4:3 conduction ratios.

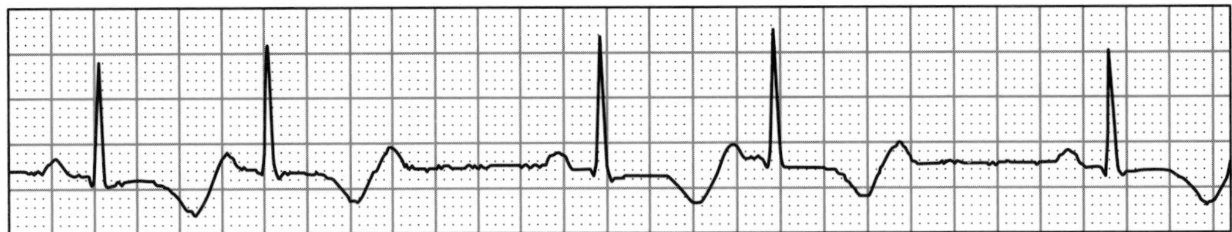

Figure 9.4 Second-degree atrioventricular block, type II (Mobitz II). Consecutive PR intervals remain the same before conduction fails. QRS complexes of normal width indicate the site of block is the bundle of His.

AV block may be confidently differentiated by the following two simple rules.

• If any two consecutive PR intervals in a cycle are of unequal length, the block is type I.

• If the PR interval of a conducted sinus beat after the pause is shorter than any PR interval before the pause, the block is type I.

It follows that second-degree AV block with constant 2:1 or 3:1 conduction ratios (Figure 9.5) poses a diagnostic problem: P waves are never conducted consecutively and therefore consecutive PR intervals are not present for inspection. In this situation, no attempt should be made to classify the block as to type.

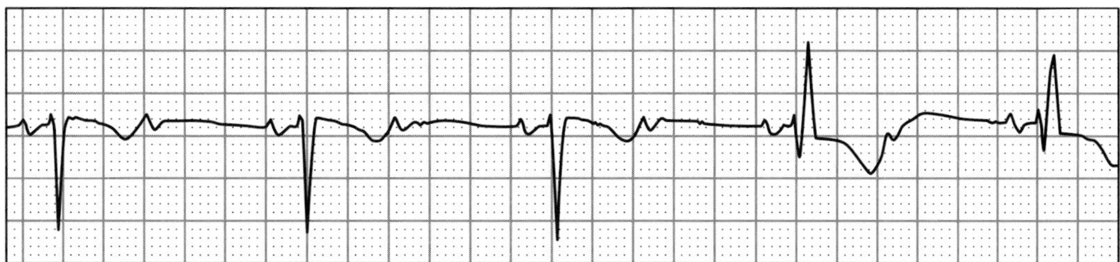

Figure 9.5 Second-degree atrioventricular block with a 2:1 conduction ratio. Intraventricular conduction switches to right bundle branch block (V1) in the final two QRS complexes.

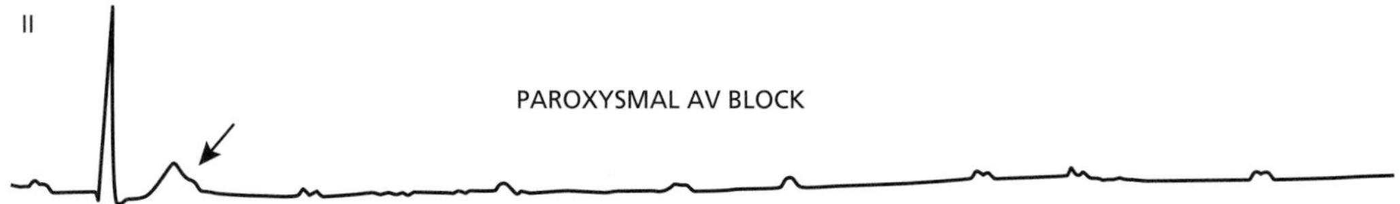

Figure 9.6 Paroxysmal atrioventricular block triggered by a premature atrial beat (*arrow*).

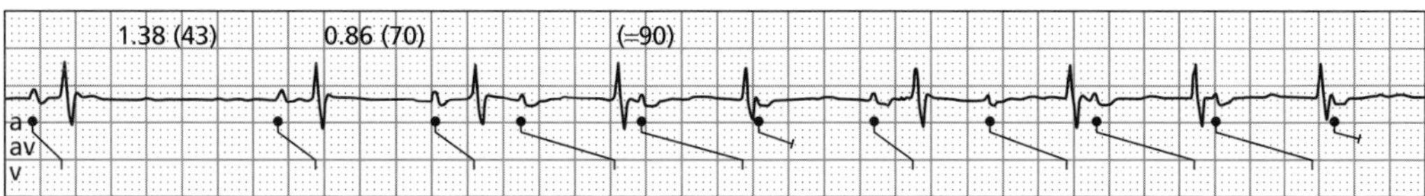

Figure 9.7 Paroxysmal atrioventricular block triggered by an increase in atrial rate.

In the majority of cases, type I AV block occurs in the atrioventricular node. In most cases of type II AV block, defective conduction is located in the His bundle or bundle branches. It is widely taught that the presence of bundle branch block confirms the diagnosis of type II AV block, but this is not the case. Either type I or type II block can be observed in the bundle of His, with or without concomitant fascicular or bundle branch block.

High-grade or *advanced second-degree AV block* occurs when three or more consecutive P waves fail to conduct. In the setting of anterior wall myocardial infarction, this finding represents a progression of type II block (bilateral bundle branch block) in most cases.

Paroxysmal atrioventricular block (PAVB) refers to sudden loss of atrioventricular conduction following a premature atrial or ventricular beat (Figure 9.6) or an increase in sinus rate (Figures 9.7). Other signs of conduction system deficits, such as fascicular block and/or bundle branch block, are generally present, and PAVB often results in prolonged periods of ventricular asystole. Atrioventricular conduction usually resumes following the eventual emergence of an escape beat. PAVB should be regarded as an equivalent of complete (third-degree) heart block.

Third-degree atrioventricular block

Third-degree (complete) atrioventricular block refers to prolonged, complete loss of conduction between the atria and ventricles that results in *atrioventricular dissociation*, i.e. independent, asynchronous atrial and ventricular activity in which P waves and QRS complexes have no fixed relationship to each other (Figure 9.8). During complete heart block the ventricles are typically controlled by a slow, regular escape rhythm. In the absence of an escape rhythm, ventricular asystole occurs (Figure 9.9).

A confident diagnosis of complete heart block usually cannot be made unless the ventricular rate is less than 45 beats per minute.

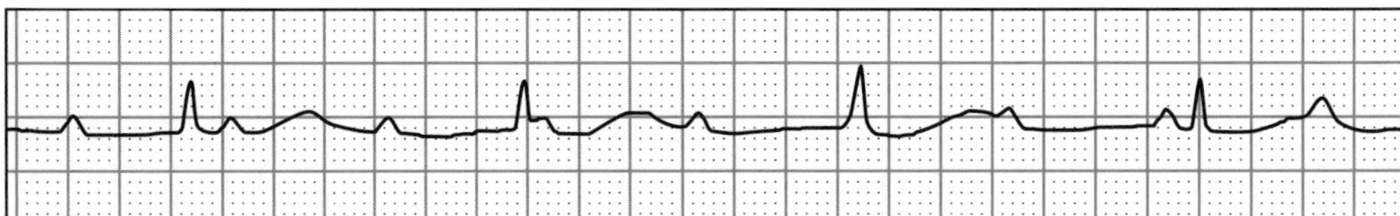

Figure 9.8 Third-degree atrioventricular block with junctional escape rhythm.

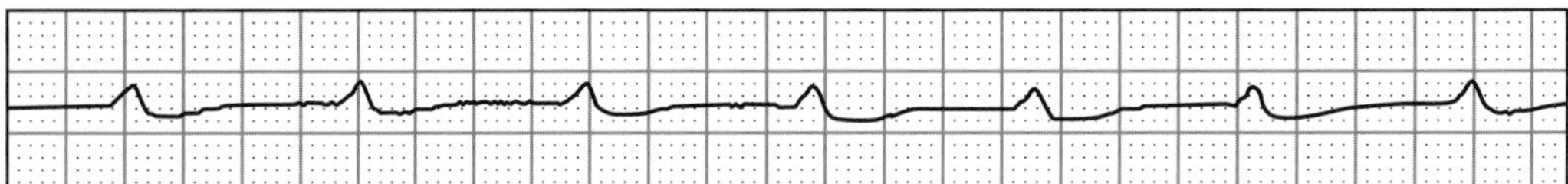

Figure 9.9 Third-degree atrioventricular block with ventricular asystole (no QRS complexes).

Complete heart block complicating inferior wall infarction is located in the AV node and is usually transient. Escape rhythms are nearly always present and the ventricular rate is generally fast enough to prevent hemodynamic collapse. In anterior wall infarctions complete AV block represents bilateral bundle branch block and may be permanent. Escape rhythms in this setting are typically absent or slow.

Third-degree AV block not complicating myocardial infarction usually represents sclerodegenerative disease of the distal conduction system (*Lenègre's syndrome*) or interruption of conduction due to calcification of the atrioventricular valve rings and related structures (*Lev's syndrome*). Complete heart block is occasionally congenital. Acquired block should prompt a search for infectious agents such as Lyme disease, Chagas' disease, valve ring abscess, rheumatic fever or viral myocarditis. Very rarely complete heart block occurs owing to cardiac or pericardial neoplasia.

Atrioventricular dissociation

Atrioventricular dissociation refers to independent asynchronous atrial and ventricular rhythms, and may be transient or sustained. Although complete heart block is an important cause of atrioventricular dissociation, the terms are not synonymous. Another common cause of independent atrial and ventricular rhythms, *isorhythmic atrioventricular dissociation*, occurs when atrial and ventricular rates are similar. In this situation atrioventricular conduction is impeded when impulses from the sinus node and an escape pacemaker enter the AV node simultaneously and cancel each other. Isorhythmic dissociation is most commonly noted when a relatively slow sinus rate coexists with an accelerated junctional rhythm, and the resulting dissociation of the upper and lower chambers is generally transitory (Figure 9.10).

Atrioventricular block of some degree often combines with an accelerated junctional rhythm to produce AV dissociation. Henry Marriott coined the useful descriptive term '*block-acceleration dissociation*' to describe this phenomenon.

Supernormal conduction

Terminology notwithstanding, there is nothing normal about 'supernormal' conduction. The phenomenon of *supernormality*, usually noted in states of severely depressed conduction, refers to impulse transmission that occurs during the so-called supernormal period, a brief period of better-than-expected conduction corresponding to the peak of the T wave. In the case of supernormal conduction, timing is everything: impulses arriving earlier or later fail to conduct (Figure 9.11).

Wenckebach periods: variations on a theme

Figure 9.12 shows sinus rhythm intermittently interrupted by short bursts of atrial tachycardia at a rate of 230 per minute. The P waves of the tachycardia are marked with dots for ease of identification and a laddergram is provided to clarify

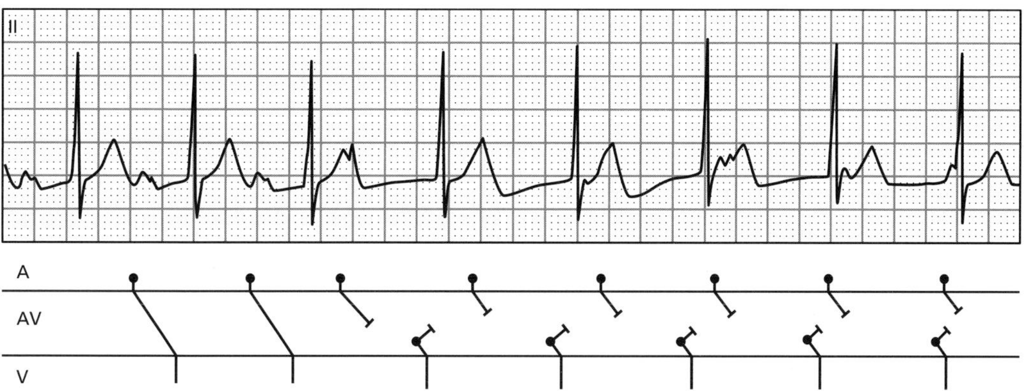

Figure 9.10 Block-acceleration dissociation: first-degree atrioventricular block combined with an accelerated junctional rhythm results in atrioventricular dissociation following a nonconducted atrial extrasystole.

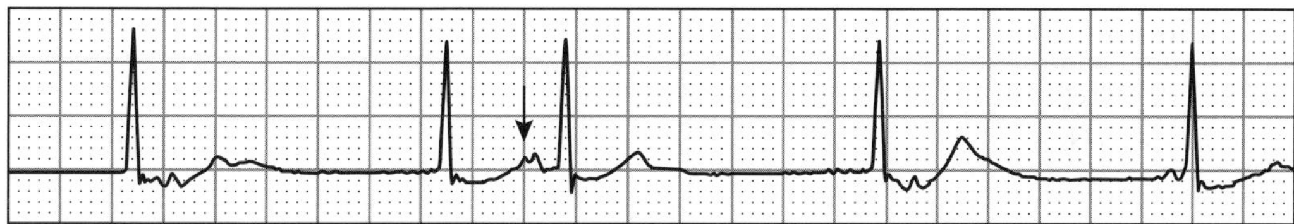

Figure 9.11 Supernormal conduction: the P wave (*arrow*) that falls on the peak of the T wave (the 'supernormal period') conducts, while P waves occurring earlier and later fail to conduct.

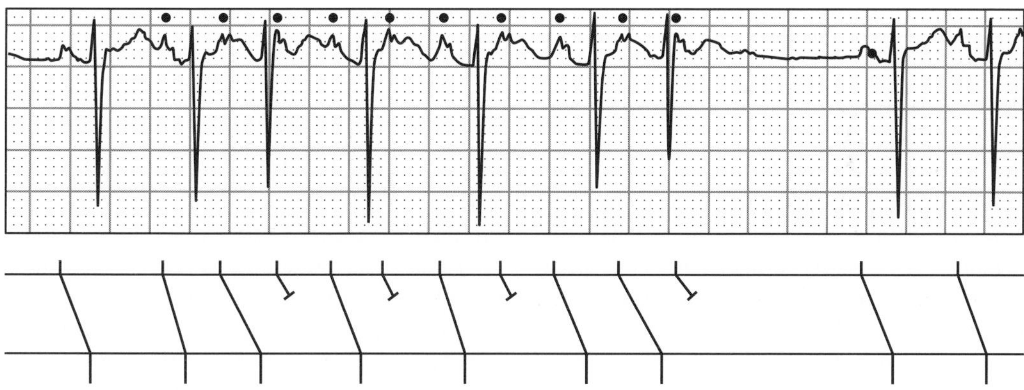

Figure 9.12 Wenckebach conduction of atrial tachycardia.

the conduction pattern. As this case illustrates, the run of tachycardia is conducted in a Wenckebach pattern in which conduction ratios vary from 2:1 to 3:2. As cycle length progressively shortens, continued 1:1 conduction eventually becomes physiologically impossible and a type I, second-degree conduction pattern ensues. The rate (cycle length) at which this occurs is called the *Wenckebach point*, which in most subjects is reached at an atrial rate of between 130 and 190 beats per minute. The tendency to shift from 1:1 conduction to a Wenckebach pattern of impulse transmission as the cycle length shortens is an example of *decremental conduction*, a characteristic of the physiology of the atrioventricular node and certain types of accessory pathways.

An understanding of conduction ratios and how they are maintained has been achieved by studying cases of atrial flutter. Although it might be expected

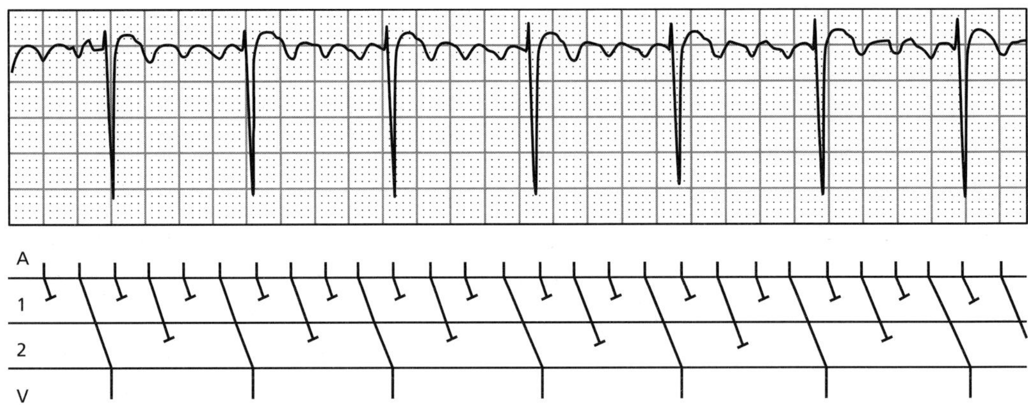

Figure 9.13 Atrial flutter with 4:1 net conduction ratio.

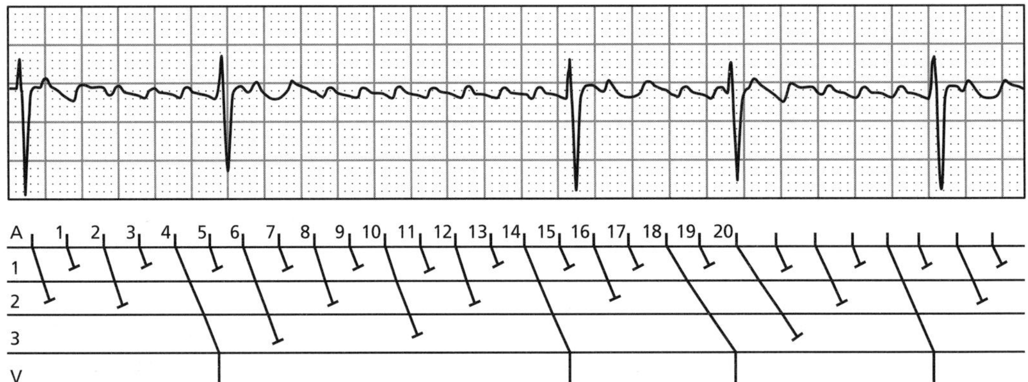

Figure 9.14 Even ratios of atrioventricular conduction (>4:1).

that even and odd conduction ratios would be equally likely, observation has proven that even ratios predominate and that sustained conduction of odd ratios is unusual. It follows that some mechanism works to maintain even ratios while excluding odd ratios.

The laddergram that accompanies the tracing of atrial flutter shown in Figure 9.13 divides the atrioventricular node into two levels (*1, 2*) each with its own conduction properties. The persistence of the even conduction ratio (4:1) can be explained if all odd-numbered impulses are blocked at the upper level and the remaining even-numbered impulses are then conducted in a 2:1 ratio. Concealed conduction into the second level produces block of the subsequent impulse at the first level.

This concept may be extended to explain the lower even ratios (6:1 to 10:1) seen in Figure 9.14. It is again assumed, as in the example already cited, that all odd-numbered beats are blocked at the first level (*1* in the laddergram). A 6:1 ratio (or lower) can then be explained by the penetration of some even-numbered impulses (*6, 10, 20*, etc.) to a third level of block (*3*), increasing the refractoriness of the conduction path so that the next even-numbered impulse is blocked at a higher level (*2*). Because all odd-numbered impulses are blocked at the first level, a 2:1 conduction ratio at the second or third level will favor the maintenance of even net ratios.

The atrial flutter shown in Figure 9.15 illustrates *Wenckebach conduction of alternate beats* (the flutter waves of several cycles have been numbered for ease of reference). The atrioventricular node is diagrammed as two-tiered: at the (proximal) upper level of conduction (*avu*), all odd-numbered impulses are blocked. At the second, middle, level (*avm*), the remaining flutter waves are conducted in Wenckebach cycles (increments of delay are

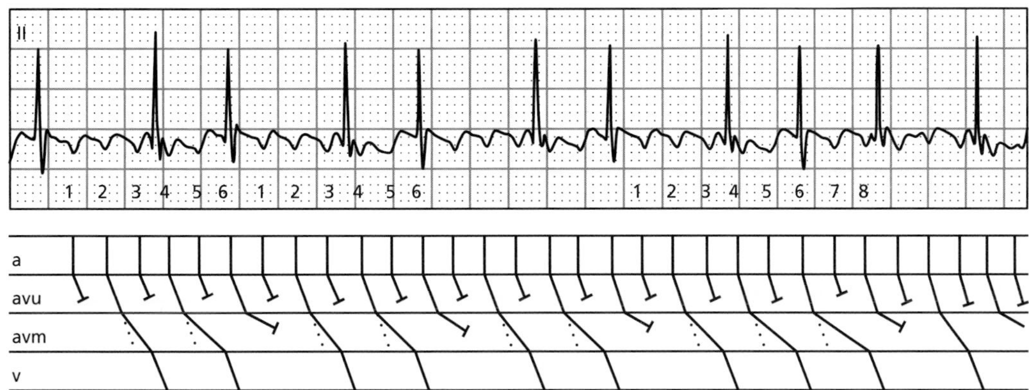

Figure 9.15 Type A Wenckebach periods of alternate beats. As in all cases of atrioventricular Wenckebach periodicity, the QRS complexes tend to cluster.

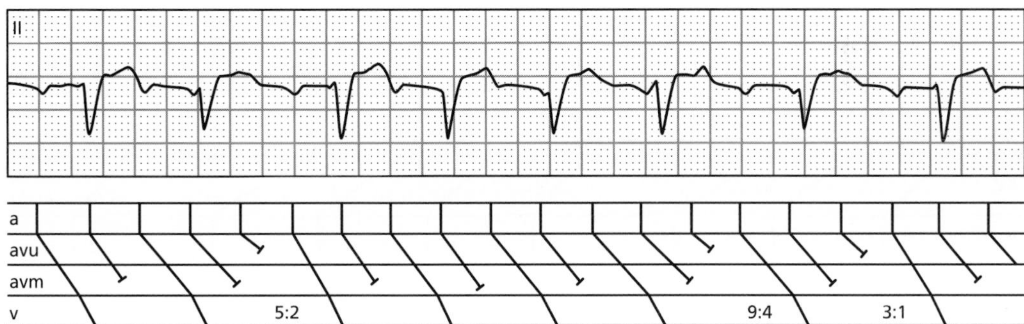

Figure 9.16 Type B Wenckebach periods of alternate beats.

indicated by *dotted lines*). This conduction pattern results in net impulse transmission expressed by the formula:

$$x = (n - 2)/2$$

in which x is the number of ventricular responses and n is the number of atrial impulses. The resulting conduction ratio identifies *Kosowsky type A* Wenckebach periods of alternate beats, indicating that the filtering of odd-numbered beats occurs proximally.

A second form of Wenckebach conduction of alternate beats, designated *Kosowsky type B*, results when the Wenckebach periods occur at the proximal level and 2:1 conduction at the second, middle, level (Figure 9.16). In these cases the net conduction ratio is predicted by the formula:

$$x = (n - 1)/2$$

The conduction ratios resulting from type A and type B Wenckebach conduction of alternate beats are given in tabular form below:

Type A *2:1/Wenckebach*	*Type B* *Wenckebach/2:1*
6:2	3:1
8:3	5:2
10:4	7:3
12:5	9:4
14:6	11:5

Very rarely, Wenckebach conduction may occur at both the proximal and distal levels. Two cycles of the laddergram accompanying Figure 9.17 are drawn to suggest that concealed re-entry from the distal level into the proximal level of conduction is responsible for this phenomenon.

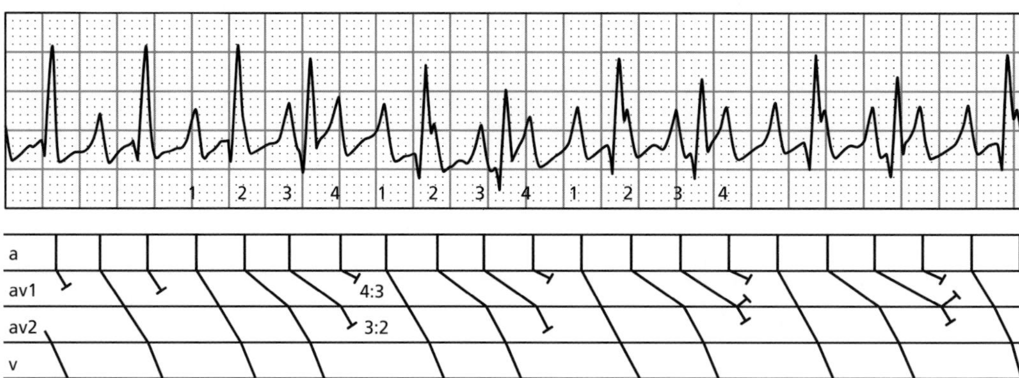

Figure 9.17 Wenckebach periods at successive levels.

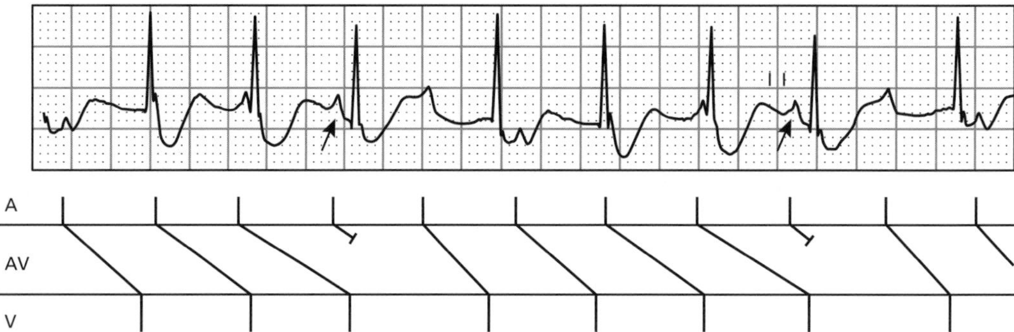

Figure 9.18 Skipped P waves: the blocked P wave (*arrow*) falls within the PR interval of a conducted P wave.

Wenckebach periodicity can probably occur in any segment of cardiac tissue that is capable of conduction. The above tracings are merely examples of the complexities that may be encountered.

Very occasionally atrioventricular conduction during Wenckebach cycles becomes so prolonged that the blocked P wave falls within the PR interval of a previously conducted sinus beat. A blocked P wave that falls within the PR interval of its conducted predecessor is called a *skipped P wave* (Figure 9.18). In addition to skipped P waves, very long conduction times during type I, second-degree block may cause some P waves to coincide with and be masked by QRS complexes. An example is shown in Figure 9.19, in which the second P wave of every 3:2 cycle is partially obscured by a QRS complex and the third P wave of each cycle is skipped (laddergram).

Concealed conduction

An impulse that only partially traverses the conduction pathway and stops before depolarizing either the atria, producing a P wave, or the ventricles, producing a QRS complex, will leave no deflection on the ECG to signal its presence. For that reason such impulses are said to be *concealed*.

Although the concealed impulse produces no ECG waveform, its presence can be inferred from its *effect on the formation or conduction of subsequent beats*. Conduction disturbance of subsequent beats occurs because the concealed impulse alters the refractory period of the portion of the pathway it has traversed. Suppression of subsequent impulse formation occurs because pacemaking sites in the wake of the concealed impulse are passively discharged and reset.

A common and easily visualized form of concealed conduction occurs when an interpolated ventricular extrasystole penetrates the atrioventricular nodal tissue in a retrograde direction, but blocks there without reaching the atria. The concealed penetration into the node prolongs its refractory period and causes delayed conduction of the subsequent sinus impulse (Figure 9.20).

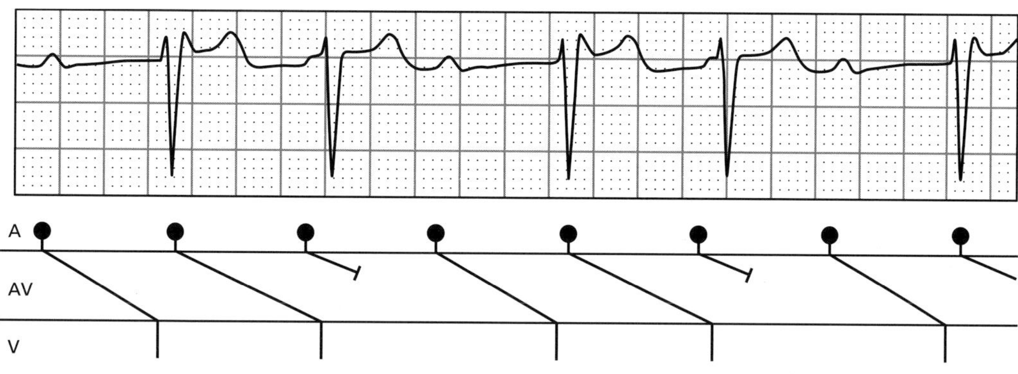

Figure 9.19 P waves coincide with QRS complexes owing to prolonged atrioventricular conduction.

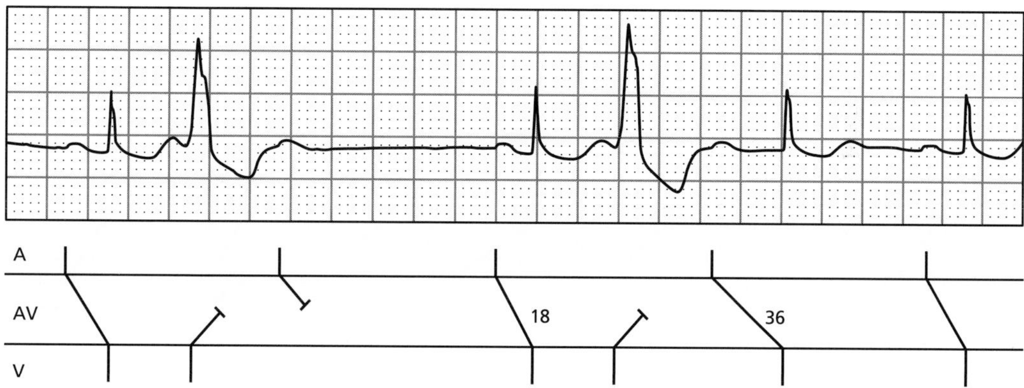

Figure 9.20 Concealed atrioventricular conduction.

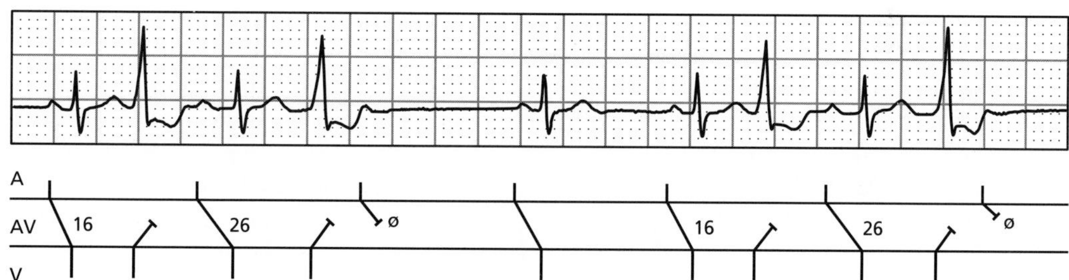

Figure 9.21 Concealed atrioventricular conduction.

Repetitive concealed conduction of interpolated extrasystoles can create a conduction sequence reminiscent of type I (Wenckebach) atrioventricular block (Figure 9.21).

Figure 9.22 illustrates an uncommon variant on the typical Wenckebach cycle: in this cycle (5:4) a sudden, unexpected increment of conduction delay (0.28 to 0.42 sec) occurs in the last PR interval before the pause. The proposed mechanism is shown in the laddergram, which depicts the atrioventricular node divided into two zones, a proximal upper common pathway (*UCP*) and a distal zone of reciprocation (*ZR*) consisting of functionally separate pathways that allow the impulse to reverse direction (reciprocate) and re-enter the upper common pathway. Repetitive *concealed re-entry* into the upper common pathway increases its refractoriness, accounting for the sudden increase in the increment of delay.

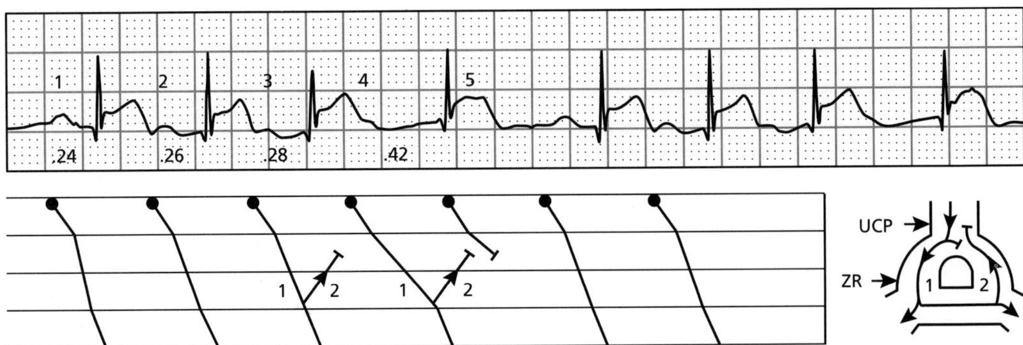

Figure 9.22 Concealed re-entry.

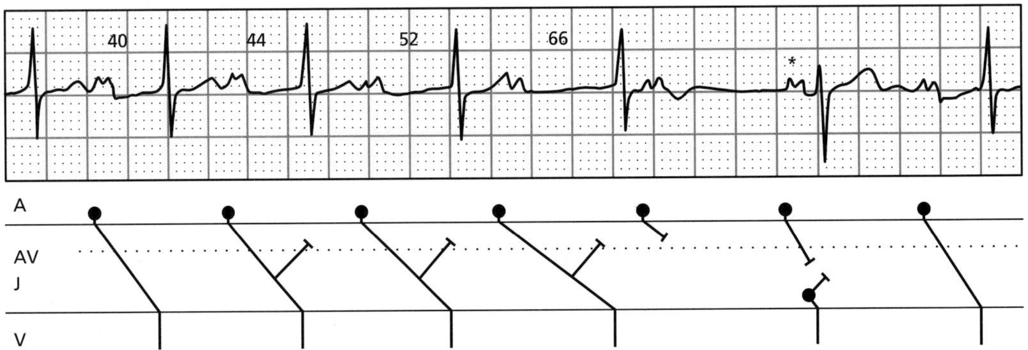

Figure 9.23 Concealed re-entry.

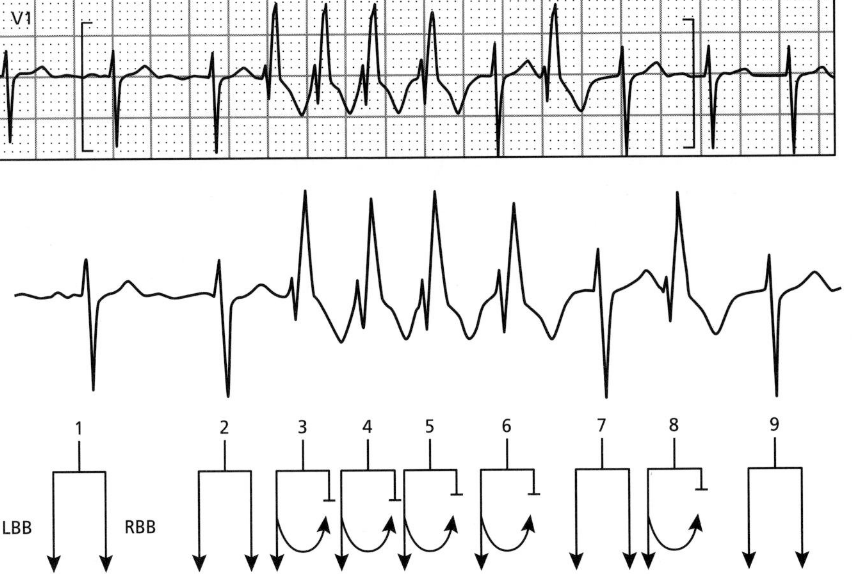

Figure 9.24 Concealed re-entry into the right bundle branch.

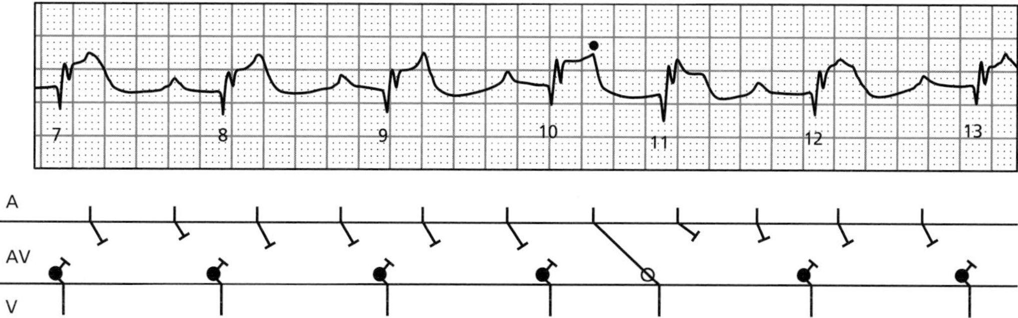

Figure 9.25 Concealed conduction into a pacemaking focus.

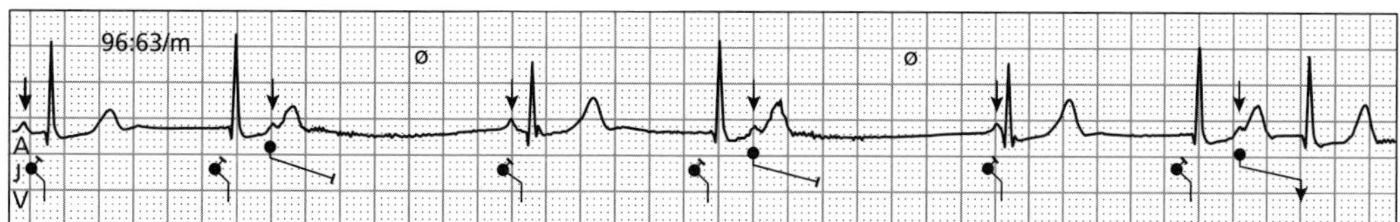

Figure 9.26 Concealed conduction of sinus impulses resets a junctional escape focus. The last sinus impulse (*6th arrow*) conducts, producing a QRS complex.

Repetitive concealed re-entry into an upper common pathway is the likely cause of the long PR intervals shown in Figure 9.23.

Figure 9.24 illustrates atrial fibrillation with varying R–R intervals. Shortening of the cycle length following the third QRS complex induces right bundle branch aberrancy that is maintained for the next three beats. The accompanying diagram indicates that subsequent fibrillation impulses are conducted trans-septally from the normally functioning left bundle branch into the right bundle branch. This repetitive concealed trans-septal conduction into the right bundle branch delays its recovery by repeatedly depolarizing it.

Figure 9.25 shows sinus tachycardia dissociated from an accelerated junctional rhythm. An occasional sinus P wave (*dot*) captures the ventricles, momentarily shortening the R–R interval. The laddergram shows that ventricular capture (*QRS 11*) by the sinus impulse passively discharges the junctional escape focus (*empty circle*), thus resetting it. The impulse that resets the junctional pacemaker is *not concealed*: it produces a QRS complex.

An example of concealed resetting of a subsidiary pacemaker is shown in Figure 9.26, in which sinus bradycardia (*arrows*) is dissociated from an accelerated junctional rhythm. Those sinus P waves falling after the QRS complexes produced by the junctional beats are able to penetrate far enough into the conduction path to reach and reset the junctional escape focus, but do not reach the ventricles to produce a QRS complex. In this case, concealed conduction of the sinus beats is inferred from the suppression of the junctional pacemaker.

10

CHAPTER 10
Atrial arrhythmias

The atrial arrhythmias are those known to originate in the atria *per se*. Supraventricular tachycardias in which atrioventricular node and atrial fibers are an obligatory part of a re-entrant circuit, as well as re-entry via anomalous atrioventricular connections, are described in a subsequent chapter. Atrial extrasystoles and four important tachyarrhythmias – atrial fibrillation, atrial flutter, atrial tachycardia and multifocal atrial tachycardia – are discussed below.

Premature atrial extrasystoles

Premature atrial extrasystoles, commonly called *premature atrial complexes* (PAC), represent the firing of an ectopic (nonsinus) atrial pacemaking focus. The resulting P wave (1) is premature, i.e. earlier than the next expected sinus P wave, and (2) has a different morphology than the sinus P wave (Figure 10.1). Ectopic P waves are sometimes called *P′* waves. Premature atrial extra-systoles usually passively discharge and reset the sinoatrial node, resulting in a pause in sinus rhythm that is *less than twice* the sinus cycle length. If the ectopic impulse fails to reset the sinus node, the extrasystole will be *interpolated*, 'sandwiched' between two sinus beats (Figure 10.2).

Because the ectopic impulse is by definition *early*, it usually finds the distal conduction system in a partially or completely refractory state. As a result, atrial extrasystoles are typically conducted to the ventricles with some measure of delay or not conducted at all. Ectopic atrial beats that fail to conduct are better called *nonconducted* PACs than the misleading 'blocked' PACs. The term 'block' implies conduction failure owing to pathology; PACs sometimes fail to conduct owing to *physiology*, a refractory distal conduction system. Because they suddenly shorten the R–R interval, premature atrial beats are common causes of aberrant ventricular conduction (Figure 10.3).

Atrial extrasystoles may occur singly, in pairs or salvos, or alternate with sinus beats (*atrial bigeminy*) and they may write an upright (positive) or inverted (negative) deflection on the ECG. The P waves of nonconducted atrial extrasystoles are frequently superimposed on the preceding T wave, creating subtle deformities that are easily overlooked. *The most common cause of pauses in sinus rhythm is nonconducted PACs* (Figure 10.4).

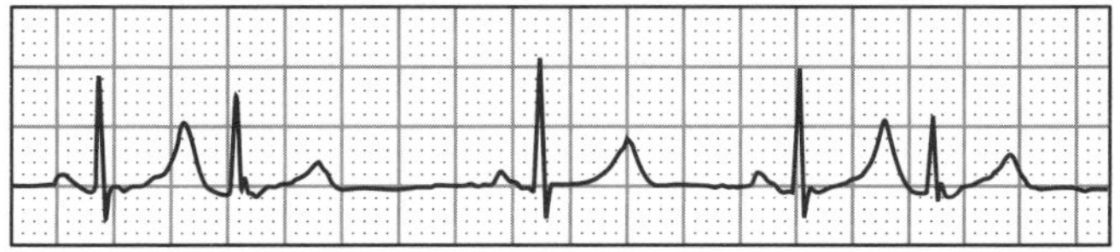

Figure 10.1 Premature atrial extrasystoles: the premature P waves fall on the T wave of the preceding sinus beats. The change in QRS morphology following the premature atrial impulses is due to aberrant ventricular conduction.

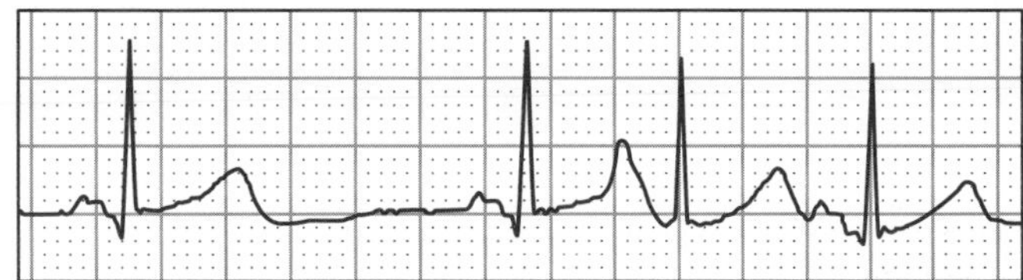

Figure 10.2 An interpolated atrial extrasystole: the premature impulse fails to penetrate the sinoatrial node and reset it. The atrial premature beat is 'sandwiched' between two sinus beats. Subtle acceleration of the sinus rate occurs in response to the extrasystole.

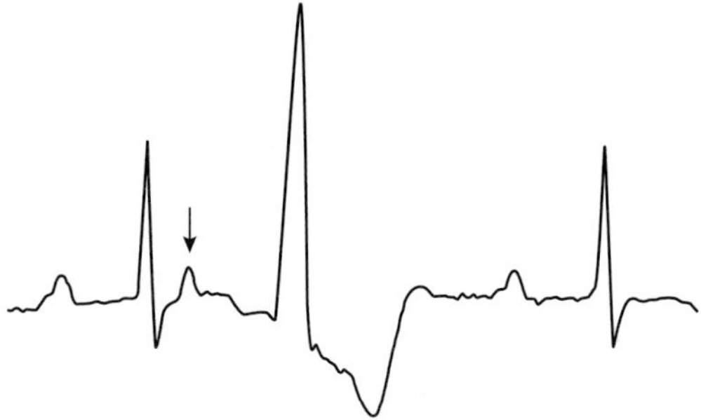

Figure 10.3 A premature atrial beat (*arrow*) triggering aberrant ventricular conduction.

Atrial fibrillation

Atrial fibrillation (AF) is the most common chronic rhythm disorder and is the most frequently treated arrhythmia in the usual hospital setting. A rapidly undulating baseline on the ECG without discretely visible P waves is characteristic (Figure 10.5). Occasionally fine to coarse 'f' waves with a rate greater than 300 per minute are visible. In many chronic cases, however, atrial activity is not clearly visible, resulting in 'flatline' atrial fibrillation.

The current consensus holds that the physiologic substrate of atrial fibrillation is multiple re-entrant circuits located in the left atrium.

The ventricular response to atrial fibrillation is invariably *irregularly irregular*; the random nature of the atrioventricular conduction of the atrial impulses is due to repetitive concealed conduction into the distal conduction structures. Multifocal atrial tachycardia, discussed below, is the only other atrial tachycardia that invariably presents with an irregularly irregular ventricular response. Many arrhythmias result in repetitive sequences of beats (*allorhythmia*), sequences which result in *regularly irregular* patterns. Atrial bigeminy and trigeminy are simple examples of allorhythms that exhibit regular irregularity. Apparent regularization of the ventricular response to atrial fibrillation may occur when atrial fibrillation coexists with complete atrioventricular block and the ventricles are being driven by a junctional pacemaking site (Figure 10.6).

Although atrial fibrillation can occur in subjects with no demonstrable cardiac disease – 'lone atrial fibrillation' – in the majority of cases atrial fibrillation is a reliable sign of heart disease. Subjects with left atrial abnormality while in sinus rhythm are particularly prone to develop AF (Figure 10.7).

The most common conditions associated with AF are (1) mitral valve disease, (2) cardiomyopathy, (3) pericarditis, particularly following open heart

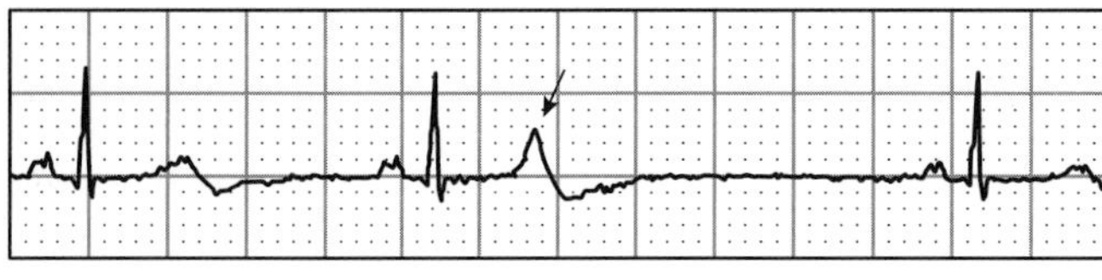

Figure 10.4 A nonconducted atrial extrasystole (*arrow*) superimposed on the T wave of the preceding beat.

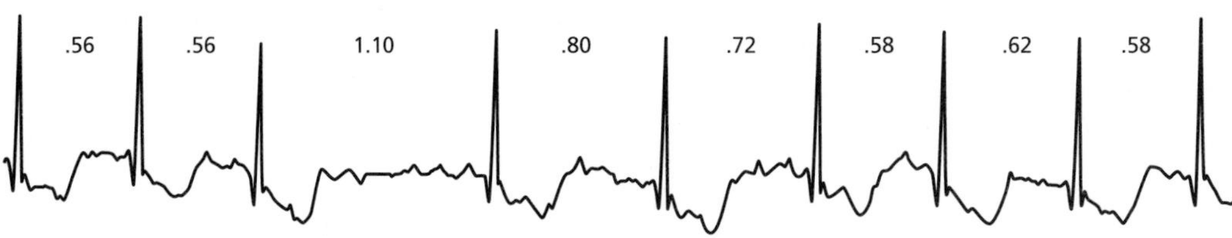

Figure 10.5 Atrial fibrillation: the R–R intervals are irregularly irregular.

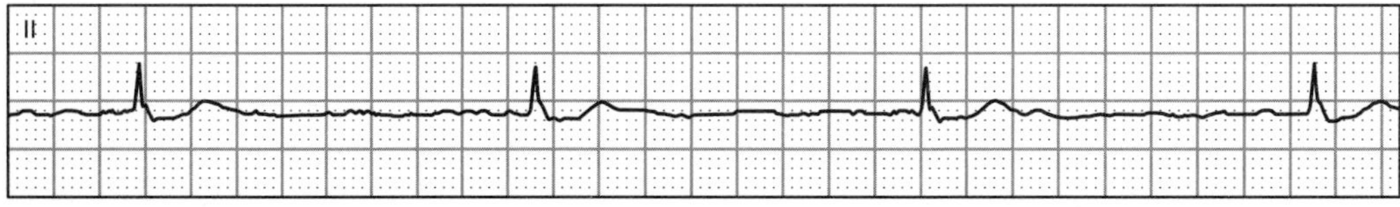

Figure 10.6 Atrial fibrillation with complete atrioventricular block: the ventricles are being driven by a regular junctional escape rhythm.

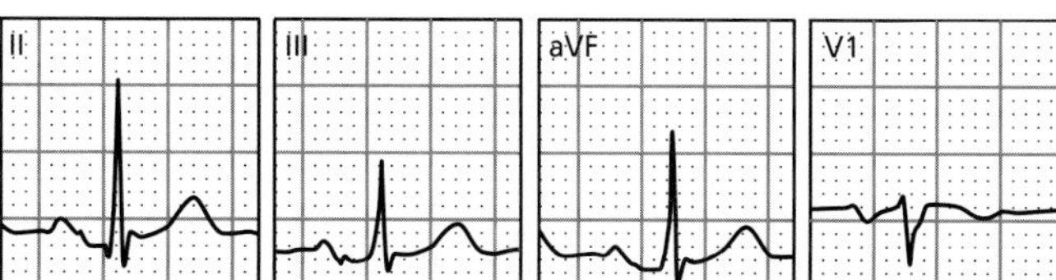

Figure 10.7 Left atrial abnormality: a wide 'double-humped' P wave in the inferior leads and a wide terminal deflection in V1.

surgery, (4) acute myocardial infarction, (5) thyrotoxicosis, and (6) acute alcohol intoxication ('holiday heart syndrome'). Atrial fibrillation is an important cause of cerebral embolism and is the arrhythmia that may provoke ventricular fibrillation in subjects with Wolff–Parkinson–White syndrome.

Atrial flutter

The ECG presentation of *atrial flutter* (AFL) consists of 'sawtooth' or 'picket fence' flutter waves (F waves), most clearly visible in the inferior leads and V1. The rate of AFL is usually from 240 to 340 per minute, with 300 per minute being most often observed (Figure 10.8). Even ratios of atrioventricular conduction are the rule in AFL. Odd ratios are typically skipped, so that 2:1 conduction (the most common ratio) jumps to 4:1 and even occasionally to 6:1 or higher. Flutter waves often obscure ('swamp') T waves, but may be difficult to see when superimposed on the QRS complex. Because 2:1 conduction is most common in new, untreated AFL, and the atrial rate is nearly always around 300 per minute, the astute clinician will always suspect AFL when confronted with a regular supraventricular tachycardia with a rate approximating 150 per minute.

Broadly speaking, atrial flutter refers to a set of arrhythmias that originate in re-entrant circuits in the right atrium. In *counterclockwise* (CCW) atrial flutter, the most common form, the re-entrant wavefront moves up the atrial septum and down the lateral wall of the right atrium, writing inverted (negative) flutter waves in the inferior leads and positive flutter waves in lead V1. In *clockwise* (CW) atrial flutter, the re-entrant wave moves down the atrial septum and back up the lateral wall. In both forms, an 'isthmus' of tissue located between the tricuspid valve and the inferior vena cava forms an essential part of the circuit and serves as the most common target for radio-frequency ablation (RFA), which permanently interrupts the arrhythmia in around 90% of cases. In fact, atrial flutter could be classified as isthmus dependent or non-isthmus dependent. Scar-related atrial flutter involves the formation of a re-entrant circuit around a (usually postoperative) scar.

Atrial flutter is also subtyped into a slower *type I variety* that can be entrained and interrupted by rapid atrial pacing, and a faster *type II variety* (340–430 per minute) that does not respond to rapid atrial pacing. Both types of AFL can be interrupted by cardioversion.

In hospitalized adults congestive cardiomyopathy and pericarditis immediately following open-heart surgery represent most of the AFL cases, but previous congenital heart defect repairs that involve the right atrium, chronic obstructive pulmonary disease (COPD), and muscular dystrophy also predispose to scar-related AFL.

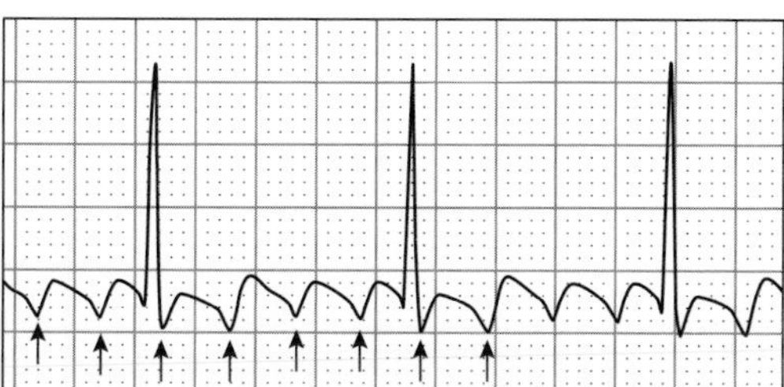

Figure 10.8 Flutter waves that coincide with QRS complexes (arrows) must be counted. The conduction ratio is 4:1, with four flutter waves for each R wave.

Atrial tachycardia

The term *tachycardia* refers to impulse formation at rates greater than 100, regardless of site. More common in children, sustained *atrial tachycardia* (AT) is a relatively uncommon arrhythmia in adults. Brief asymptomatic runs of atrial tachycardia are, however, quite commonly observed in adults in monitored critical care units (Figure 10.9). Atrial tachycardia is characterized by P waves of uniform morphology that are sometimes similar to sinus

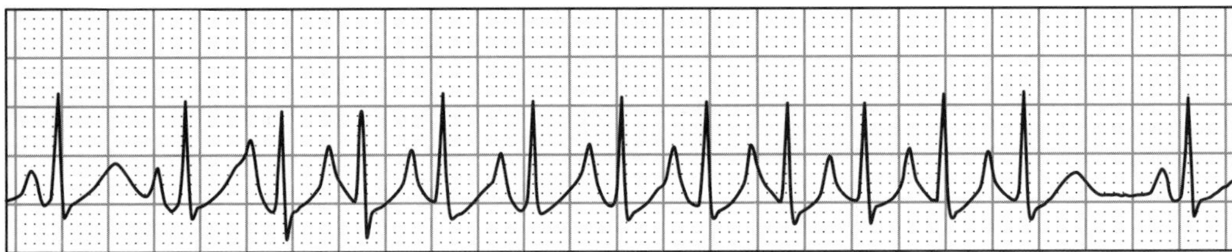

Figure 10.9 A short burst of atrial tachycardia.

P waves. Rate acceleration ('warm up') at the beginning of the tachycardia is frequently noted. Atrioventricular conduction ratios less than 1:1 are common – 2:1 ratios and Wenckebach patterns of conduction are frequently seen.

The rate of AT is quite variable, with a range of 120–280 seen in adults and even faster rates in children. Paroxysmal AT, usually conducted in Wenckebach periods to the ventricles, is most often encountered in adults with advanced cardiac or pulmonary disease, or previous atrial surgery, and is a particularly well-known manifestation of digitalis toxicity. In children, chronic AT is an important cause of tachycardia-mediated cardiomyopathy.

The term *rhythm* refers to impulse formation at rates less than 100 per minute, regardless of site. *Ectopic atrial rhythms* are occasionally seen, but since the P waves are often inverted, these arrhythmias are usually classified as 'junctional.'

Multifocal atrial tachycardia

Multifocal (or multiform) *atrial tachycardia* (MAT) is characterized by (1) discretely visible P waves that exhibit three or more morphologies, (2) an atrial rate greater than 100 per minute, and (3) an irregularly irregular atrial impulse formation and ventricular response (Figure 10.10). If the atrial rate

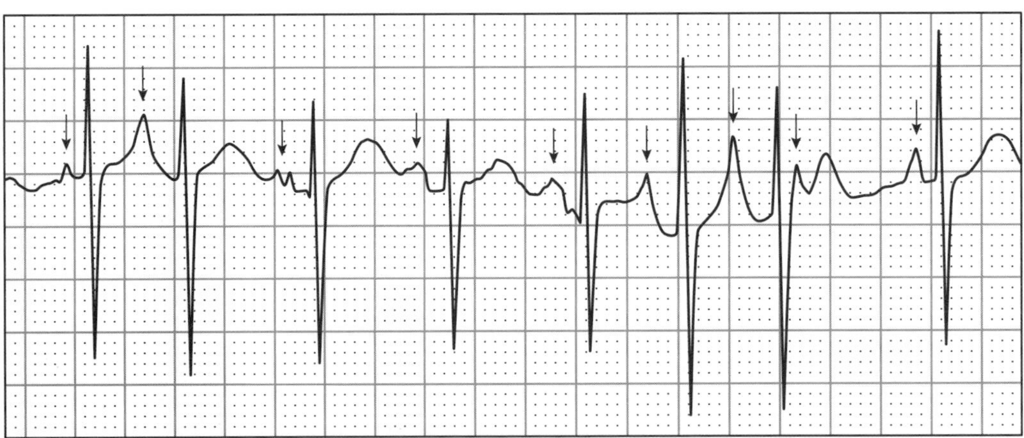

Figure 10.10 Multifocal atrial tachycardia. Note that the baseline is flat between atrial complexes, a feature that distinguishes atrial tachycardia from atrial fibrillation.

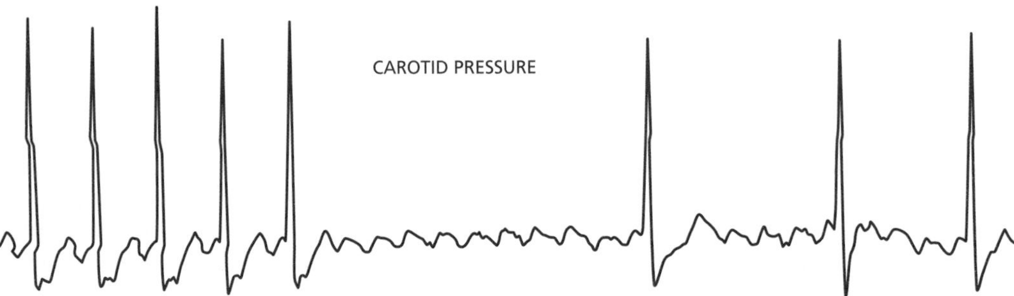

Figure 10.11 Carotid pressure momentarily reveals atrial flutter with a rapid ventricular response.

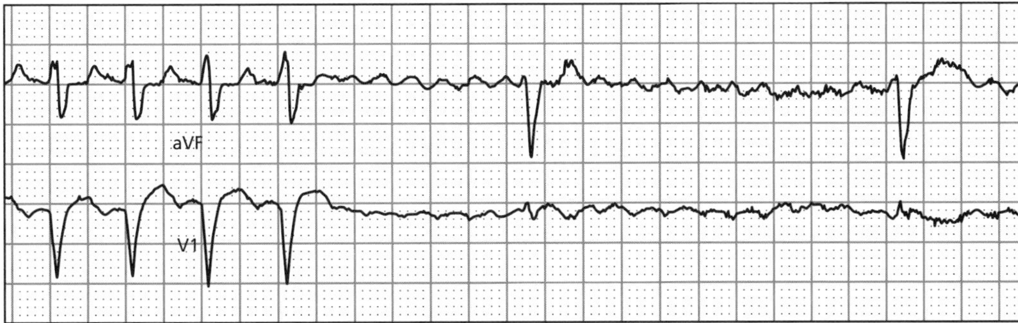

Figure 10.12 A rapid bolus of adenosine reveals low-amplitude atrial flutter.

is less than 100 per minute, *multifocal atrial rhythm* is diagnosed. The multiform ectopic P waves, usually easiest to visualize in the inferior leads and lead V1, may be upright or inverted, rounded or pointed, narrow or wide, flat or tall, bifid or biphasic. Each change in morphology is accompanied by a change in rate, and nonconduction of early P waves is common. The arrhythmia is often seen in subjects with exacerbation of severe pulmonary disease.

Multifocal atrial tachycardia is often mistaken for atrial fibrillation, but established atrial fibrillation usually presents with an undulating baseline without discrete P wave activity. Unlike AF, MAT has isoelectric intervals between discrete P waves. Atrial flutter exhibits uniform morphology as does established atrial tachycardia.

Diagnostic maneuvers

A rapid ventricular response to atrial arrhythmias may produce a picture so obscure that accurate diagnosis is difficult. Several maneuvers may be attempted to clarify the nature of the arrhythmia. *Carotid sinus massage*, which triggers baroreceptors that produce a reflex slowing of atrioventricular conduction, is a time-honored technique for transiently revealing atrial rhythms (Figure 10.11).

An effect similar to carotid massage can be achieved by rapid injection of adenosine. This method is safer for patients, particularly those with carotid artery disease. The transitory atrioventricular conduction block will often unmask the underlying atrial rhythm (Figure 10.12).

Clarification of atrial activity can also be attempted by changing lead placement in a way that enhances the amplitude of atrial complexes. The

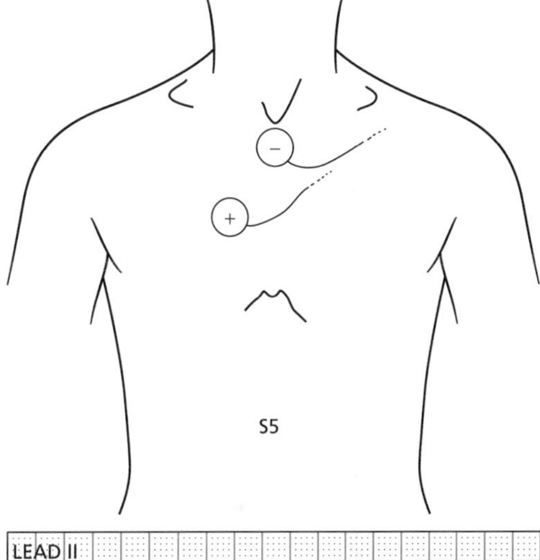

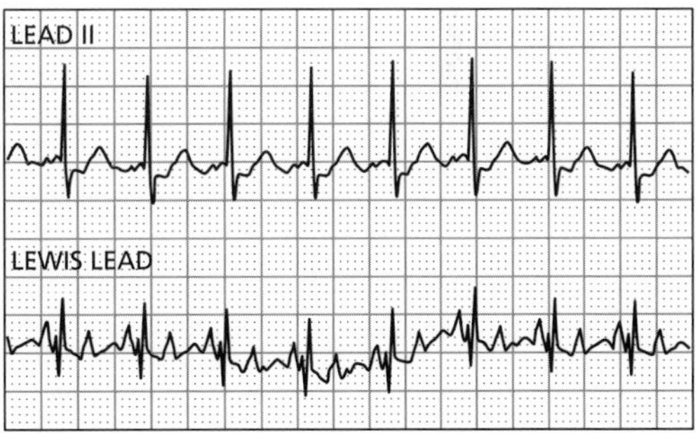

Figure 10.13 The Lewis lead used to clarify atrial activity. The rhythm is atrial flutter with 2:1 conduction.

application of the *Lewis lead* or *S5 lead* is illustrated in Figure 10.13. A negative electrode is placed over the upper manubrium and a positive electrode is placed to the right of the midsternal border. In patients with temporary atrial pacing wires in place, atrial activity may be visualized on the monitor by connecting the atrial wires to monitor cables.

Self-Assessment Test Four

Identify the abnormalities in the following 45 tracings.

4.1.

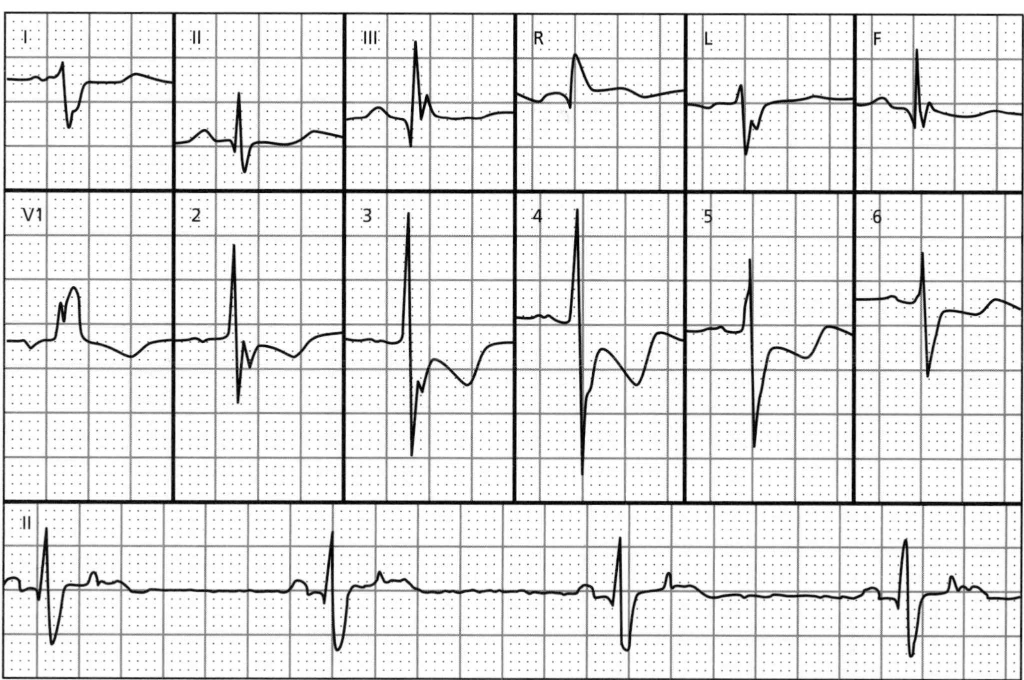

4.2.

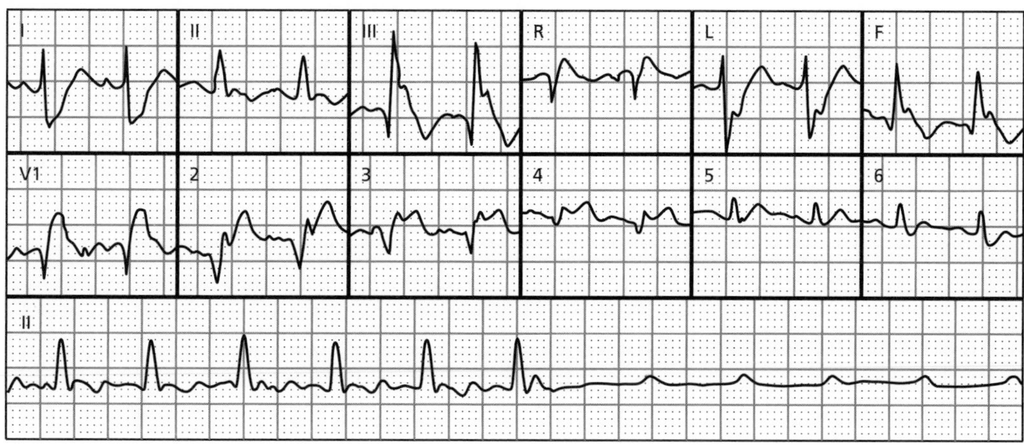

4.3.

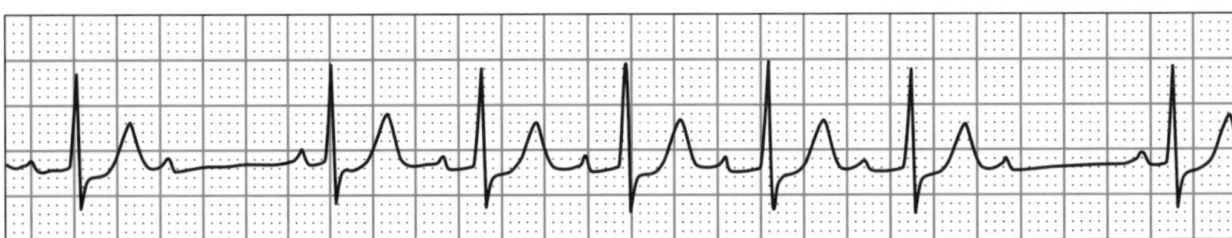

4.4.

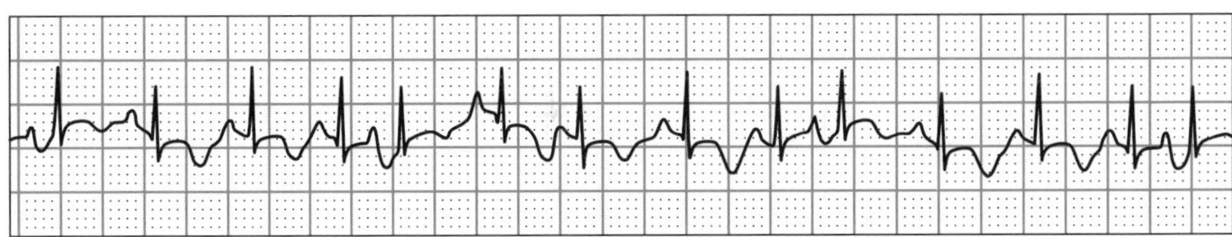

4.5.

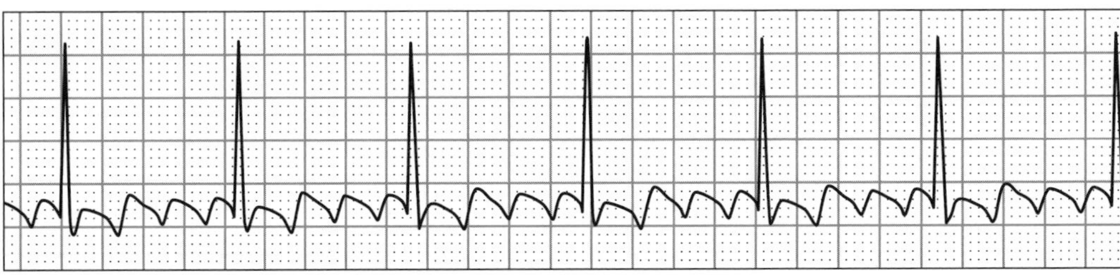

4.6.

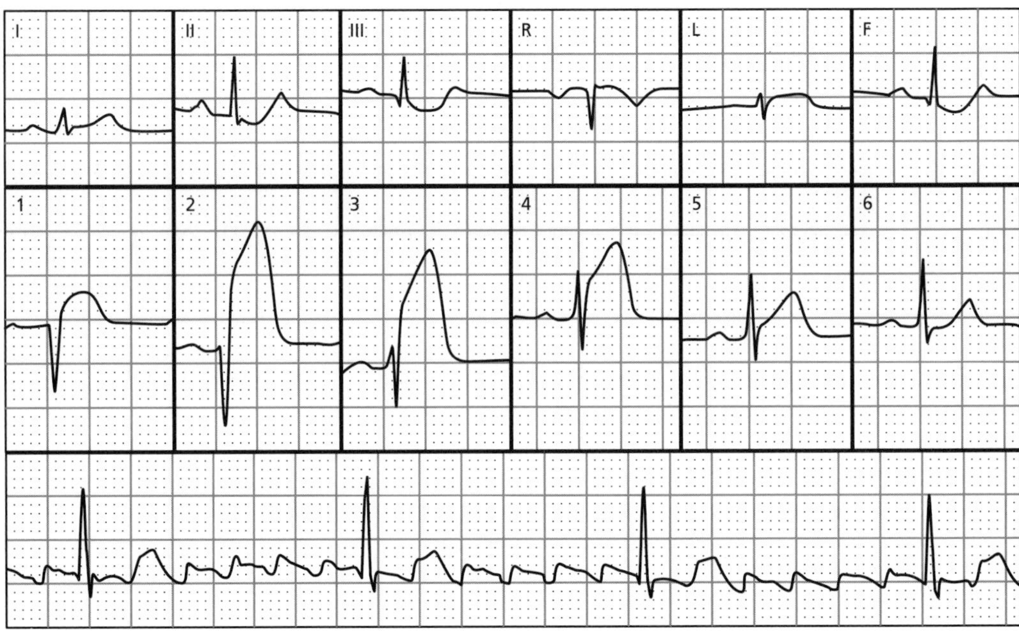

4.7.

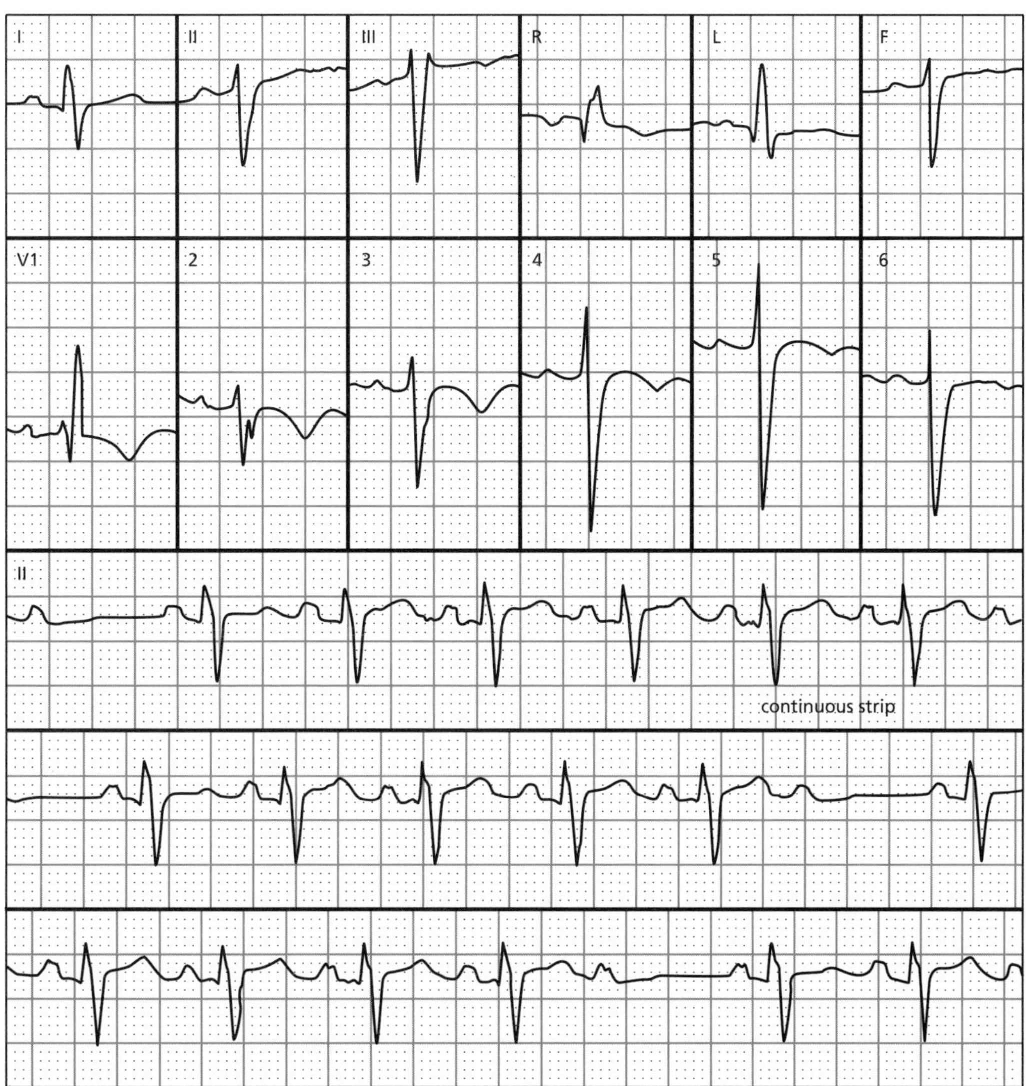

4.8.

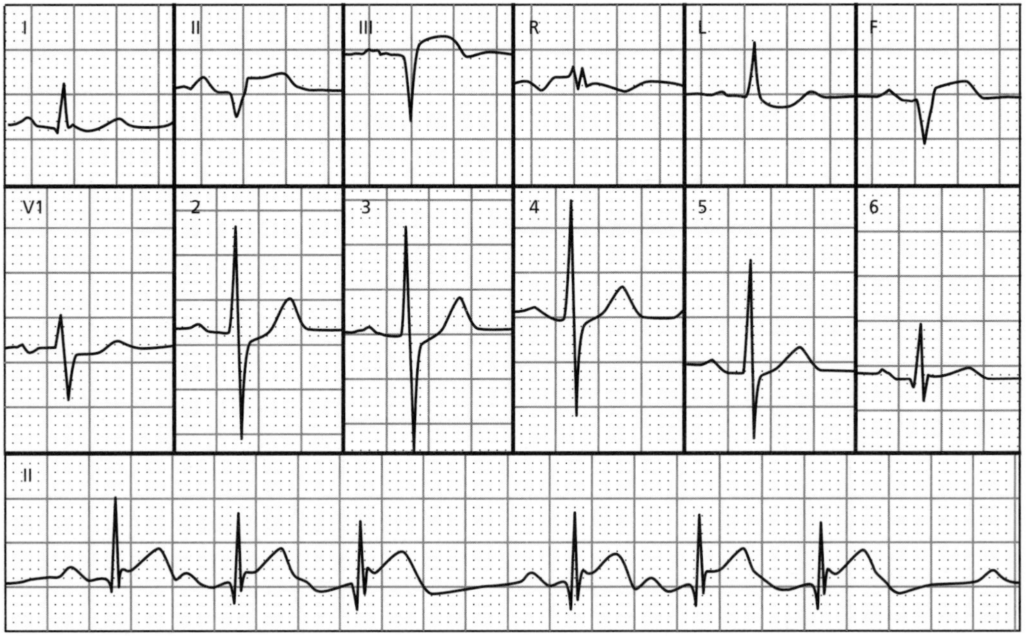

4.9.

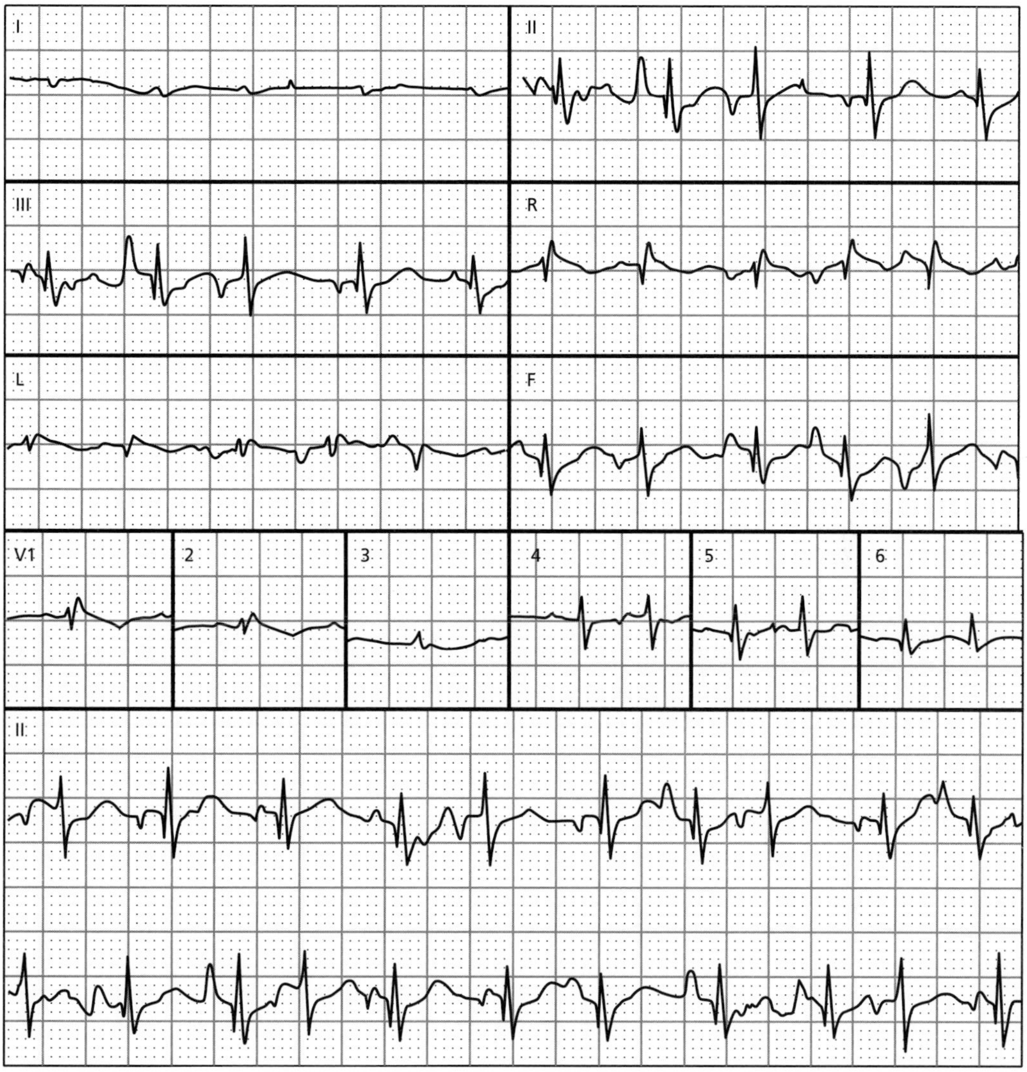

4.10.

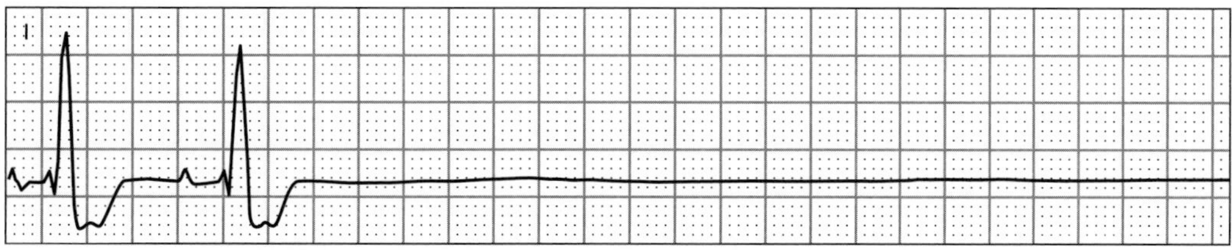

4.11.

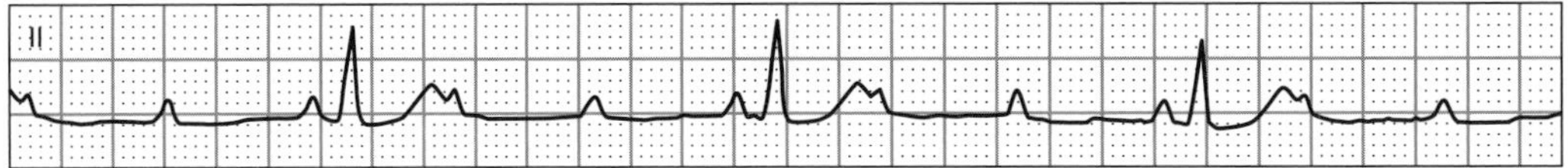

4.12.

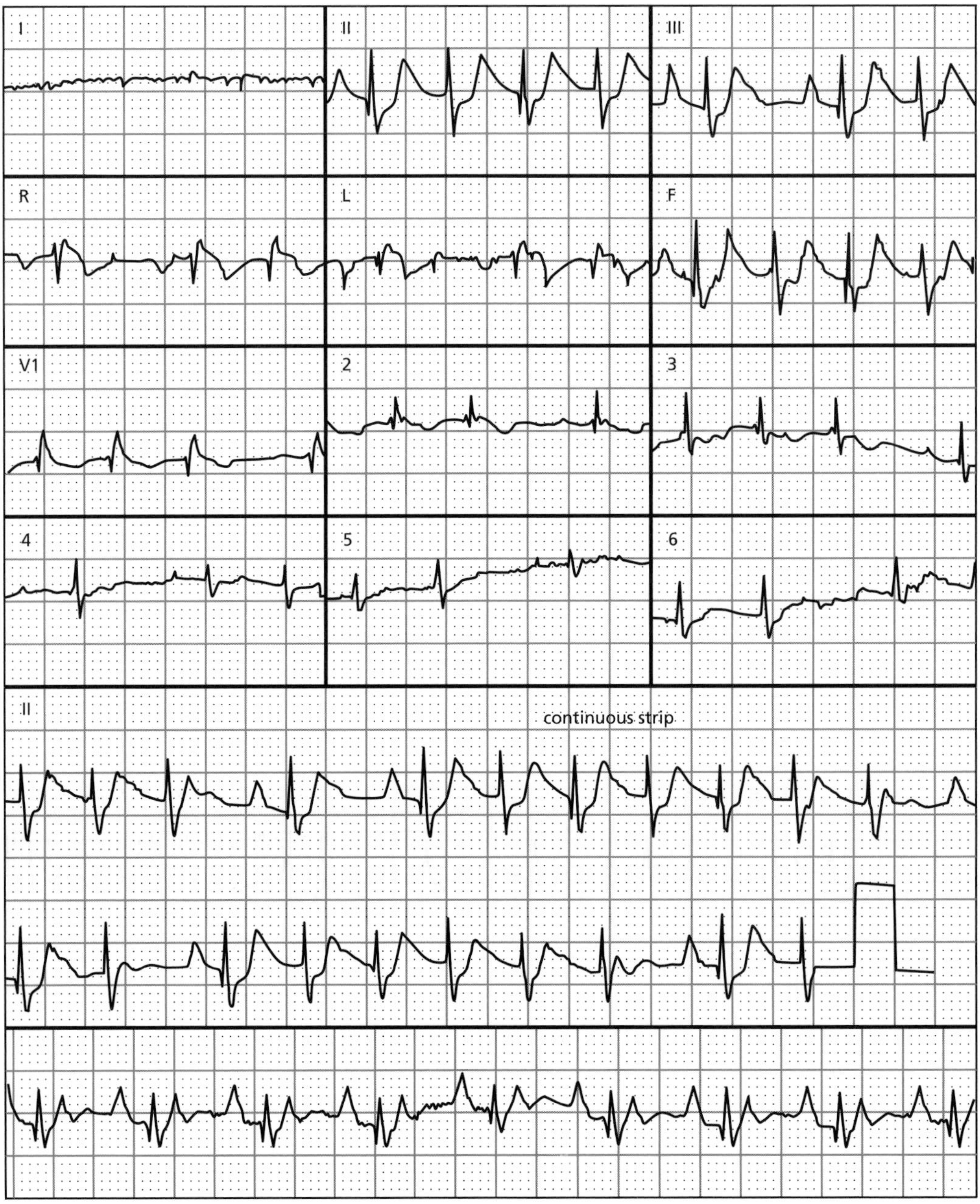

4.13.

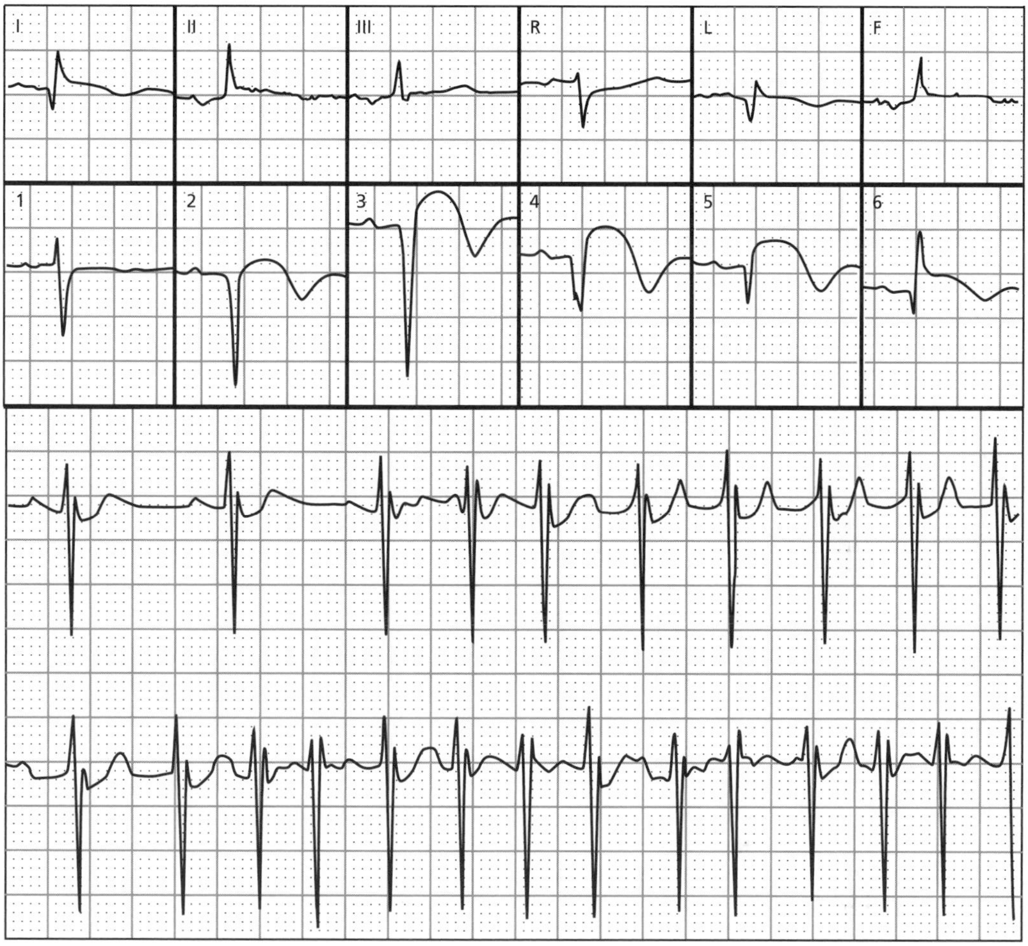

4.14.

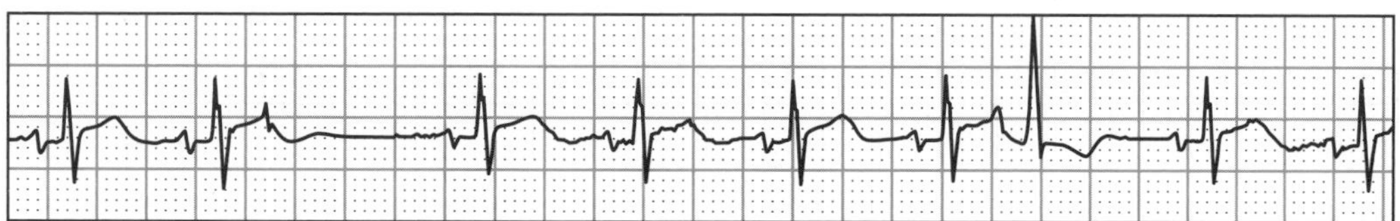

4.15.

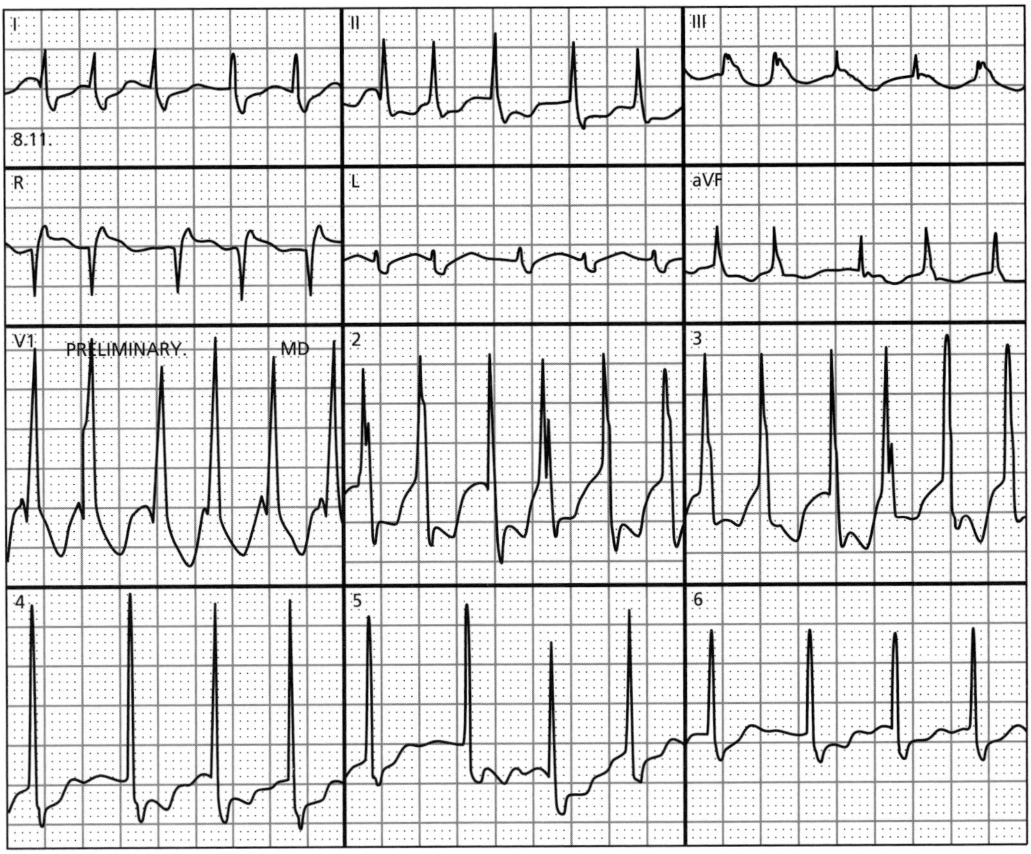

4.16.

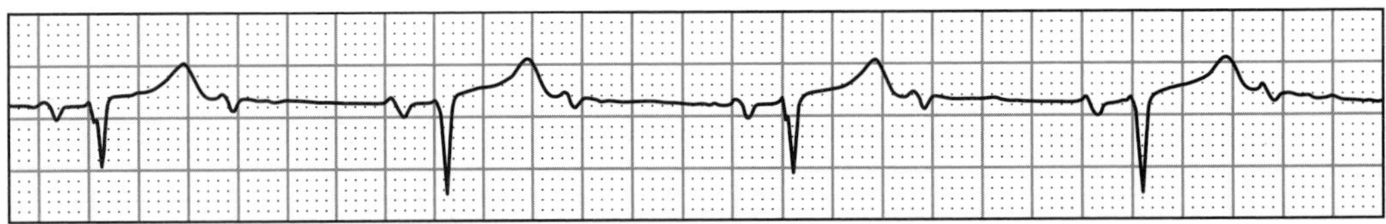

4.17.

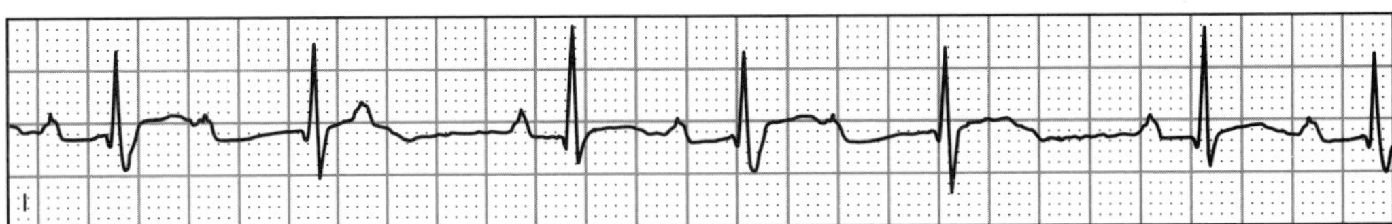

4.18.

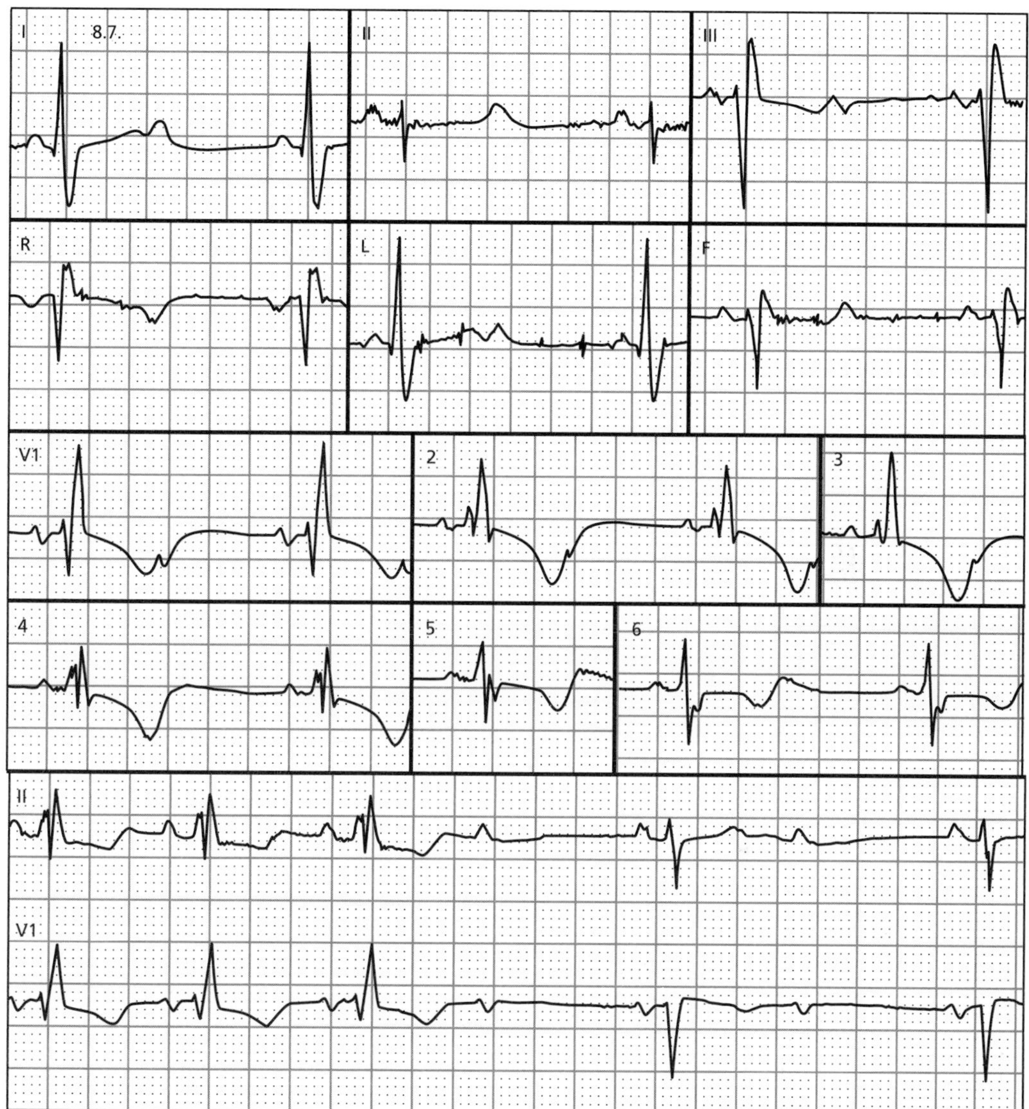

4.19.

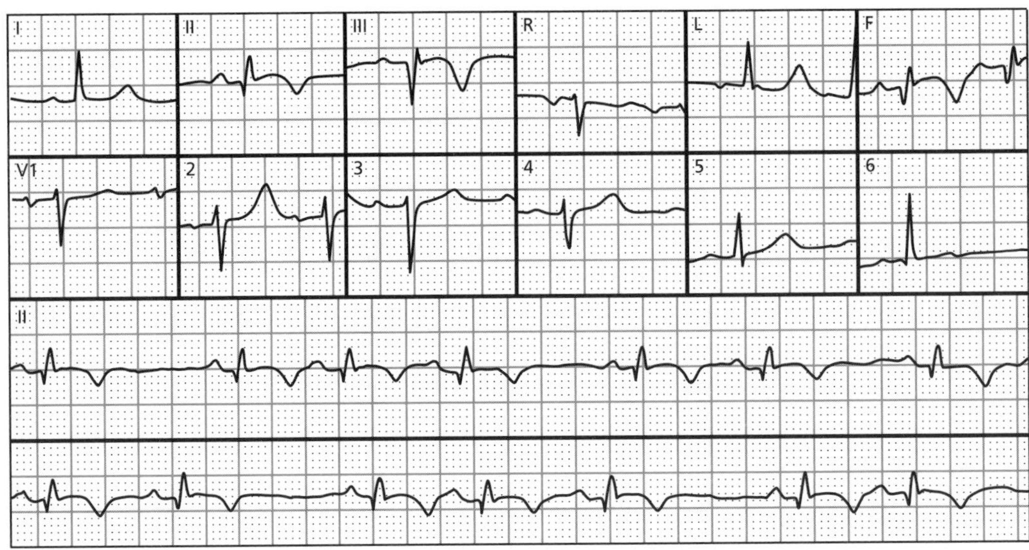

4.20.

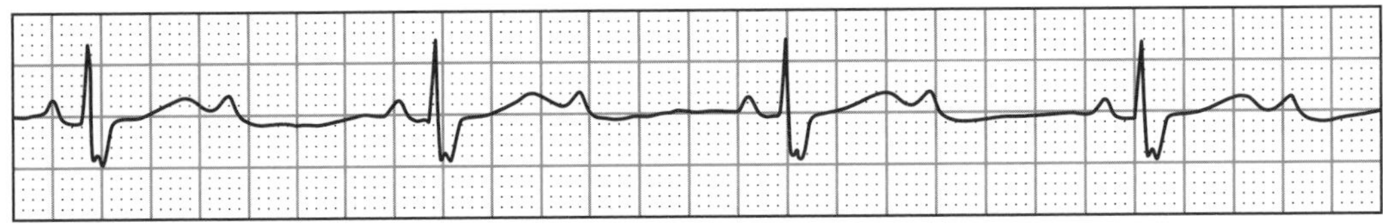

4.21.

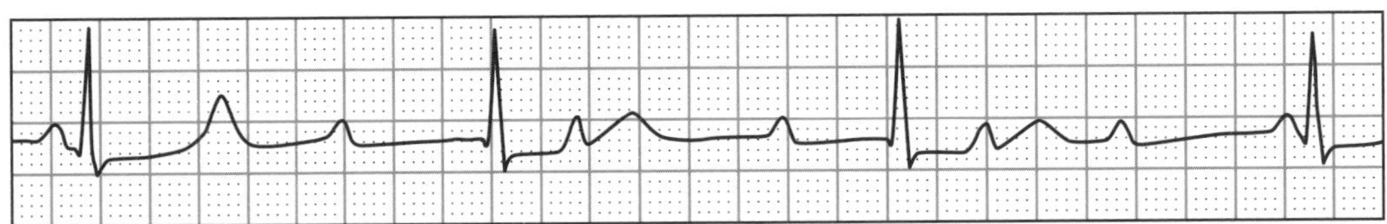

4.22.

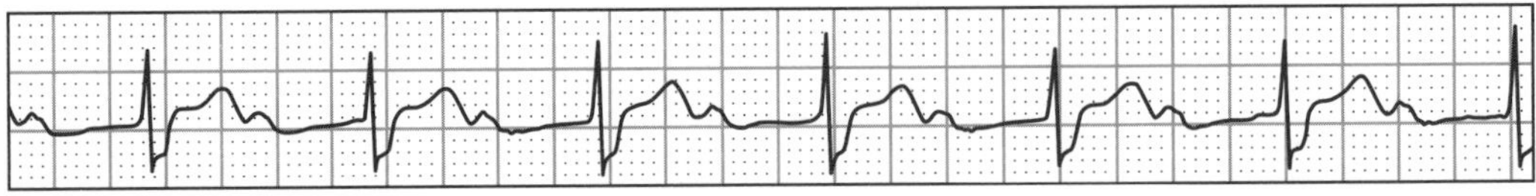

4.23.

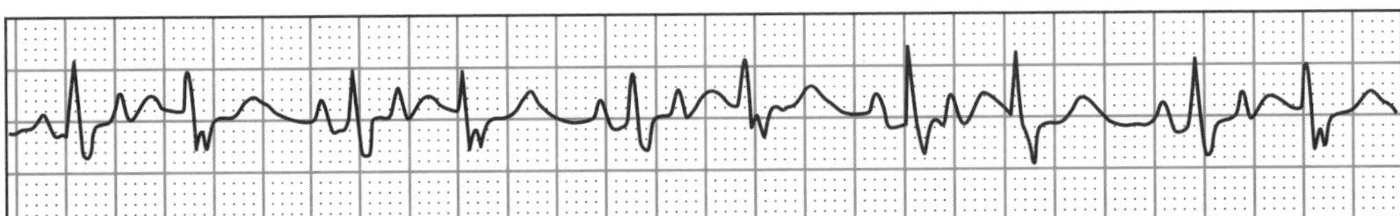

4.24.

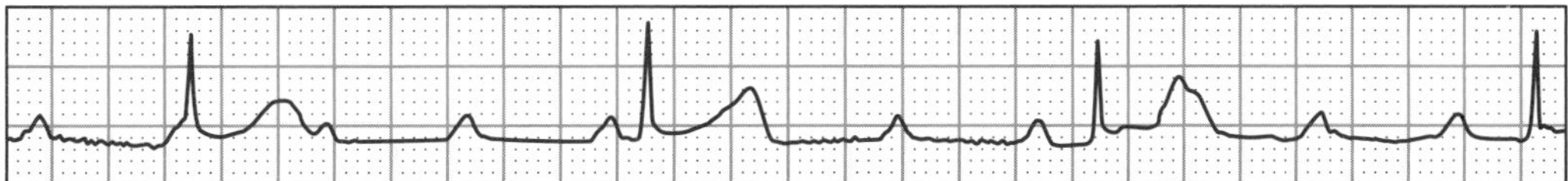

4.25.

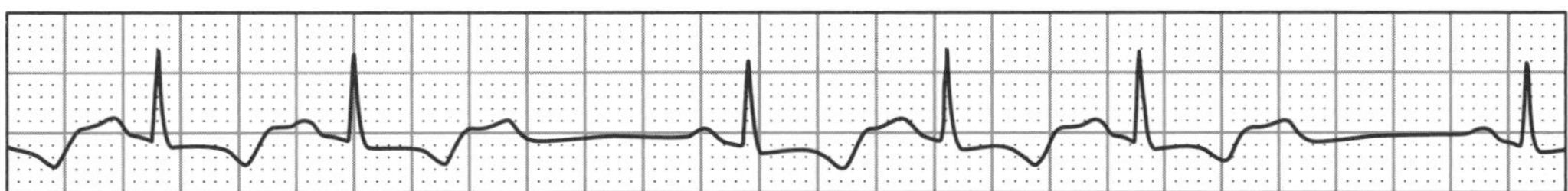

4.26.

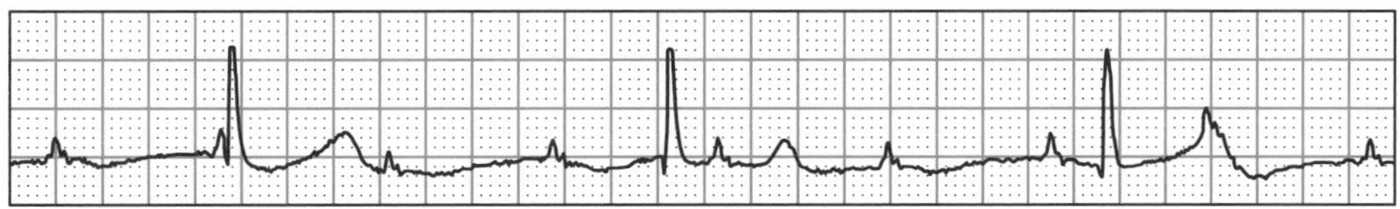

4.27.

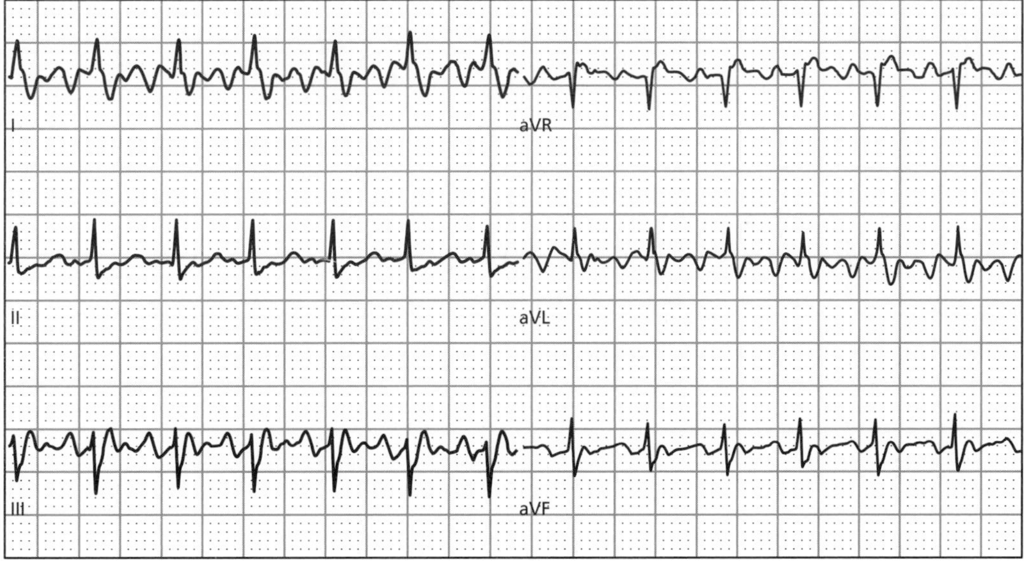

4.28.

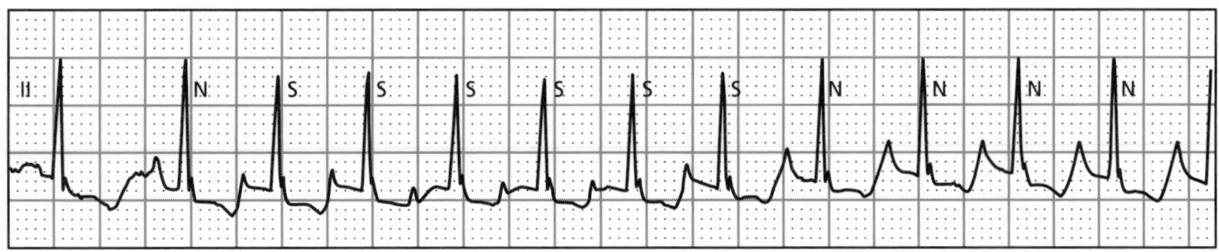

4.29.

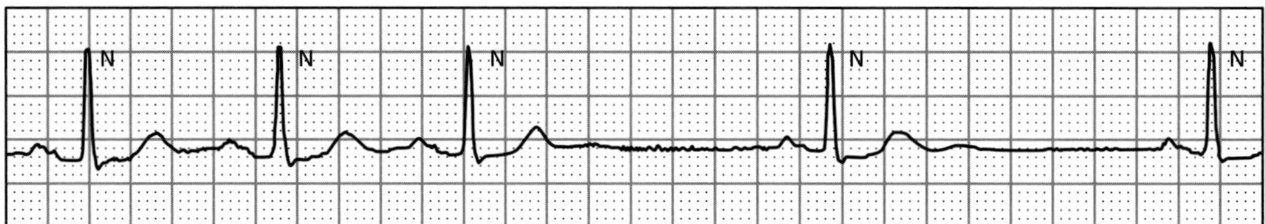

4.30.

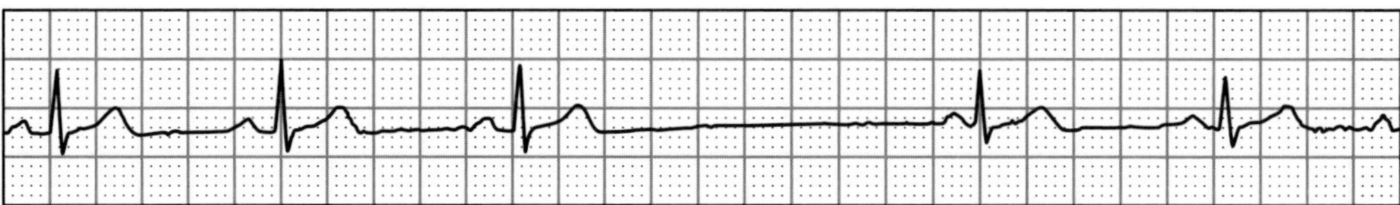

4.31.

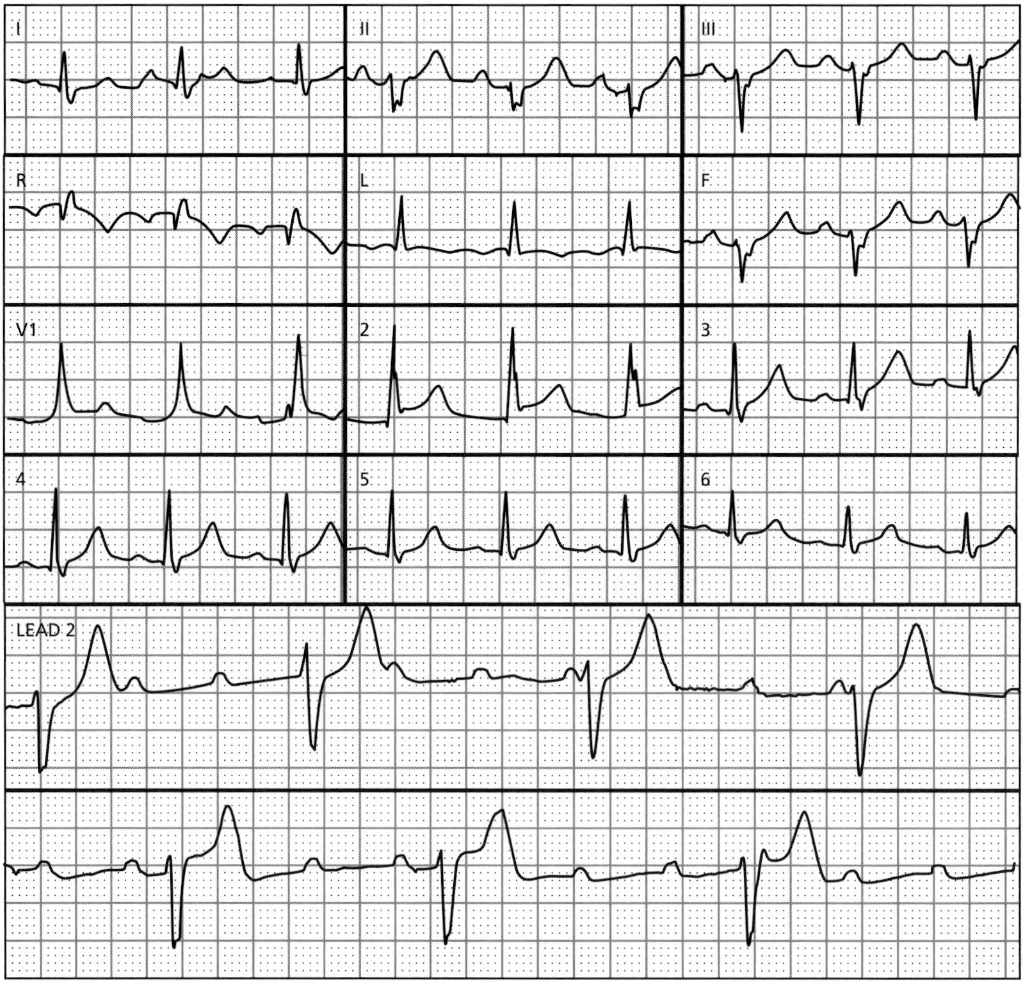

4.32.

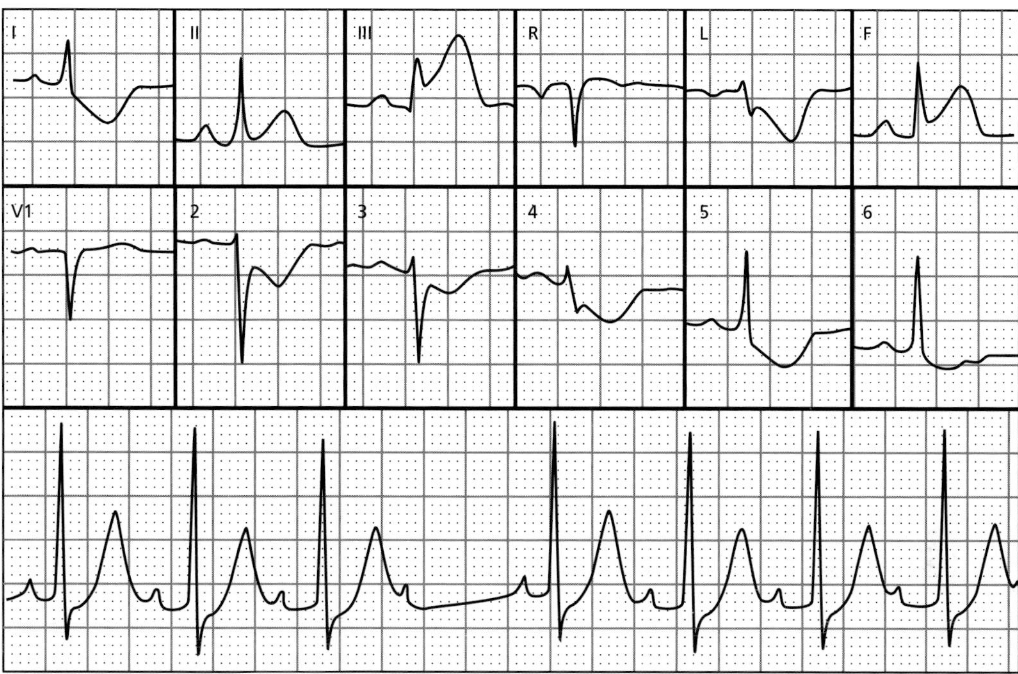

4.33.

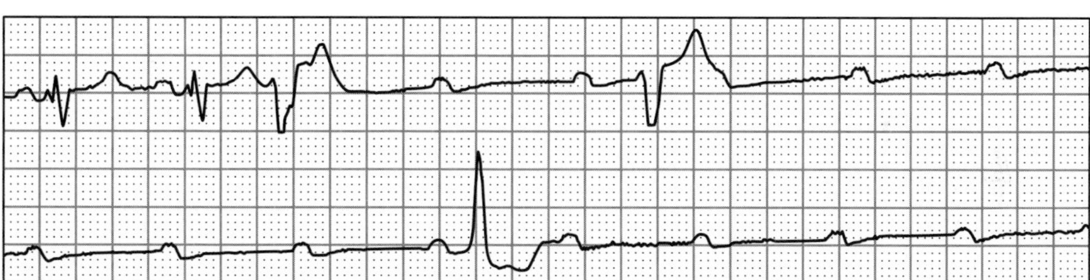

4.34.

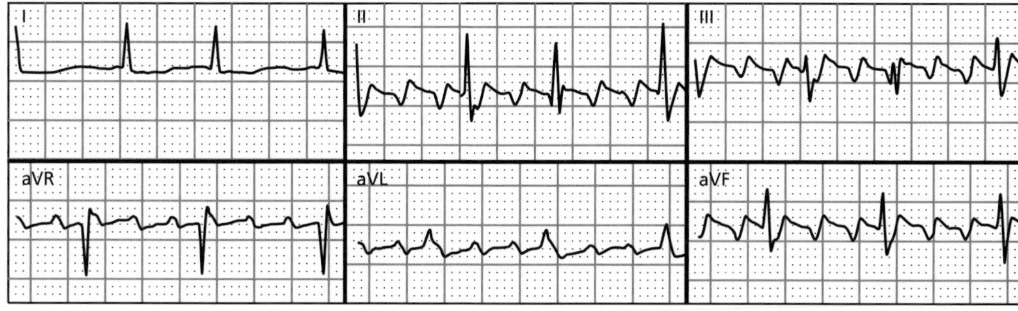

4.35.

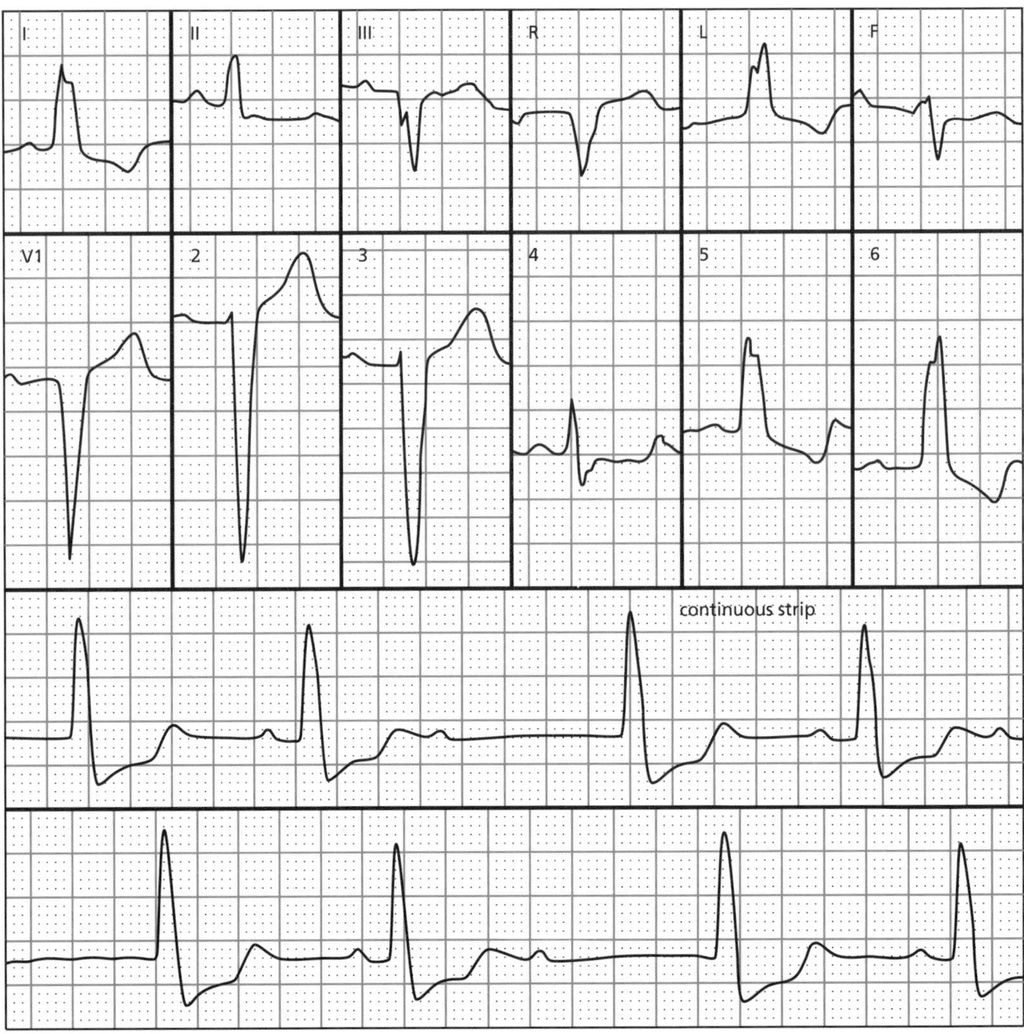

4.36.

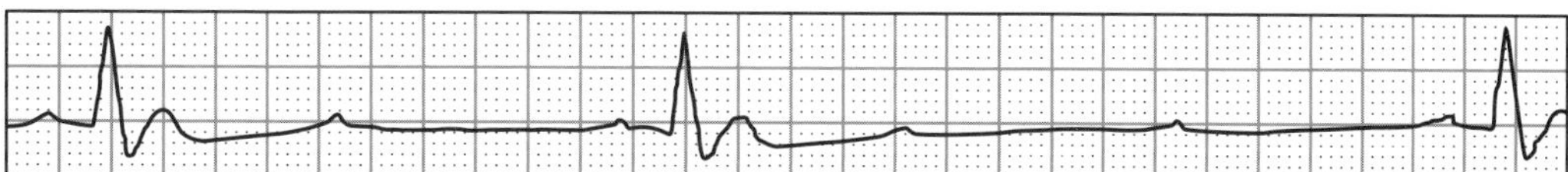

4.37.

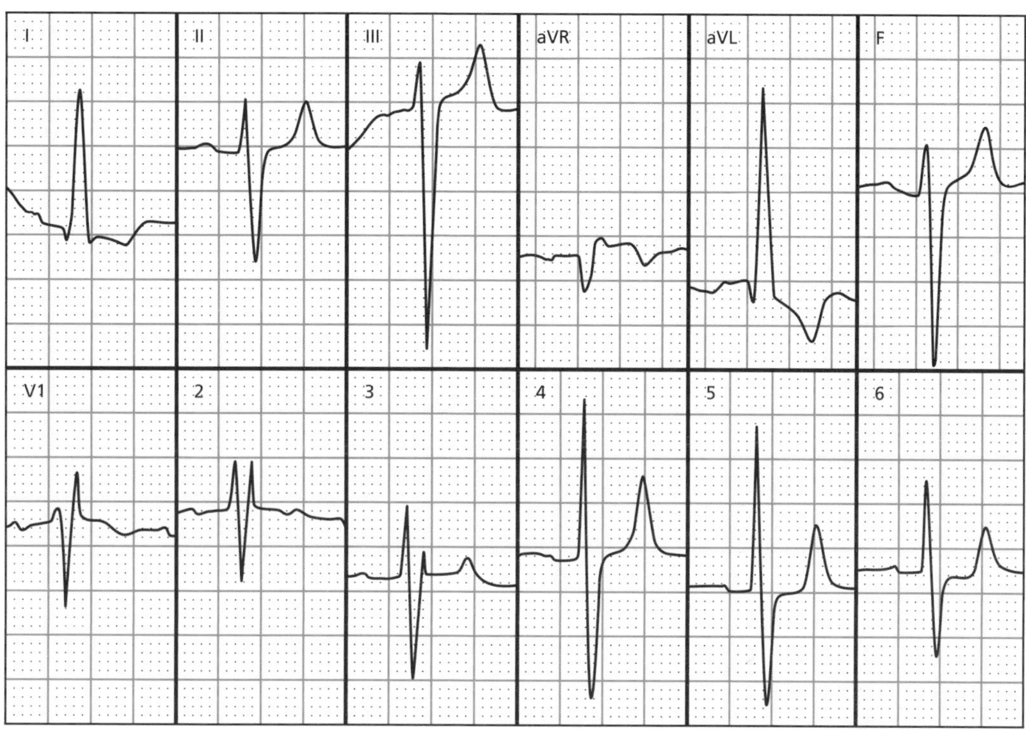

4.38.

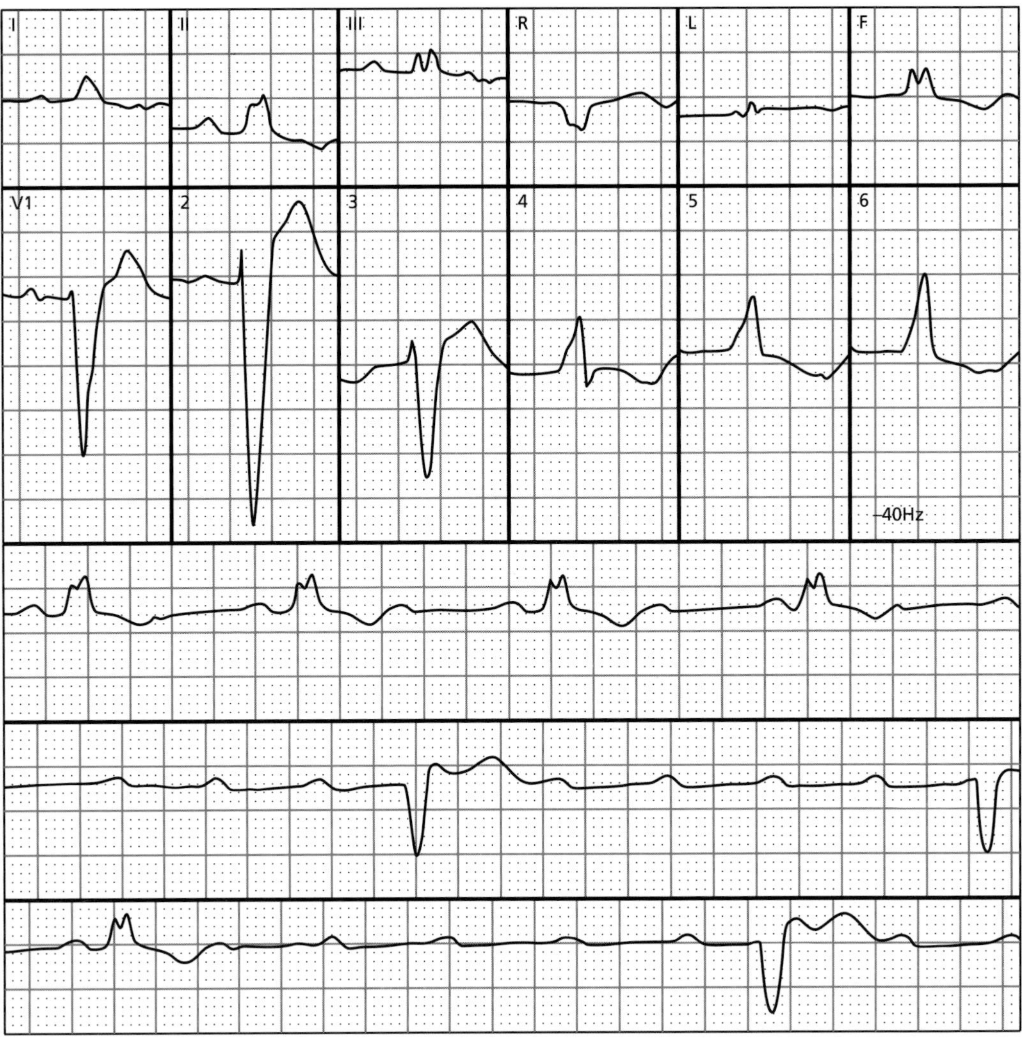

4.39.

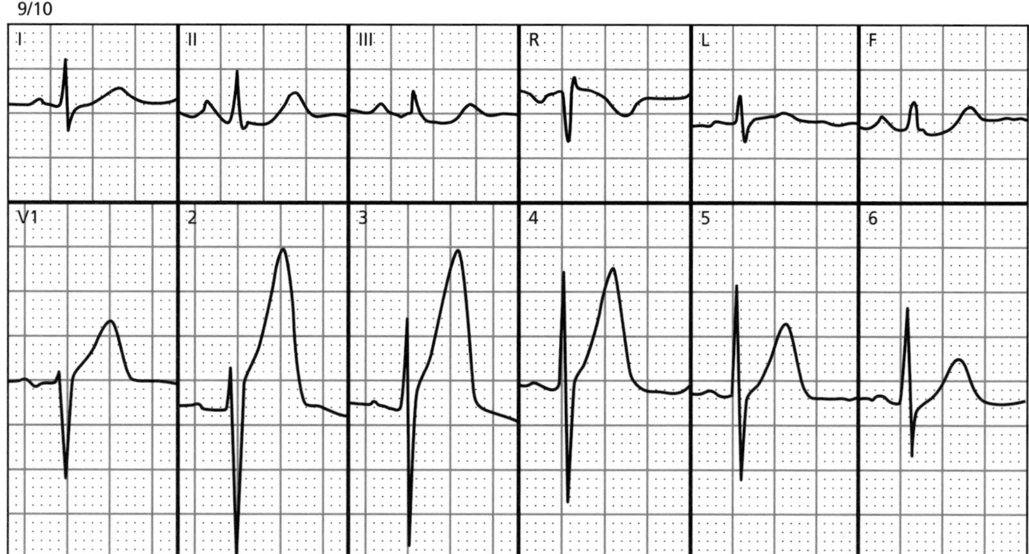

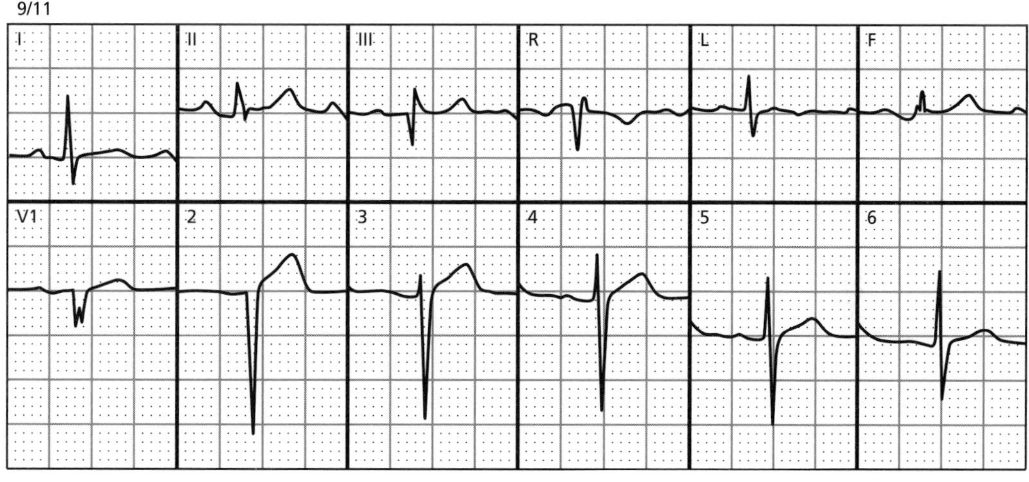

4.40.

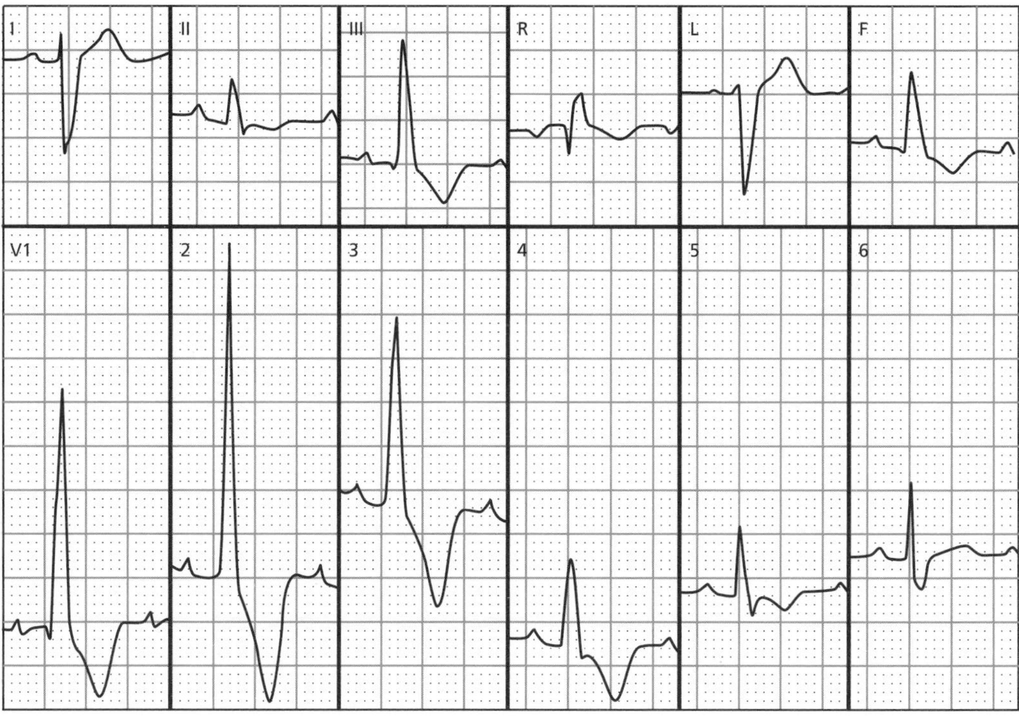

4.41.

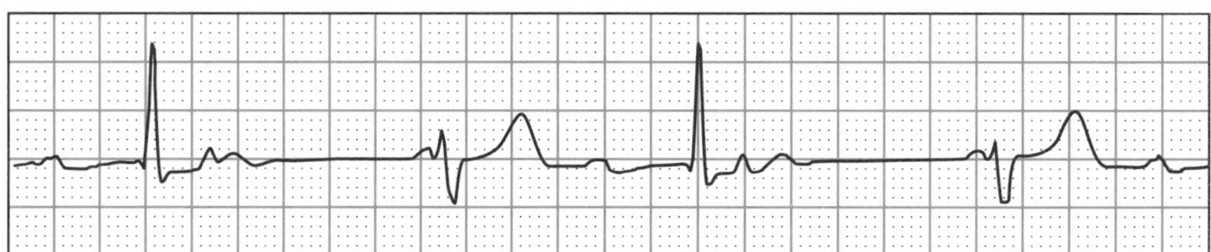

4.42.

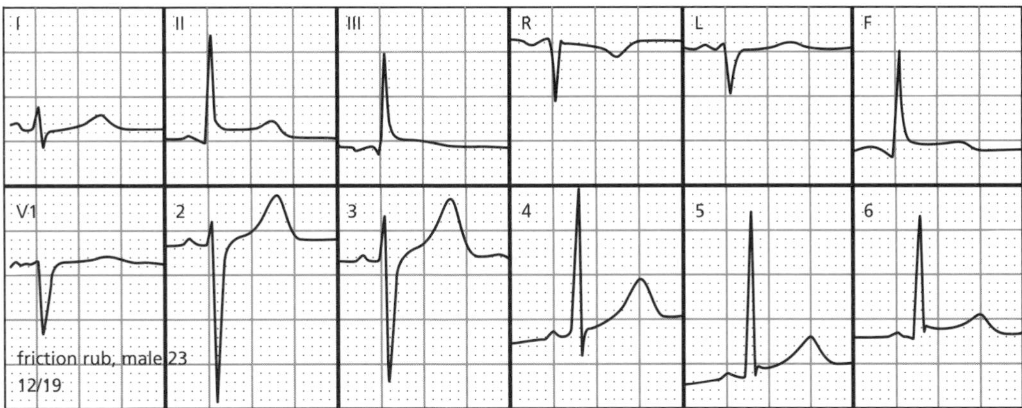
I
II
III
R
L
F
V1
2
3
4
5
6
friction rub, male 23
12/19

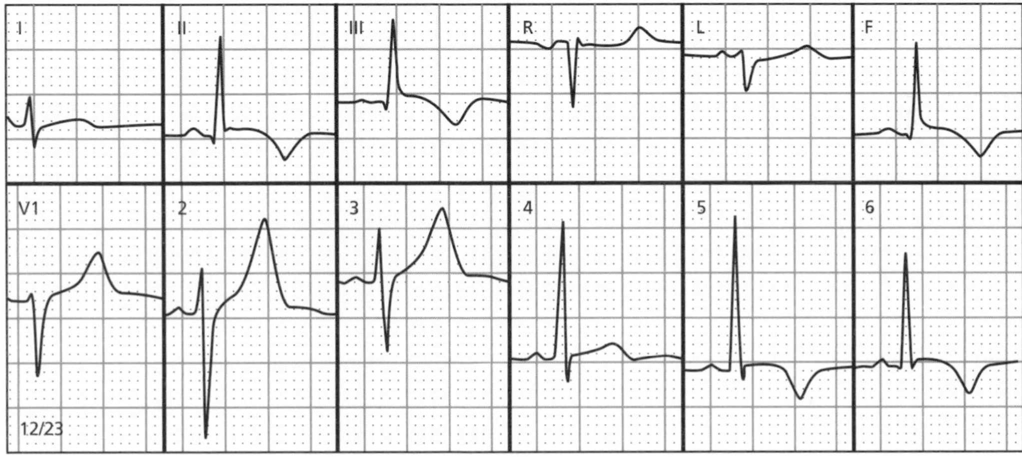
I
II
III
R
L
F
V1
2
3
4
5
6
12/23

4.43.

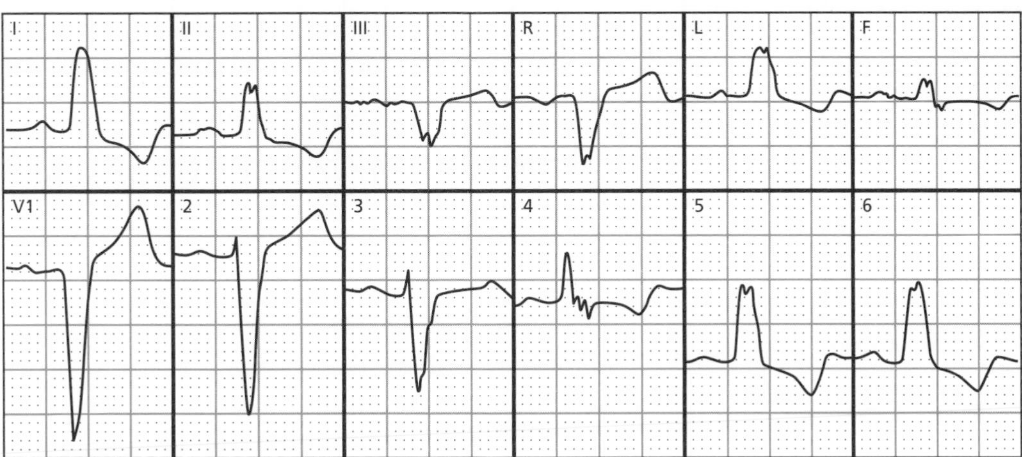
I
II
III
R
L
F
V1
2
3
4
5
6

4.44.

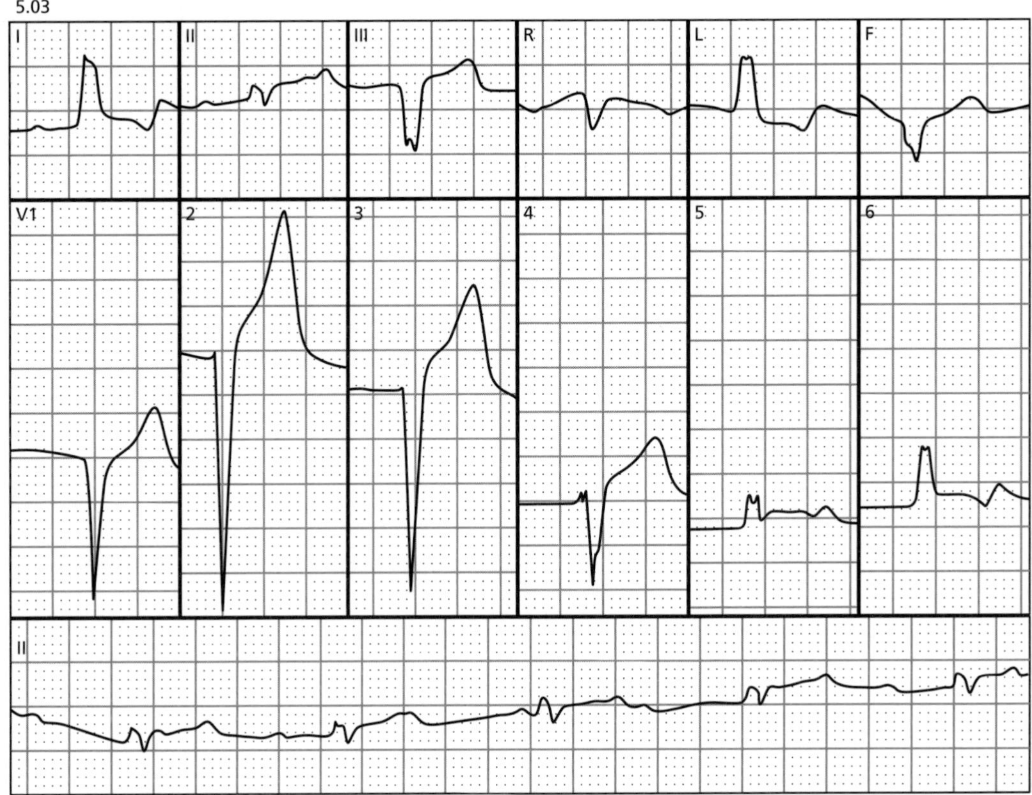

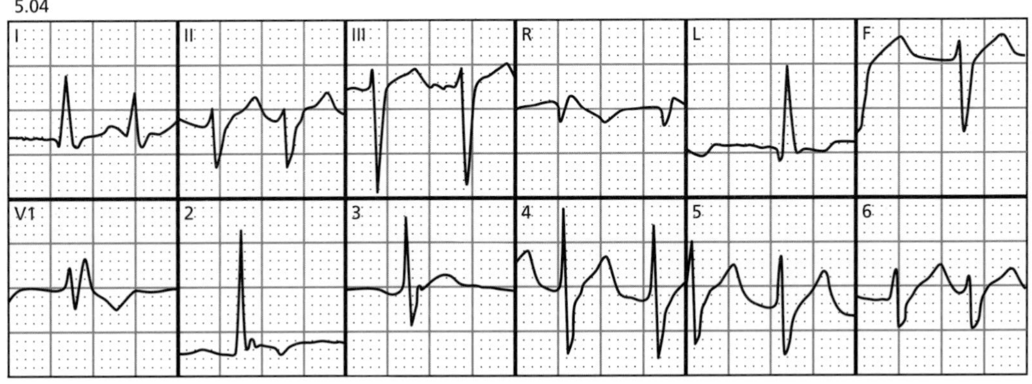

4.45.

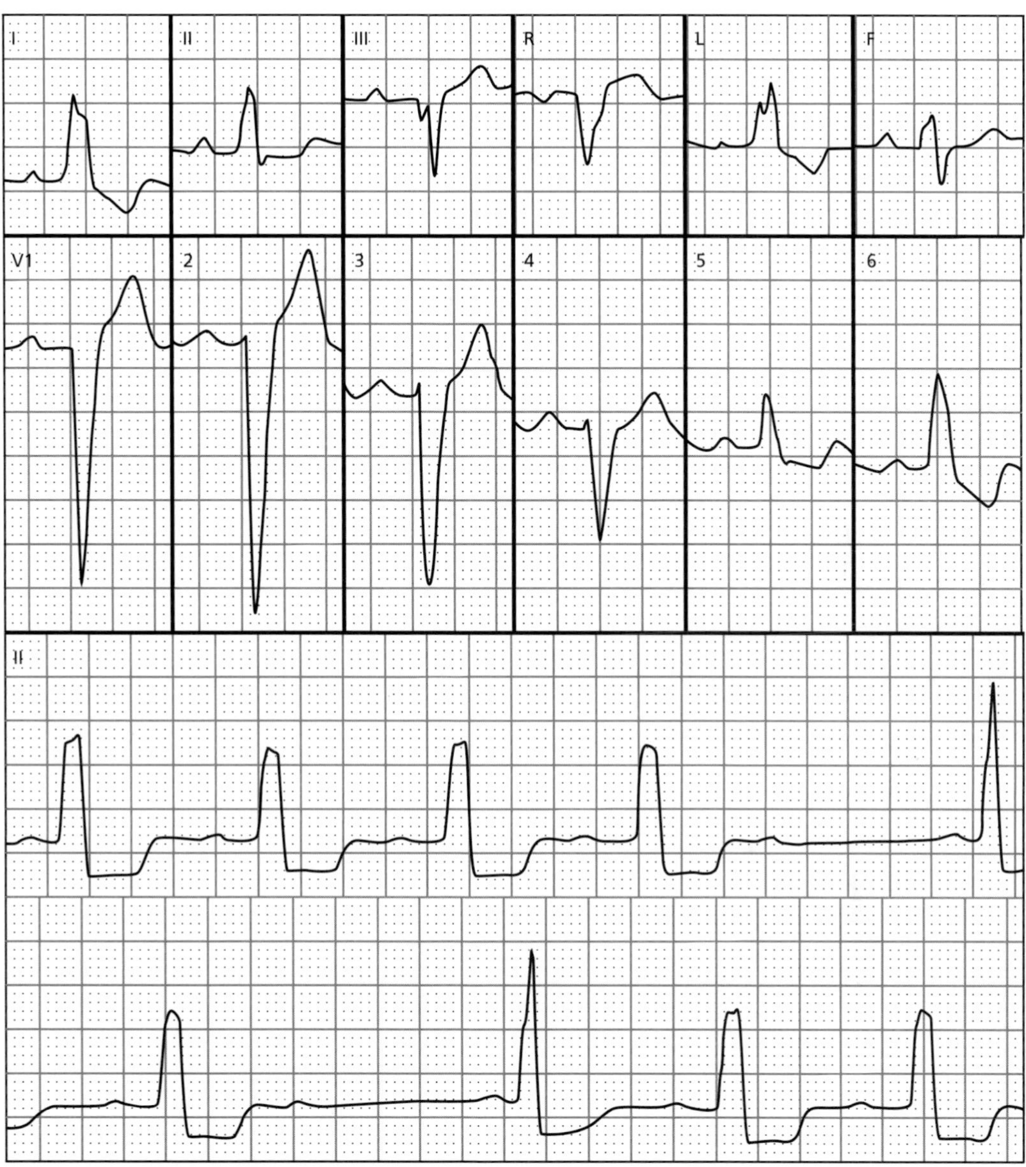

11

CHAPTER 11

Supraventricular re-entrant tachycardia

Re-entry, or *reciprocation*, occurs when an impulse travels away from its point of origin using one pathway, and then reverses direction and returns to the point of origin by means of a second pathway. Three preconditions are required for re-entry.

(1) Two functionally or anatomically separate pathways must form a circuit.

(2) Conduction in one of the pathways must initially exhibit unidirectional block.

(3) Prolonged conduction in the second pathway must be of sufficient duration to permit recovery of the first pathway.

These preconditions exist as the substrate of several common and uncommon forms of supraventricular re-entrant tachycardia.

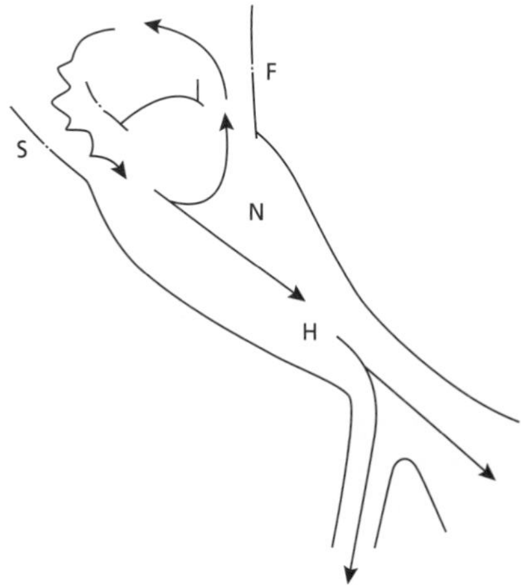

Figure 11.1 The mechanism of slow–fast AVNRT: F: fast pathway, H: bundle of His, N: atrioventricular node, S: slow pathway.

Atrioventricular nodal re-entrant tachycardia

In some subjects the atrioventricular node and adjacent atrial myocardium are anatomically or functionally dissociated into two or more pathways with differing conduction properties. A rapidly conducting fast pathway (FP), located in the anterior atrial septum, and a slowly conducting pathway (SP), located in the posterior atrial septum, form a circuit that results in *atrioventricular nodal re-entrant tachycardia* (AVNRT).

AVNRT is typically initiated by a premature atrial extrasystole that finds the fast (anterior septal) pathway refractory, but is conducted to the atrioventricular node via the slow (posterior septal) pathway (Figure 11.1). Slow conduction in the posterior pathway allows for recovery of the fast pathway. The impulse then 're-enters' the fast anterior limb of the circuit. Repetition of this mechanism results in tachycardia. The slow–fast variant of AVNRT typically begins with a premature atrial complex conducted with delay, which initiates a narrow-QRS complex tachycardia without visible P waves (Figure 11.2).

In this instance the criteria for re-entry are met when (1) functionally dissociated atrial fibers

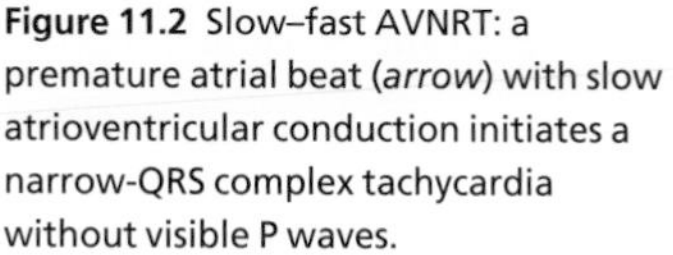
Figure 11.2 Slow–fast AVNRT: a premature atrial beat (*arrow*) with slow atrioventricular conduction initiates a narrow-QRS complex tachycardia without visible P waves.

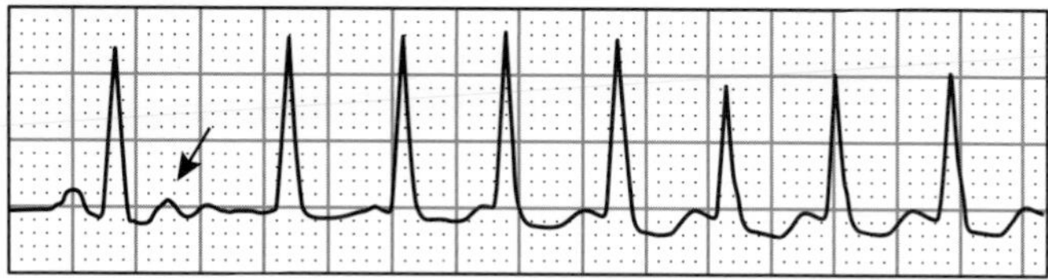

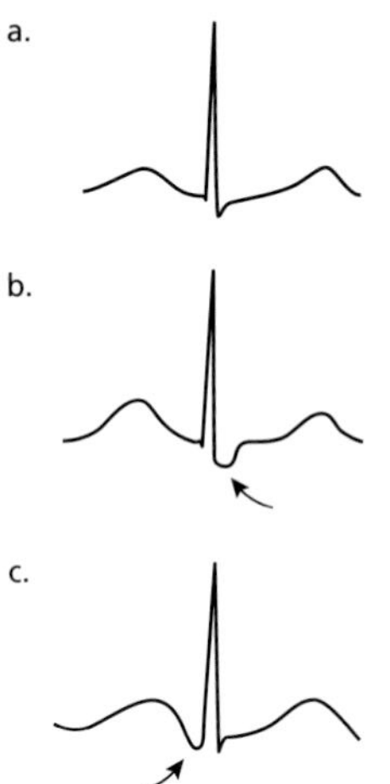

Figure 11.3 Retrograde P waves during AVNRT.

connecting to the AV node form a circuit, (2) a premature atrial systole is initially blocked in the fast anterior pathway because of its longer refractory period, and (3) prolonged conduction in the slow posterior pathway permits recovery of the anterior pathway, making it available to conduct the impulse back again to the fast pathway. The resulting tachycardia is the *slow–fast* variant of AVNRT.

Because the rapidly conducting pathway is utilized for retrograde conduction in the circuit, P waves (if visible) will generally be inverted (negatively inscribed) in leads II, III and aVF, and positive in lead V1, but in most cases atrial and ventricular depolarization are nearly simultaneous and P waves are obscured by QRS complexes (a, Figure 11.3). In some cases atrial depolarization lags slightly behind ventricular depolarization so that an inverted P wave appears in the terminal portion of the QRS complex, resulting in a *pseudo S wave* (b). Rarely, atrial activation slightly precedes ventricular activation, resulting in a *pseudo Q wave* (c).

The slow–fast variant accounts for about 80% of atrioventricular nodal re-entrant tachycardias.

A less common form of AVNRT, the *fast–slow variant*, results when antegrade conduction occurs over the faster anterior pathway and slow conduction occurs over the slower posterior pathway. Because atrial activation occurs over the slow pathway, atrial activation follows ventricular activation and retrograde (inverted) P waves are noted following each QRS complex. The differential diagnosis of the fast–slow variant of AVNRT includes atrial tachycardia and atrioventricular re-entrant tachycardia due to bypass tracts (see below). The fast–slow variant accounts for about 5% of atrioventricular nodal re-entrant tachycardias.

In some subjects, two slowly conducting pathways, located in the posterior atrial septum, form the re-entrant circuit. This form of AVNRT is known as the *slow–slow* variant. Because retrograde conduction occurs over a slow pathway, during tachycardia P waves typically fall behind the QRS complex. The slow–slow variant is therefore difficult to distinguish from the fast–slow variant using tracings recorded from the body surface. The slow–slow variant may account for up to 15% of atrioventricular nodal re-entrant tachycardias.

In an important subset of individuals, multiple functioning pathways exist. In these subjects, differing sets of pathways may be utilized during re-entrant tachycardia.

Atrioventricular re-entrant tachycardia

In a significant fraction of the population, electrical isolation of the atria and ventricles by the annulus fibrosus is incomplete owing to the persistence of myocardial strands that bridge the atrioventricular sulcus. If such anomalous accessory connections are capable of antegrade (atrioventricular) conduction during sinus rhythm, they may produce a ventricular fusion complex that is the hallmark of the Wolff–Parkinson–White syndrome.

However, many such accessory connections or *bypass tracts* conduct only in a retrograde (ventriculoatrial) direction. Consequently there is no evidence of pre-excitation on the surface electrocardiogram during sinus rhythm. Anomalous connections in which only ventriculoatrial conduction occurs are called 'concealed bypass tracts.' In these cases, the bypass tract (BT) functions as the retrograde limb of a circuit during *atrioventricular re-entrant tachycardia* (AVRT), resulting in P waves that typically fall in the ST segments of preceding QRS complexes (RP < PR). The normal conduction pathway through the atrioventricular node and bundle of His serves as the antegrade limb of the circuit (Figure 11.4).

In the less common form of AVRT, the anomalous connection exhibits slow conduction

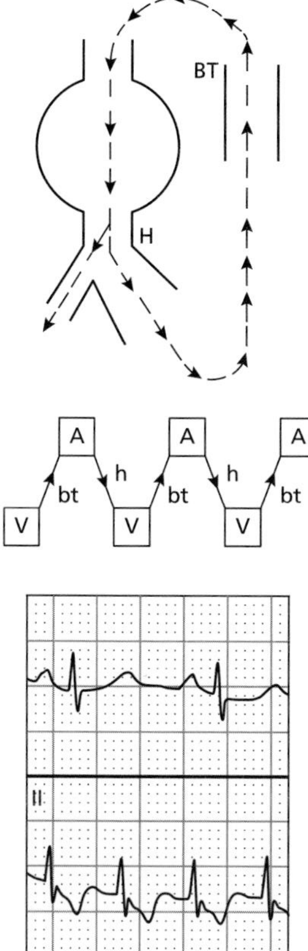

Figure 11.4 Atrioventricular re-entrant tachycardia (AVRT): negatively inscribed P waves are visible in the ST segment following each QRS complex (RP < PR). A: atria, BT: bypass tract, H: bundle of His, V: ventricles.

properties (Figure 11.5), a so-called 'sick bypass tract.' As a result, the inverted P waves are displaced even further from the preceding QRS complex (RP > PR) as illustrated in Figure 11.6.

Differing mechanisms of re-entrant tachycardia are differently distributed both by age and by sex. Atrioventricular nodal re-entrant tachycardia (AVNRT) occurs almost twice as frequently in women. Subjects with re-entrant tachycardias regardless of mechanism usually experience their

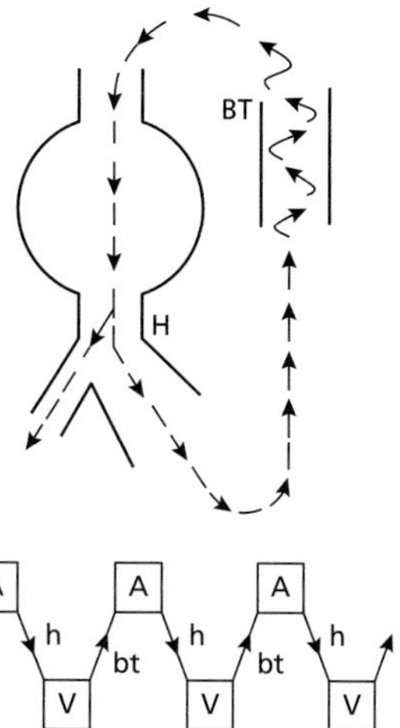

Figure 11.5 A slowly conducting ('sick') bypass tract. A: atria, BT: bypass tract, H: bundle of His, V: ventricles.

first arrhythmic episodes in their teens or early twenties.

Differential diagnosis: AVNRT versus AVRT

Unless the patient's hemodynamic status precludes it, an ECG during tachycardia should be obtained and compared with the ECG in sinus rhythm, with particular attention paid to QRS and ST segment morphology in various leads. Subjects with slow–fast AVNRT may exhibit *pseudo S waves* in leads II, III and aVF and *pseudo R′ waves* in lead V1.

The mode of initiation of a supraventricular tachycardia provides clues to the underlying mechanism. Most slow–fast AVNRT is initiated by premature atrial complexes (PACs) and rarely by premature ventricular complexes (PVCs) because refractoriness of the distal conduction system makes it unlikely that a premature ventricular impulse will penetrate the AV node. Premature ventricular beats may, however, trigger AVRT or fast–slow AVNRT (Figure 11.7). Termination of a re-entrant

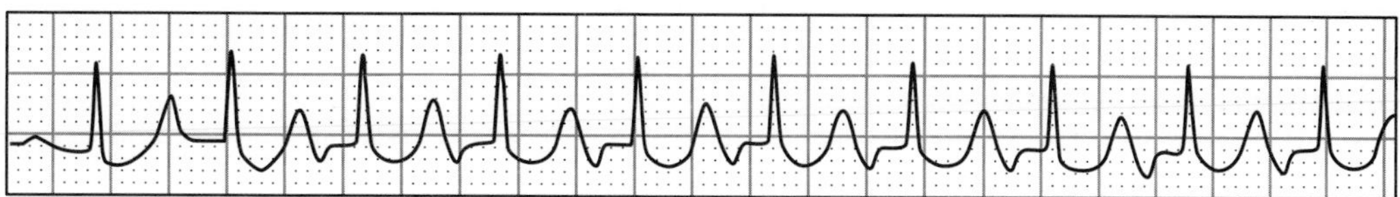

Figure 11.6 Atrioventricular re-entrant tachycardia (AVRT) with a slowly conducting accessory pathway. Negatively inscribed P waves appear far behind each QRS complex (RP > PR).

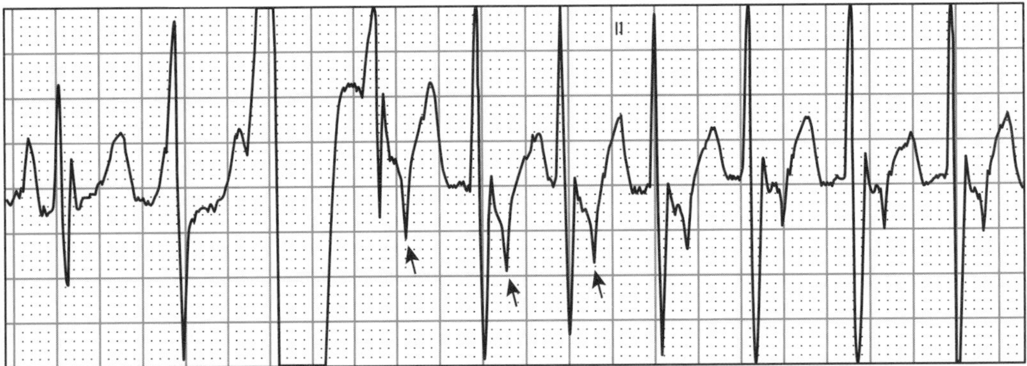

Figure 11.7 A pair of premature ventricular complexes initiate AVRT. Retrograde P waves (*arrows*) fall within the ST segment following each QRS complex.

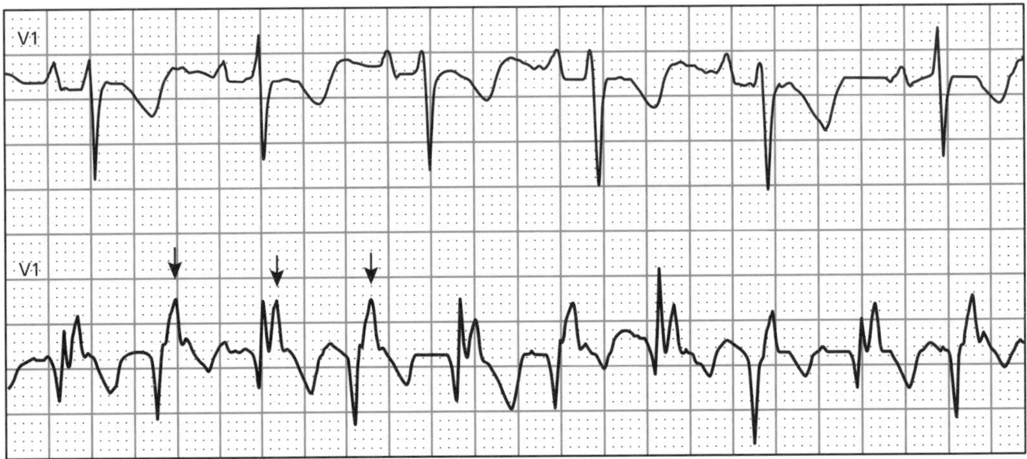

Figure 11.8 Electrical alternans during AVRT: QRS complexes alternate between a biphasic and negative morphology. Retrograde P waves (*arrows*) fall in the ST segment following each QRS complex.

tachycardia by a premature ventricular beat indicates that the retrograde limb of the circuit is probably an accessory pathway.

A beat-to-beat change in QRS morphology is the most common form of *electrical alternans*. Electrical alternans is most directly related to the rate of a tachycardia (Figure 11.8). Even sinus tachycardia can exhibit alternans.

Variable atrioventricular conduction is commonly noted during atrial flutter and atrial tachycardia and is the rule during atrial fibrillation. In the case of AVRT, both the atria and ventricles are indispensable parts of the re-entry circuit, so that any conduction ratio less than 1:1 rules out AVRT as a mechanism. Very rarely AVNRT briefly exhibits 2:1 atrioventricular conduction ratios, particularly at the beginning of the tachycardia (Figure 11.9). In these cases, P waves will be noted spaced equidistantly between the remaining QRS complexes. Resumption of 1:1 conduction will

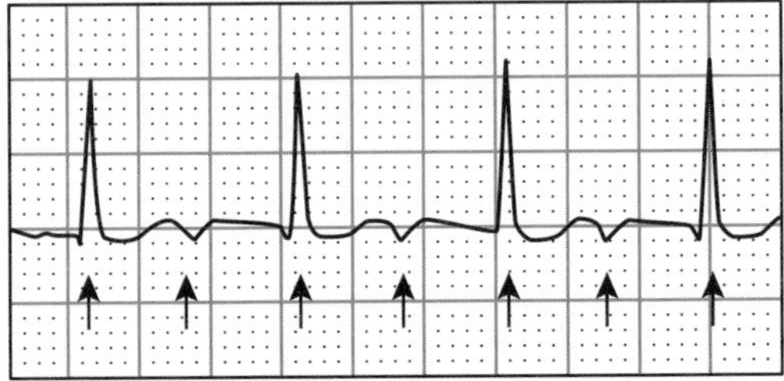

Figure 11.9 AVNRT with transient 2:1 conduction distal to the re-entry circuit: every other retrograde P wave (*arrows*) is unmasked by momentary 2:1 conduction.

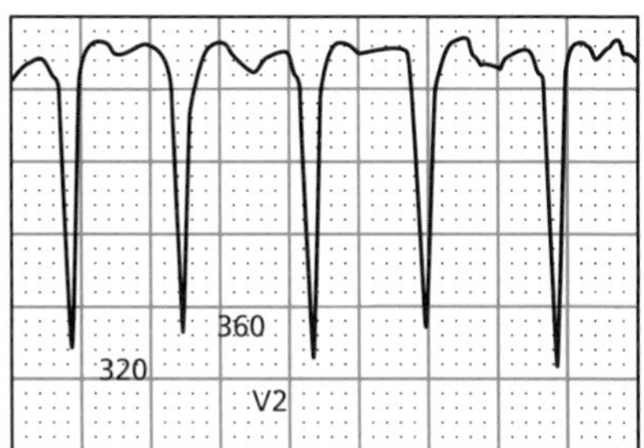

Figure 11.10 Alternating R–R intervals during AVRT. The R–R intervals are in milliseconds.

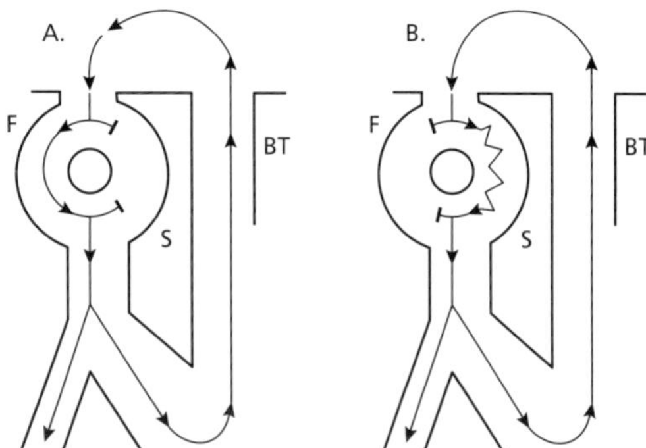

Figure 11.11 One mechanism of changing R–R intervals during AVRT: antegrade conduction alternates over fast and slow AV nodal pathways.

typically mask atrial activity, causing the P waves to disappear into the simultaneously occurring QRS complexes.

Aberrant ventricular conduction (rate-related bundle branch block) can occur with either AVNRT or AVRT, but aberrant ventricular conduction is rare with AVNRT because antegrade conduction through the slow pathway allows time for the distal conduction system to completely repolarize. If aberrant conduction does occur, it does not alter the rate of AVNRT or atrial tachycardia, and the rate-related block is nearly always in the right bundle branch.

Re-entrant *supraventricular tachycardia* (SVT) with left bundle branch aberrancy results from AVRT in 90% of cases. Because the ventricle is an essential part of the re-entry circuit, development of bundle branch block *on the same side as the bypass tract* ('ipsilateral bundle branch block') will produce measurable slowing of the tachycardia owing to lengthening of the circuit. Therefore an increase in cycle length that develops concomitantly with bundle branch block is diagnostic of AVRT.

Sudden cycle length changes without simultaneous bundle branch block during re-entrant tachycardia indicate that more than one accessory pathway is being utilized for conduction. Coexisting multiple pathways are fairly common; up to 30% of patients with Wolff–Parkinson–White syndrome are thought to have multiple anomalous atrioventricular connections. *Alternating R–R intervals* during supraventricular re-entrant tachycardia (Figure 11.10) can be due to (1) alternating antegrade conduction over dual atrioventricular nodal pathways (Figure 11.11), (2) alternating conduction over dual accessory pathways with differing conduction properties, or (3) retrograde conduction that alternates between the anterior and posterior fascicles of the left bundle branch. *Alternating R–P intervals* can be produced by (1) alternating retrograde conduction over two different accessory pathways with differing conduction properties, or (2) retrograde conduction alternating between the anterior and posterior fascicles of the left bundle branch.

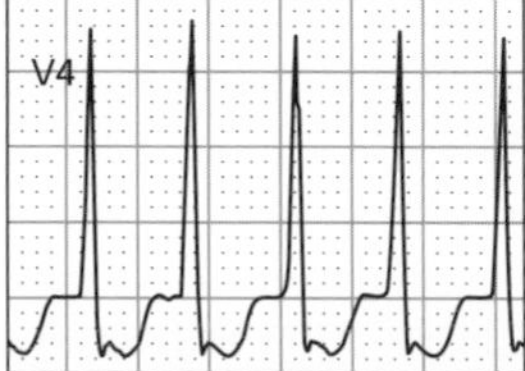

Figure 11.12 Depression of the ST segment during AVRT.

Depression of the ST segment is often noted during AVRT (Figure 11.12). It is related to the increased rate and usually carries no prognostic significance.

Carotid sinus massage or drugs such as adenosine will stop most re-entrant tachycardias by producing block in the antegrade limb of the circuit. If the run of tachycardia ends with a P wave, the block has occurred in the atrioventricular node. If the tachycardia ends with a QRS complex, block has occurred in the accessory pathway (Figure 11.13).

In Figure 11.14, an atrial extrasystole initiates atrial tachycardia with prolonged atrioventricular conduction (*arrows*). A critical degree of conduction delay in the atrioventricular pathway permits

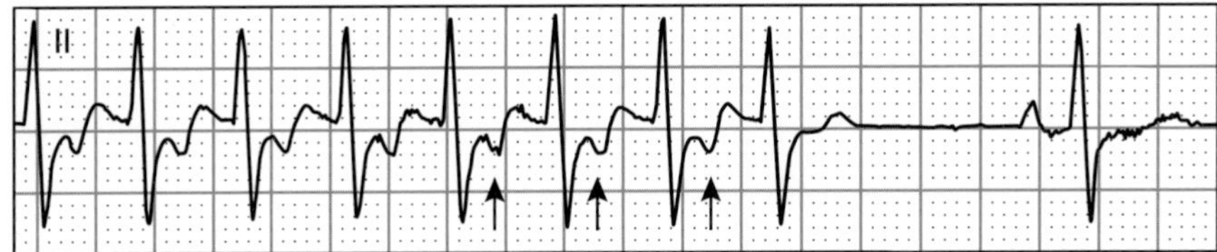

Figure 11.13 Atrioventricular re-entrant tachycardia (AVRT). Retrograde P waves (*arrows*) follow each QRS complex. The tachycardia ends with a QRS complex: block has occurred in the accessory pathway.

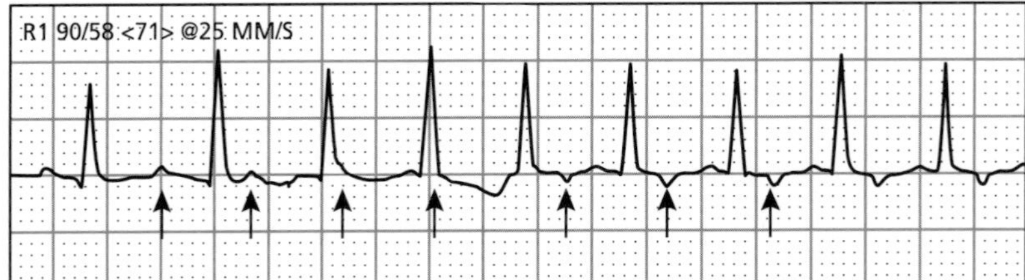

Figure 11.14 Atrial tachycardia switches to AVRT.

ventriculoatrial conduction to begin over a second, accessory pathway. This shift in conduction is announced by the appearance of an inverted P wave in the ST segment following the fifth QRS complex and every QRS complex thereafter (*vertical arrows*).

Permanent junctional reciprocating tachycardia

First described in France by Coumel and his associates in 1967, *permanent junctional reciprocating tachycardia* (PJRT) was at first thought to be a form of fast–slow AVNRT (Figure 11.15). It was subsequently determined that this form of bypass tract-mediated tachycardia generally utilizes a slowly conducting pathway located in the posterior interatrial septum, although other sites for such slowly conducting pathways are well documented. The accessory pathway responsible for PJRT exhibits AV node-like physiology that includes responsiveness to autonomic tone.

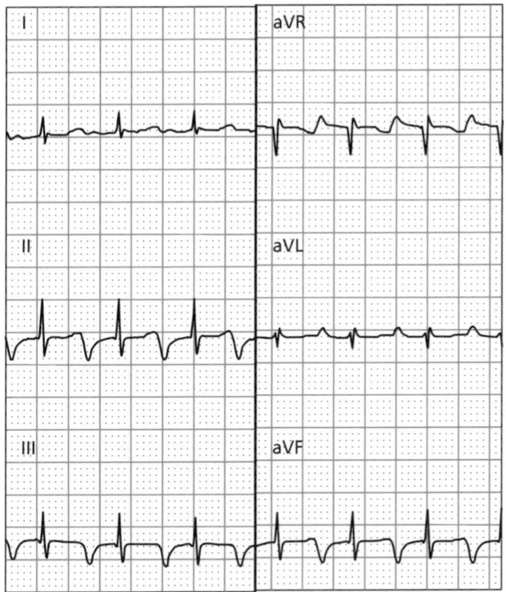

Figure 11.15 Permanent junctional reciprocating tachycardia (PJRT).

Although PJRT can present in maturity, it is most often recognized in children and young adults. In this population it is an important cause of *tachycardia-induced cardiomyopathy*. The incessant nature of the arrhythmia leads to left ventricular dysfunction, which may result in severe, irreversible congestive failure. In young subjects, the arrhythmia must be distinguished from *ectopic atrial tachycardia*.

The ECG manifestations of PJRT include (1) incessant tachycardia interrupted by short periods of sinus rhythm, (2) initiation of the tachycardia by changes in sinus rate, (3) increased tachycardia rate in response to exercise, (4) slowing of the rate

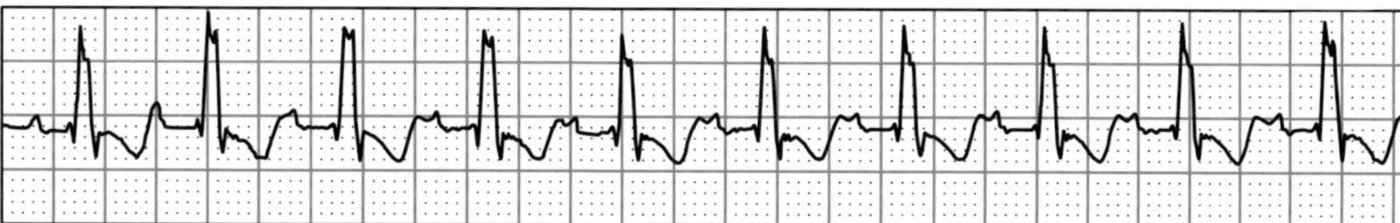

Figure 11.16 Sinoatrial re-entrant tachycardia (SART) in a subject with right bundle branch block. Note the prolongation of the PR interval during tachycardia.

in response to increased vagal tone, (5) inverted P waves in leads II, III and aVF, (6) RP > PR interval, and (7) absence of pre-excitation during sinus rhythm (the accessory pathway remains concealed).

Sinoatrial re-entrant tachycardia

The sinoatrial node and adjacent atrial myocardium form the limbs of the re-entry circuit that results in *sinoatrial re-entrant tachycardia* (SART). The diagnostic criteria include (1) P waves that are identical or very similar to sinus P waves, and (2) paroxysmal initiation (Figure 11.16). During tachycardia prolongation of the PR interval may occur. SART tends to occur in an older age group than other re-entrant tachyarrhythmias and unless sustained or unusually rapid (>120 per minute), is usually asymptomatic.

Multiple pathways

Two anatomically separate pathways with differing conduction physiology can result in (1) atrioventricular re-entry, (2) echo beats, (3) two different PR or RP intervals, or (4) dual ventricular response.

Figure 11.17 illustrates a common mechanism of the echo beat: in panel A, a ventricular premature beat conducts in retrograde manner to the atria, producing an inverted P wave. In panel B, the retrograde P wave is followed by a second, narrow QRS indicating that the retrograde impulse has entered a second pathway and returned to the ventricles to produce a *ventricular echo beat*.

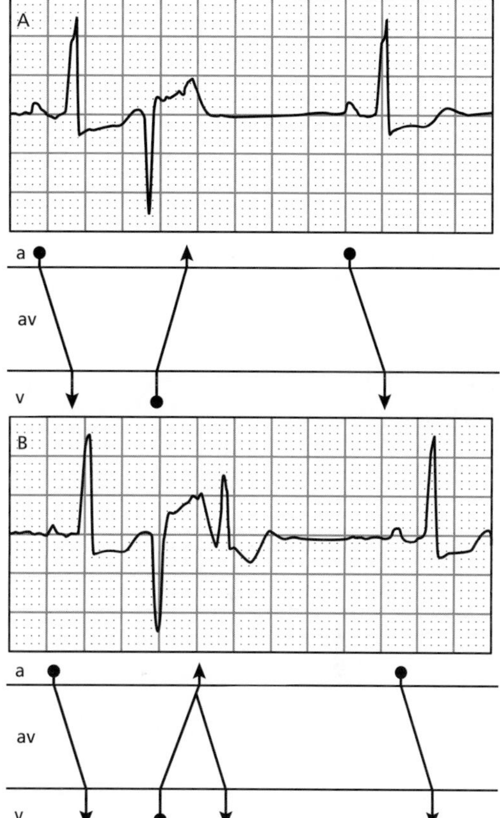

Figure 11.17 Re-entry producing a ventricular echo beat.

In many cases the presence of a second pathway becomes evident only after a critical degree of conduction delay occurs in the first pathway. In Figure 11.18 ventricular complexes followed by inverted P waves with RP intervals of 0.24 sec are noted. The second ventricular impulse in each set is also followed by an inverted P wave with an RP interval of 0.42 sec. The longer ventriculoatrial conduction time permits recovery of the first pathway, resulting in ventricular echo beats.

An example of *differing PR intervals* is shown in Figure 11.19. Sinus rhythm with a prolonged PR interval (240 msec) is interrupted by a premature atrial extrasystole (*arrow*). Subsequent conduction times lengthen to 360 msec. The shift to the pathway with slower conduction occurs because the faster, primary pathway has a longer refractory

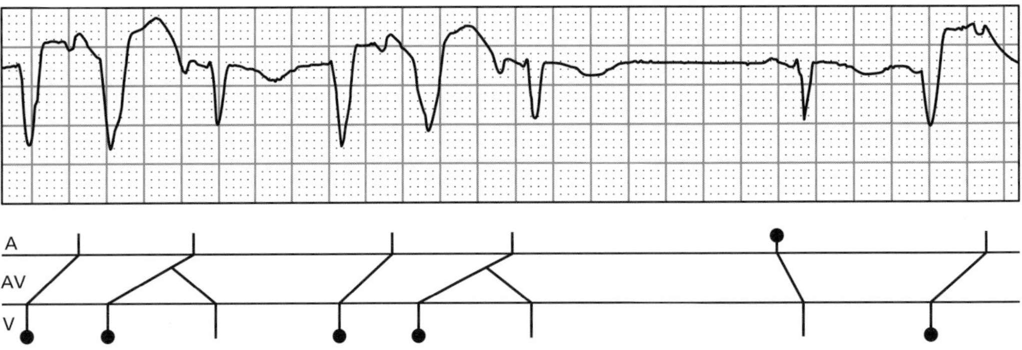

Figure 11.18 Dual pathways: ventricular echo beats.

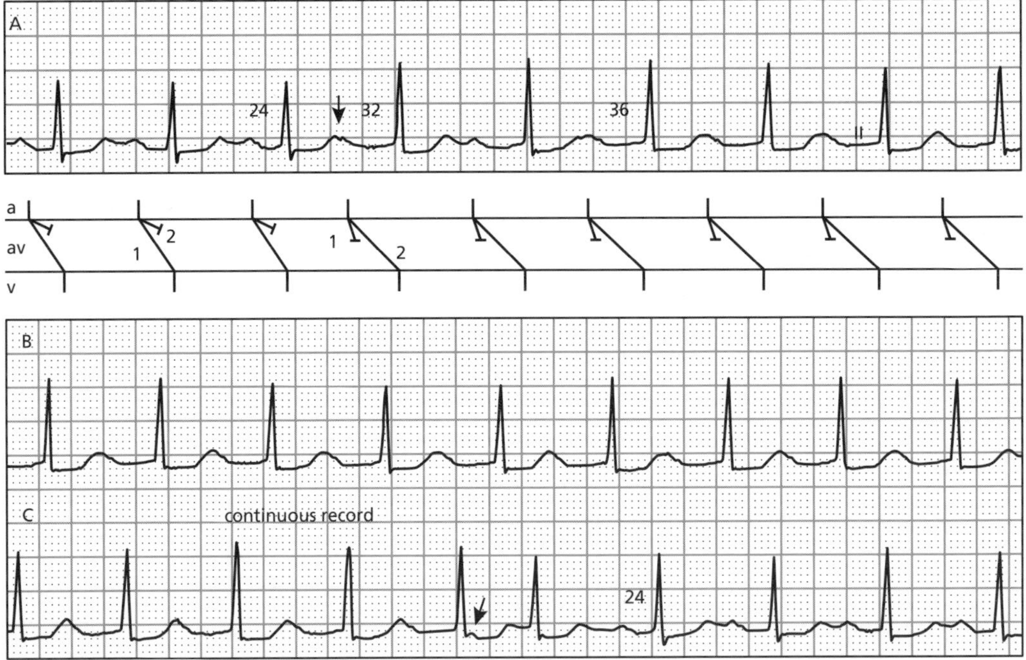

Figure 11.19 Dual pathways: two PR intervals.

period, causing the premature atrial impulse to block in that pathway. In the second strip, another premature extrasystole is noted (arrow), which depolarizes the slow pathway and shifts conduction back to the faster pathway, restoring the PR interval to its previous value (240 msec).

An example of *differing RP intervals* caused by dual pathways is shown in Figure 11.20. The P waves have been numbered for ease of reference. The first P wave in the strip (1) is a sinus P wave conducted via the fast pathway (a in the laddergram) with a PR interval of 140 msec (0.14 sec). The sinus impulse is followed by a ventricular extrasystole with retrograde conduction to the atria resulting in a P wave (*2*) that is conducted back to the ventricles with an RP interval of 360 msec (0.36 sec), revealing the presence of a slower, second pathway (b in the laddergram). A ventricular echo beat results. The echo beat is followed by another ventricular extrasystole with retrograde conduction over the faster (a) pathway as evidenced by the shorter RP interval (140 msec). As shown by the laddergram, this

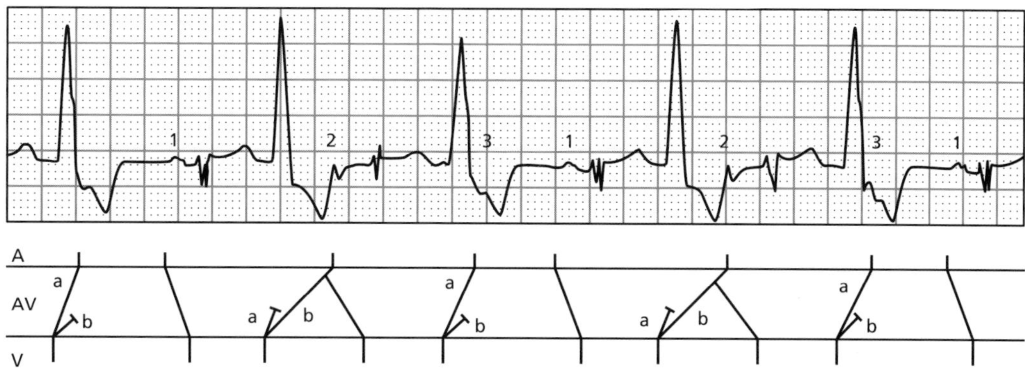

Figure 11.20 Dual pathways: two RP intervals.

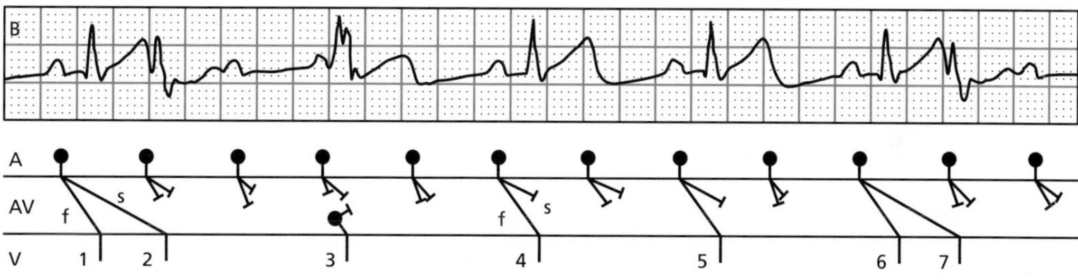

Figure 11.21 Dual pathways: dual ventricular response. QRS complexes 1, 2, 6 and 7 represent dual response to a single sinus impulse.

sequence of conduction through alternating slow and fast retrograde pathways occurs repeatedly, establishing a complex *allorhythmia*.

Dual ventricular response is an unusual manifestation of dual pathways. An example is shown in Figure 11.21, in which sinus rhythm with 2:1 atrioventricular conduction is seen. The first QRS complex (1, laddergram) is closely followed by a second QRS complex (2) that exhibits right bundle branch block aberrancy. The next QRS complex (3), which is wide and bizarre, represents an escape beat.

12

CHAPTER 12

The Wolff–Parkinson–White syndrome

In early fetal life the atrial and ventricular myocardia are continuous, but after the first month of gestation the formation of the annulus fibrosus begins the anatomical and electrical separation of the atria and ventricles, leaving the atrioventricular node and His bundle as the only electrical connection between the upper and lower chambers. In approximately three out of every 1000 individuals this process is incomplete, and unobliterated myocardial strands persist that create an electrically conductive bridge between the atrial and ventricular myocardium. These congenitally anomalous fibers, known variously as *accessory pathways*, *bypass tracts* or *Kent bundles*, may be located anywhere around the atrioventricular sulcus or septum, but are most commonly found along the left lateral ventricular free wall or in a posteroseptal location. In around 10% of subjects with accessory pathways, more than one functioning anomalous connection is found to exist.

Most anomalous pathways are found in otherwise structurally normal hearts, but of the various congenital cardiac defects, right-sided defects – Ebstein's anomaly in particular – are especially prone to coexist with functional accessory pathways.

The classic ECG manifestations of the *Wolff–Parkinson–White syndrome* (WPW), named for the cardiologists who described it in 1930, include (1) a PR interval less than 120 msec in duration, (2) a QRS complex equal to or greater than 120 msec, and (3) an initial slurring of the QRS complex called a *delta wave* or *pre-excitation component* (Figure 12.1), and (4) tachycardia. Many cases of WPW syndrome do not precisely conform to these criteria, presenting with PR intervals and QRS complexes of normal or nearly normal duration and very subtle delta waves. These cases often remain undiagnosed until other factors, such as supraventricular arrhythmias or symptoms such as syncope or palpitations, prompt careful scrutiny of the ECG. Abnormalities of the ST segment and T wave are also commonly noted in subjects with WPW syndrome.

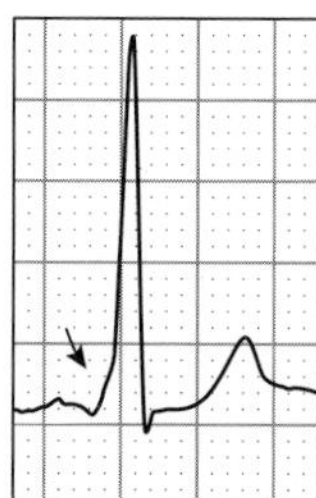

Figure 12.1 The diagnostic triad of WPW syndrome: (1) short PR interval, (2) wide QRS complex, and (3) delta wave (*arrow*).

The WPW syndrome is the classic example of *pre-excitation*: because the sinus impulse is able to bypass the slowly conducting atrioventricular node and reach the ventricle by means of the rapidly conducting anomalous connection, ventricular depolarization begins at the ventricular insertion of the accessory pathway, inscribing the *delta wave* on the ECG. The polarity of the delta wave in the various leads thus becomes a clue to the location of the accessory path (see below).

Depending on its conduction properties and distance from the sinoatrial node, the accessory path may contribute relatively little to ventricular depolarization, producing a small delta wave ('minimal pre-excitation'), or conversely, most of the ventricular activation may occur via the accessory connection, producing a wide QRS ('maximally pre-excited') complex in which the pre-excitation component predominates. In either case, the resulting QRS complex is a *fusion beat*, a morphological hybrid that results when ventricular activation starts from two

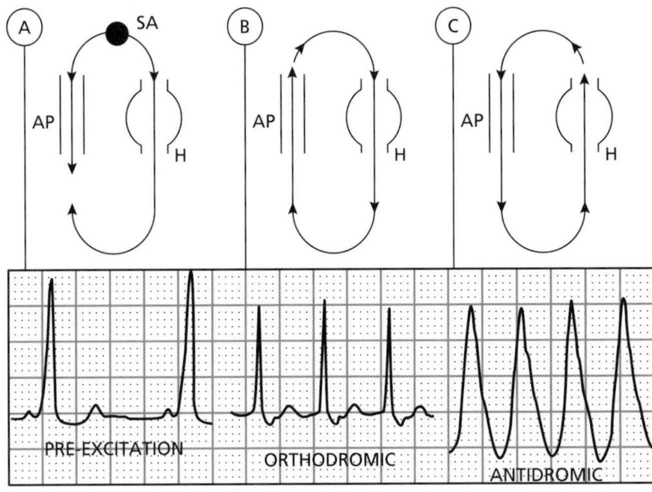

Figure 12.2 Mechanisms of re-entry in the WPW syndrome: AP: accessory pathway, H: bundle of His, SA: sinoatrial node.

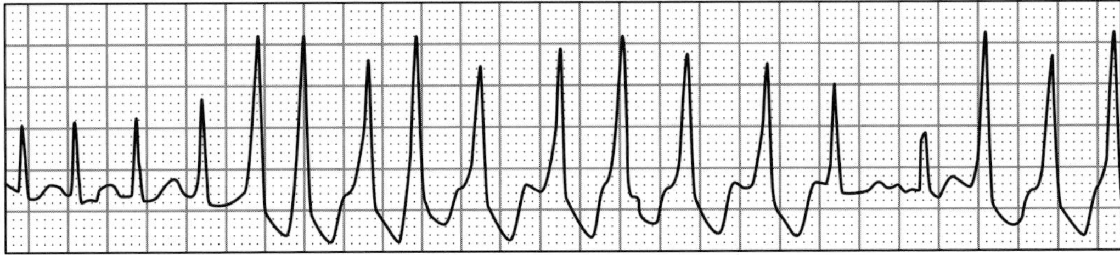

Figure 12.3 Atrial fibrillation in a patient with WPW syndrome: the narrow QRS complexes result from normal conduction over the His bundle, the wide QRS complexes result from conduction over the accessory pathway.

points of origin: the insertion of the anomalous connection and the normal conduction system (A in Figure 12.2). The degree of pre-excitation, reflected in both the duration of the PR interval and the width of the delta wave, may vary from time to time or even from beat to beat, or may fluctuate in cyclical fashion–the *concertina effect*. Pre-excitation may be intermittent, present in some beats but not in others (Figure 12.3), or in some tracings but not in others.

In subjects with slowly conducting bypass tracts, conduction through the accessory pathway may be lost altogether as the person ages. In others, the accessory connection may conduct only in a retrograde, ventriculoatrial direction. Because such pathways cannot produce signs of pre-excitation to signal their presence, they are called *concealed pathways*. Although capable of producing atrioventricular re-entrant tachycardia (AVRT), these subjects do not, technically speaking, have WPW syndrome, in which evidence of pre-excitation is the distinguishing feature.

Mechanism and incidence of tachyarrhythmias

Among subjects with WPW syndrome, as many as 80% are estimated to have associated tachyarrhythmias due to re-entry: the accessory path creates a circuit between the atria and ventricles, which consists of the His bundle as one limb and the bypass tract as the other. A fortuitously timed premature impulse may encounter *unidirectional block* in one pathway (usually the accessory path), and *slow conduction* in the other limb of the circuit (the AV node–His bundle), which permits recovery of the secondary limb (the accessory path) of the circuit.

In the majority of cases, antegrade conduction during re-entrant tachycardia occurs through the His bundle (*H*) and retrograde conduction back to the atria occurs over the accessory path (*AP*), producing a narrow-complex or *orthodromic* tachycardia (B, Figure 12.2). During orthodromic tachycardia, antegrade conduction occurs exclusively over the normal conduction pathway, so the resulting QRS

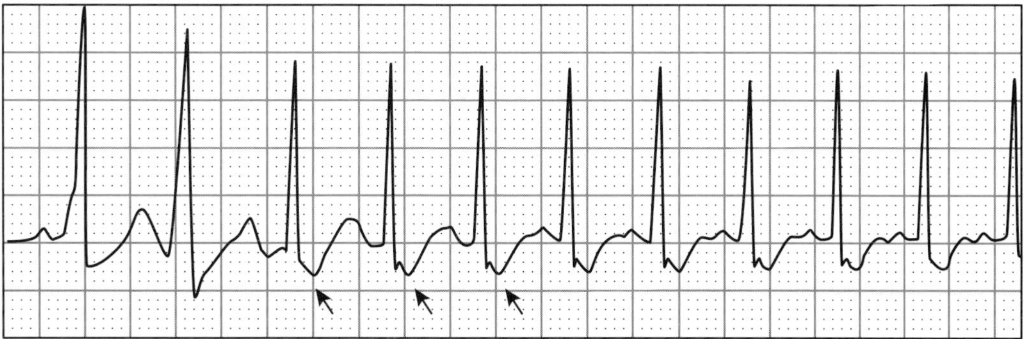

Figure 12.4 Orthodromic tachycardia: note the retrograde P waves (*arrows*) following the QRS complexes.

complexes are narrow and *lack evidence of pre-excitation*, and because the resulting tachycardia is due to atrioventricular re-entry, inverted P waves are usually visible in the ST segment following each QRS complex (Figure 12.4).

In the case of antidromic tachycardia (C, Figure 12.2), impulse re-entry takes the reverse route: antegrade conduction occurs over the accessory path (*AP*) and retrograde conduction through the His bundle (*H*). Because ventricular activation occurs from the insertion point of the accessory pathway and not over the normal conduction path, the resulting QRS complexes are wide.

Atrial fibrillation accounts for a significant percentage of the supraventricular tachycardias encountered in patients with WPW syndrome. Atrial fibrillation does not involve re-entrant conduction using the His bundle and accessory path to form a circuit. Because the accessory pathway typically lacks the slower conduction inherent in the AV nodal tissue, atrial fibrillation impulses are preferentially conducted over the accessory path. Ventricular rates of 300 per minute or more can result and at such rates ventricular fibrillation may supervene. An example of WPW syndrome with atrial fibrillation is shown in Figure 12.5. Because

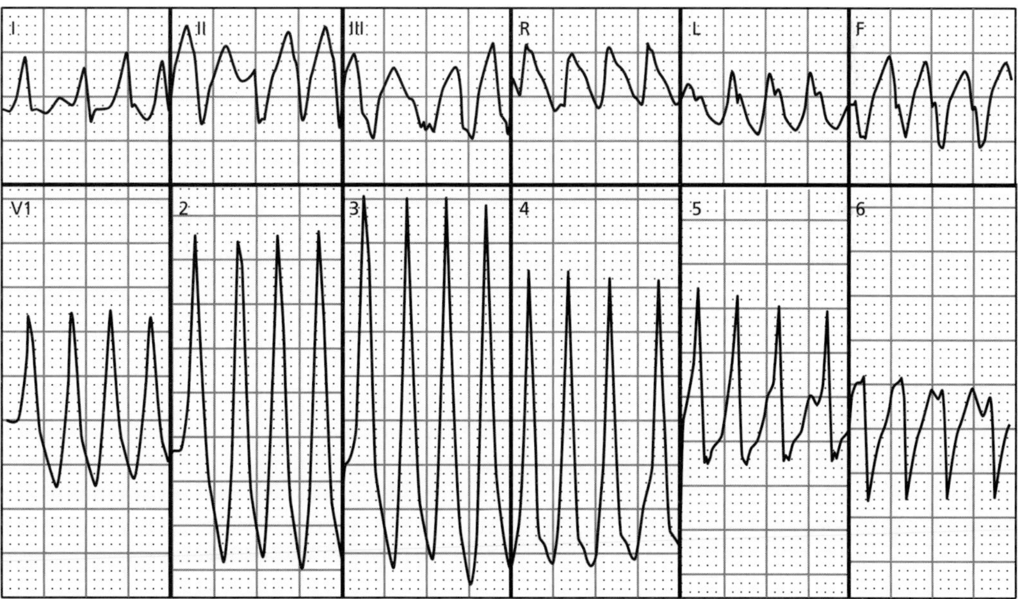

Figure 12.5 Atrial fibrillation in WPW syndrome: atrioventricular conduction occurs exclusively over the accessory pathway, resulting in an irregular wide-QRS tachycardia.

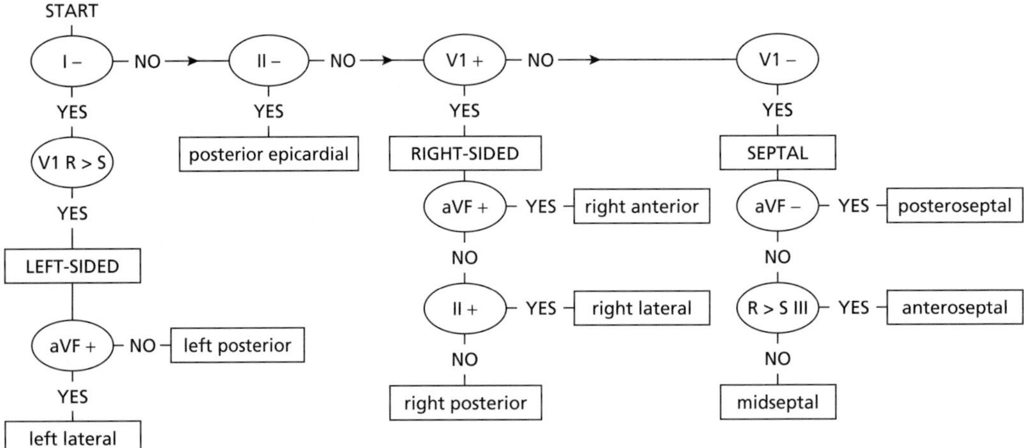

Figure 12.6 An algorithm for locating the accessory pathway based on the polarity of the delta wave and the R:S ratios in lead V1.

conduction of the fibrillation impulses occurs exclusively over the accessory pathway, an irregularly irregular wide-QRS complex tachycardia results.

Localization of the accessory pathway

Ablation of accessory pathways carries a significant advantage over medical management, so the ability to generally localize the ventricular insertion site of an anomalous pathway before the initiation of an invasive procedure is of obvious benefit. An algorithm for such identification is shown in Figure 12.6. The decision tree is based on (1) delta wave polarity in the various leads and (2) the R:S wave ratio in leads V1 and III. Examination of lead V1 yields an approximate location of the ventricular end of the accessory pathway: a *positive delta wave* in V1 is indicative of a right-sided pathway, a *negative delta wave* in V1 indicates a septal location, and an *R wave* > *S wave* configuration in V1 indicates that the connection is left-sided.

An application of the algorithm is shown in Figure 12.7, in which the accessory pathway (*AP*) is in the left lateral ventricular free wall. A second example, in which the accessory pathway is midseptal in location, is given in Figure 12.8.

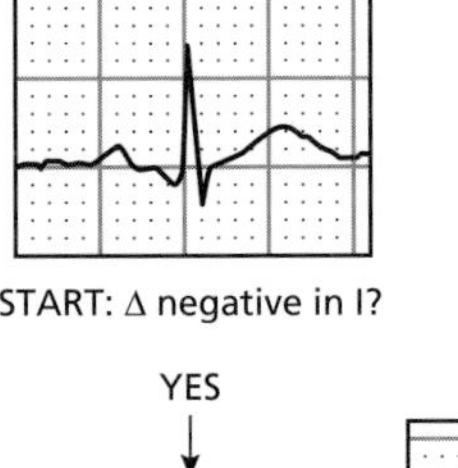

START: Δ negative in I?

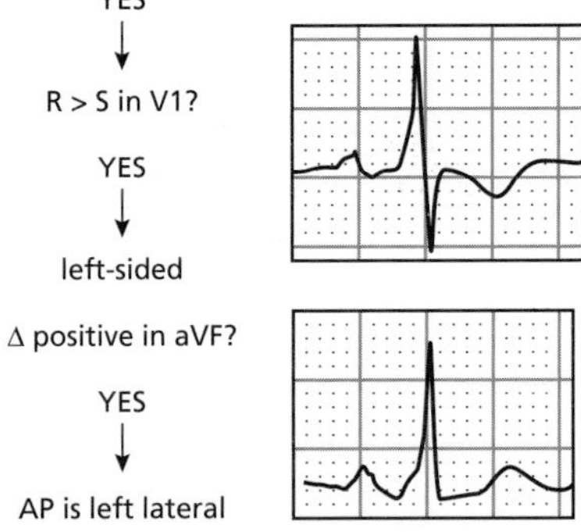

Figure 12.7 Algorithm: a left lateral pathway.

Risk stratification

Since the short refractory period of the accessory pathway can lead to very high rates of ventricular response of atrial fibrillation in patients with WPW syndrome, identification of those most at risk for this development is highly desirable. A positive response to any of the following tests or observations implies, *but by no means guarantees*, that the accessory connection has a relatively long refractory period and that the risk of dangerously fast ventricular response to atrial fibrillation is low.

1. Pre-excitation is intermittent.
2. Pre-excitation disappears during exercise.
3. The QRS complex normalizes following IV injection of ajmaline or procainamide.

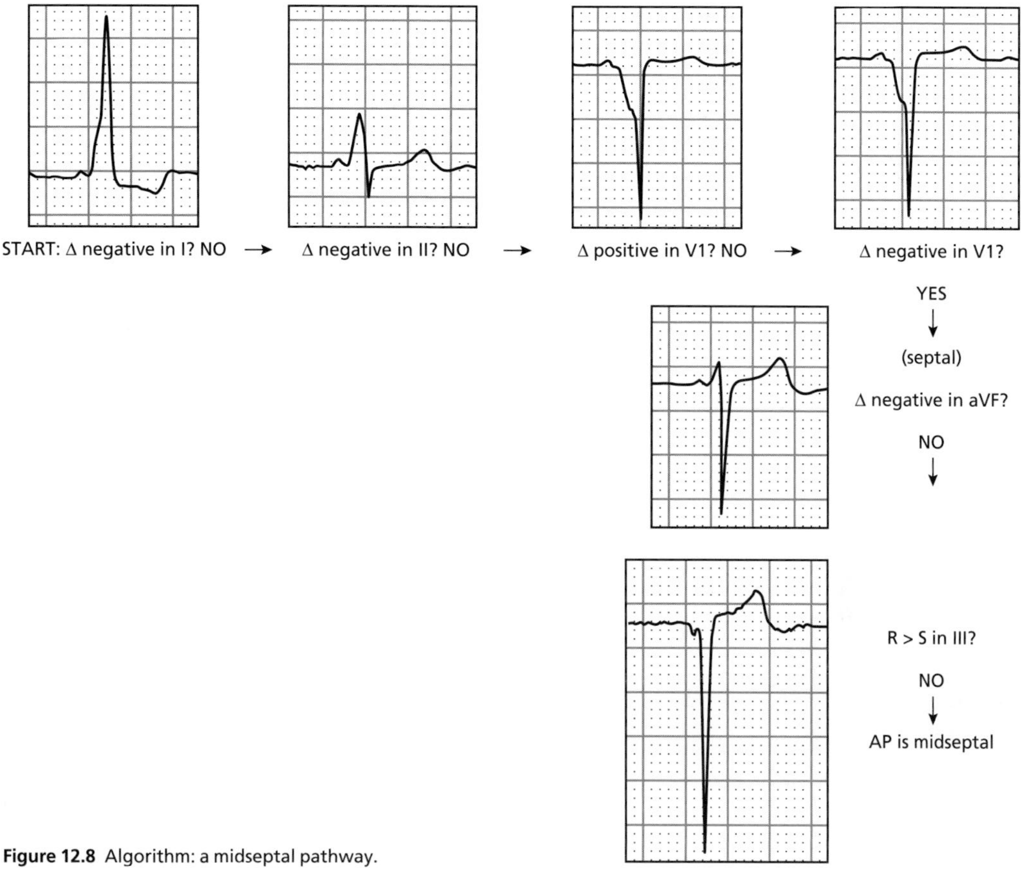

START: Δ negative in I? NO → Δ negative in II? NO → Δ positive in V1? NO → Δ negative in V1?

YES
↓
(septal)
Δ negative in aVF?

NO
↓
R > S in III?

NO
↓
AP is midseptal

Figure 12.8 Algorithm: a midseptal pathway.

Correspondingly, patients in whom pre-excitation is a permanent feature are at greater risk and require more precise risk stratification.

Mahaim (atriofascicular) tachycardia

The term *Mahaim tachycardia* refers to a group of re-entrant tachycardias caused by an accessory pathway originating in the right atrium and terminating in the right ventricular free wall in or near the right bundle branch (Figure 12.9). Because ventricular activation begins in the right ventricle, the ECG recorded during tachycardia has left bundle branch block morphology. These unusual *atriofascicular pathways*, which account for about 3% of accessory pathway-mediated tachycardias, exhibit antegrade conduction only and physiologic properties similar to AV nodal tissue. The baseline

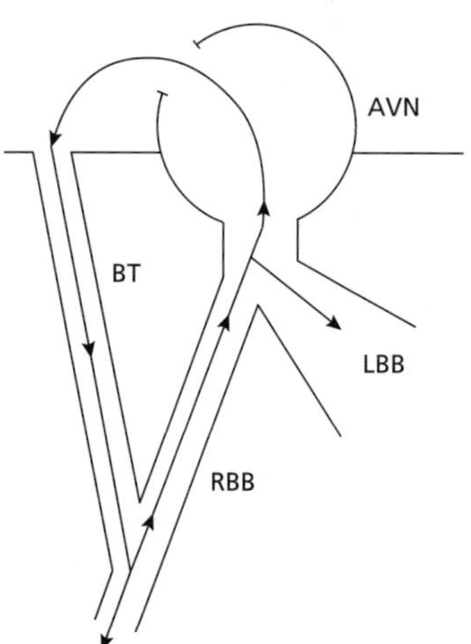

Figure 12.9 A common mechanism of Mahaim fiber tachycardia.

ECG in most patients shows only subtle signs of pre-excitation at best, such as absence of a septal q wave in leads I and V6, with an rS complex in lead III.

Antidromic tachycardia in which the His bundle serves as the retrograde limb of the re-entry circuit is typical, resulting in a regular tachycardia exhibiting left bundle branch block morphology with a rapid, smooth descent of the S wave in V1, a feature that tends to distinguish Mahaim tachycardia from ventricular tachycardia with left bundle branch block morphology. The inverted P waves resulting from retrograde atrial activation are usually buried in the QRS complexes and therefore not visualized.

Self-Assessment Test Five

5.1. Identify the abnormality in the following tracing.

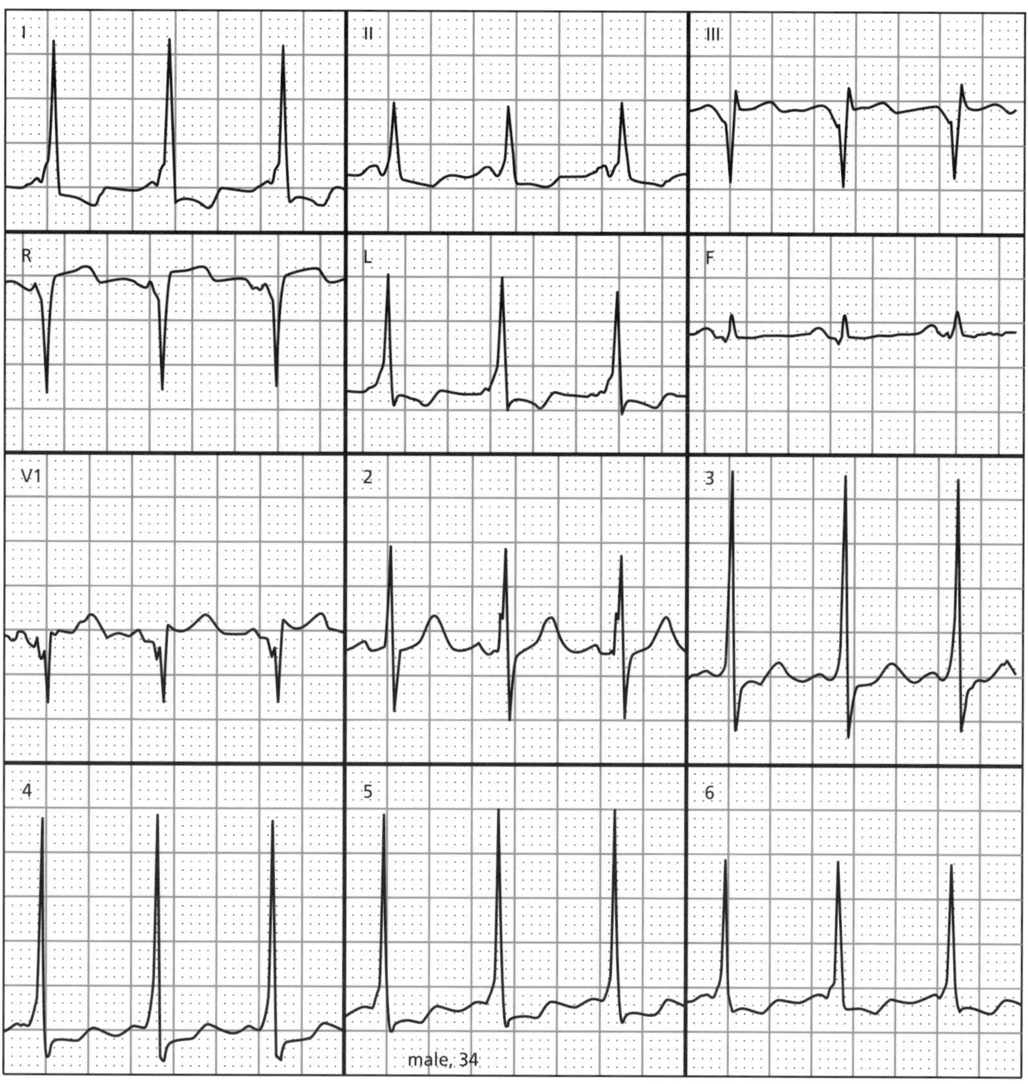

5.2. The most common form of re-entrant tachycardia is . . .

a. fast–slow atrioventricular nodal re-entrant tachycardia
b. atrioventricular re-entrant tachycardia
c. permanent junctional reciprocating tachycardia
d. slow–fast atrioventricular nodal re-entrant tachycardia

5.3. The anatomical substrate of the Wolff–Parkinson–White syndrome is . . .

a. a Mahaim (atriofascicular) fiber
b. a Kent bundle
c. a His bundle
d. a James fiber

Identify the abnormalities in the following 36 tracings.

5.4.

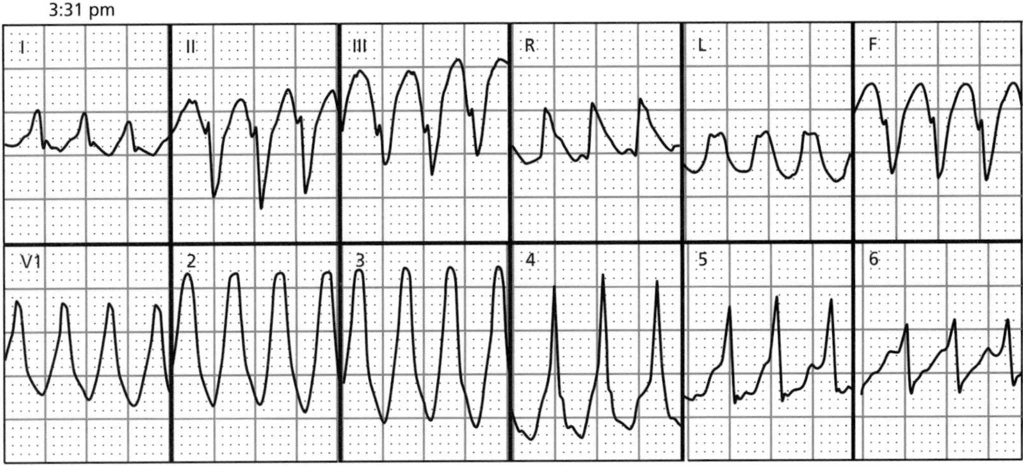

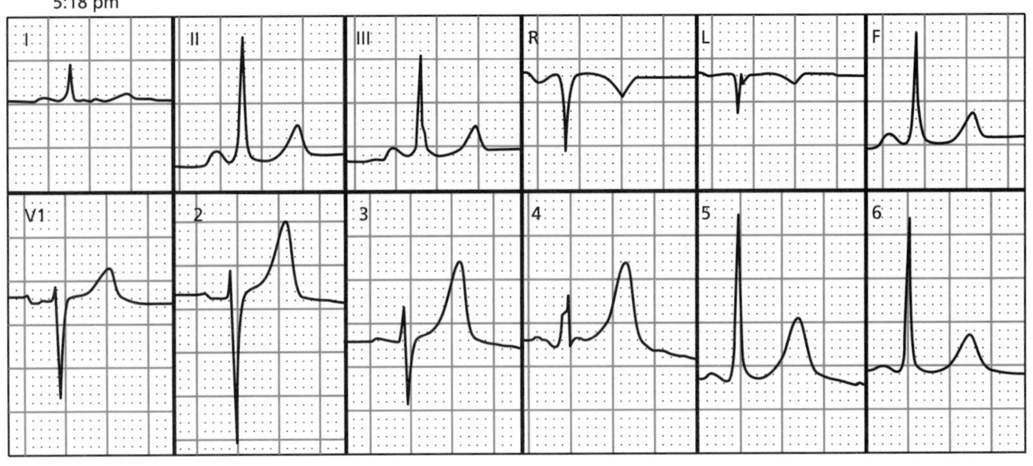

5.5.

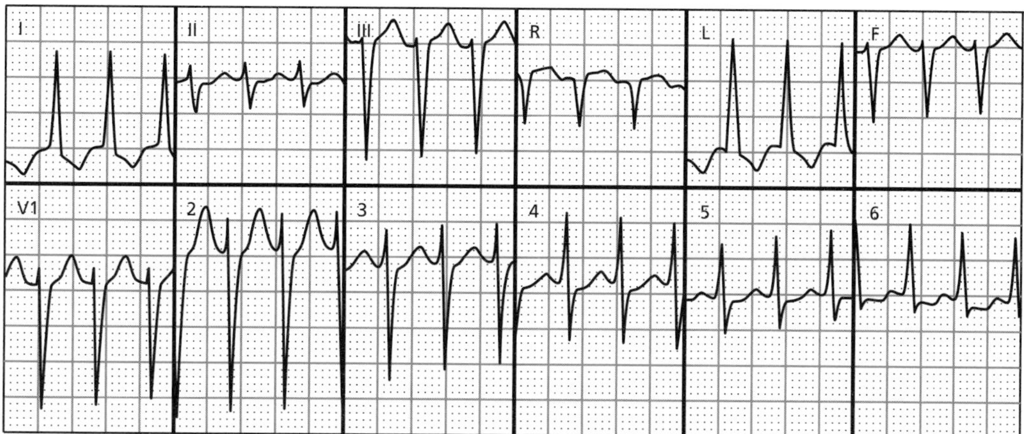

5.6.

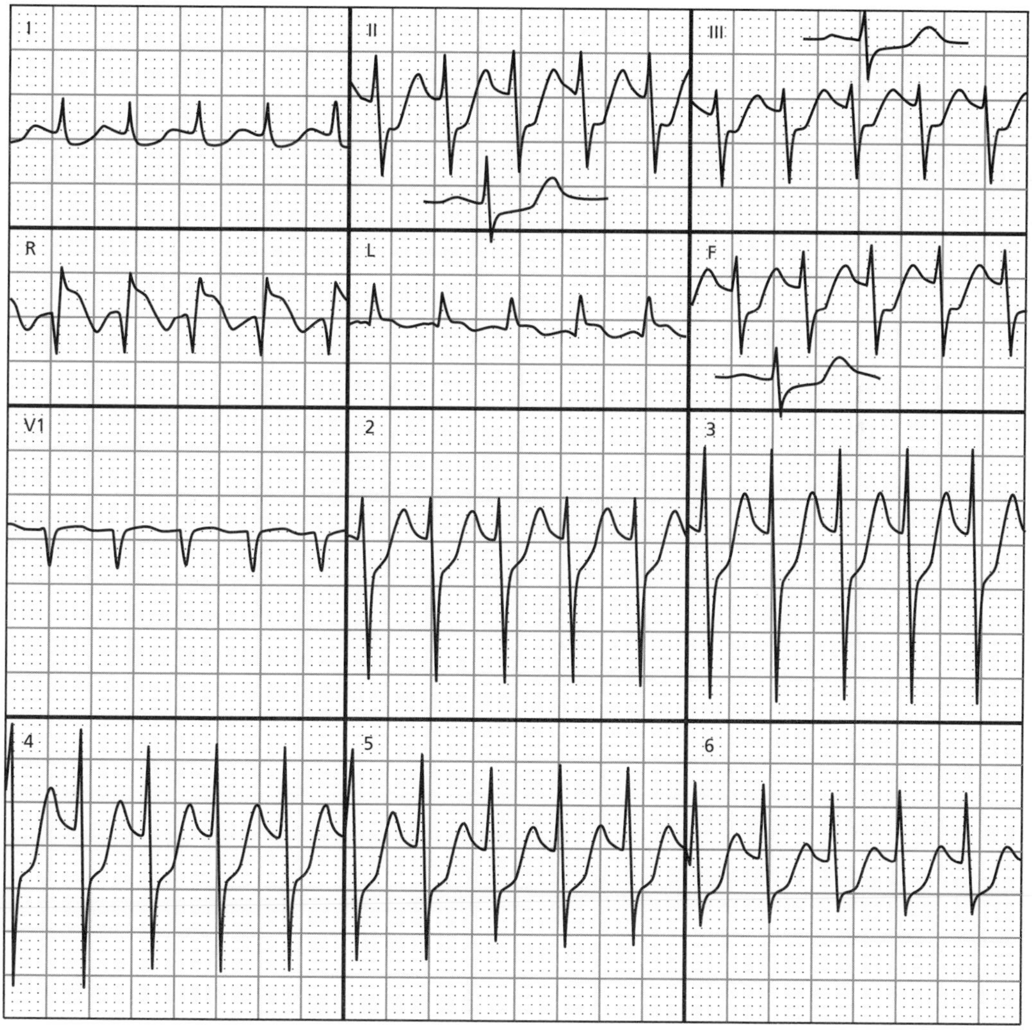

5.7.

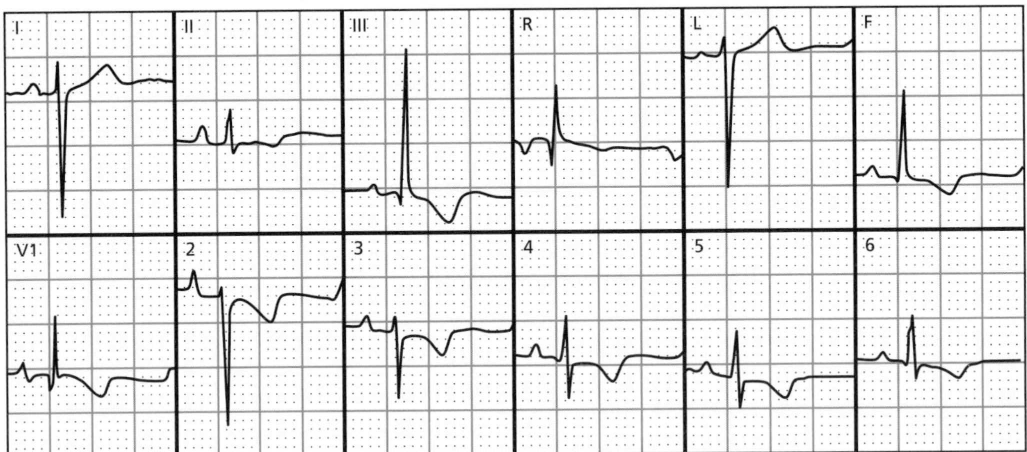
I
II
III
R
L
F
V1
2
3
4
5
6

5.8.

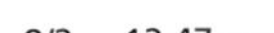
8/2 12:47 am

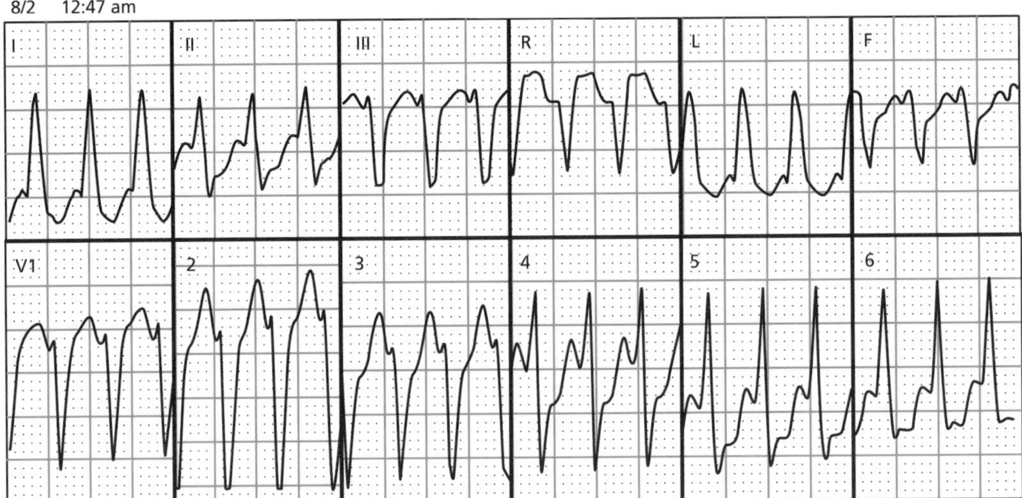
I
II
III
R
L
F
V1
2
3
4
5
6

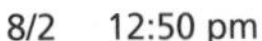
8/2 12:50 pm

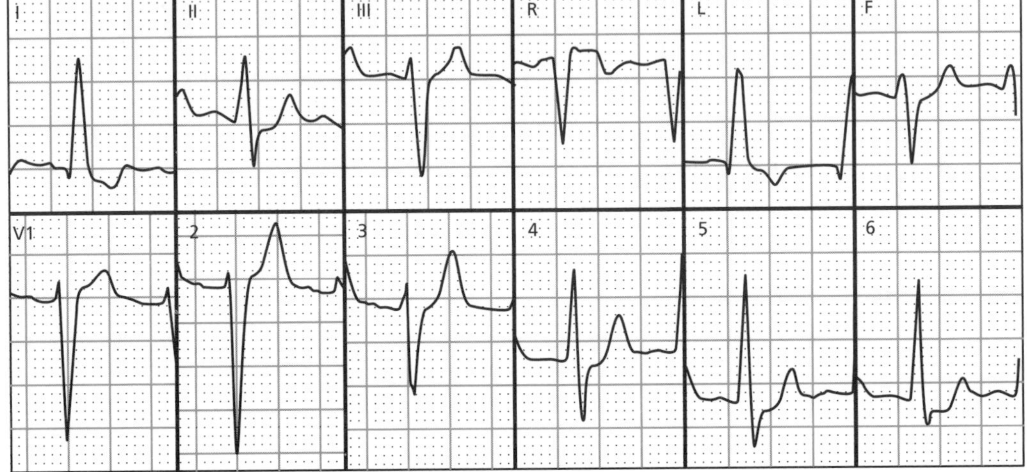
I
II
III
R
L
F
V1
2
3
4
5
6

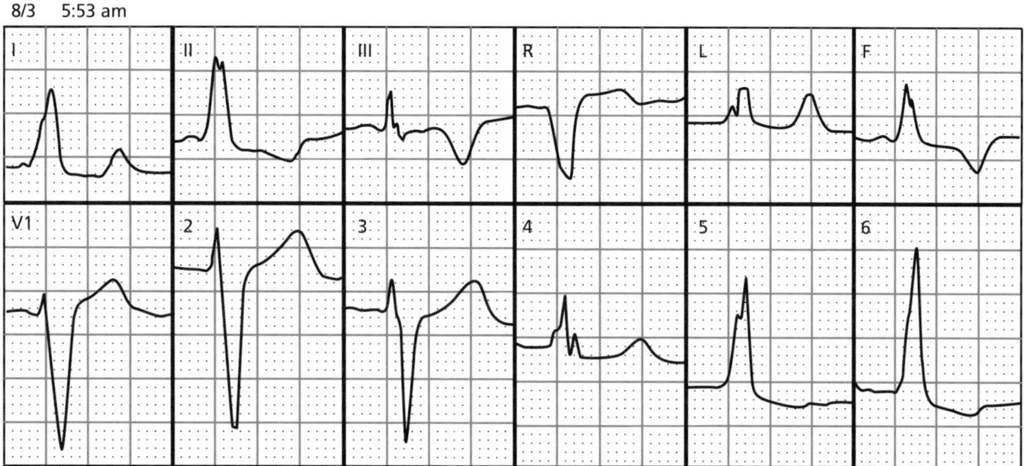

5.9.

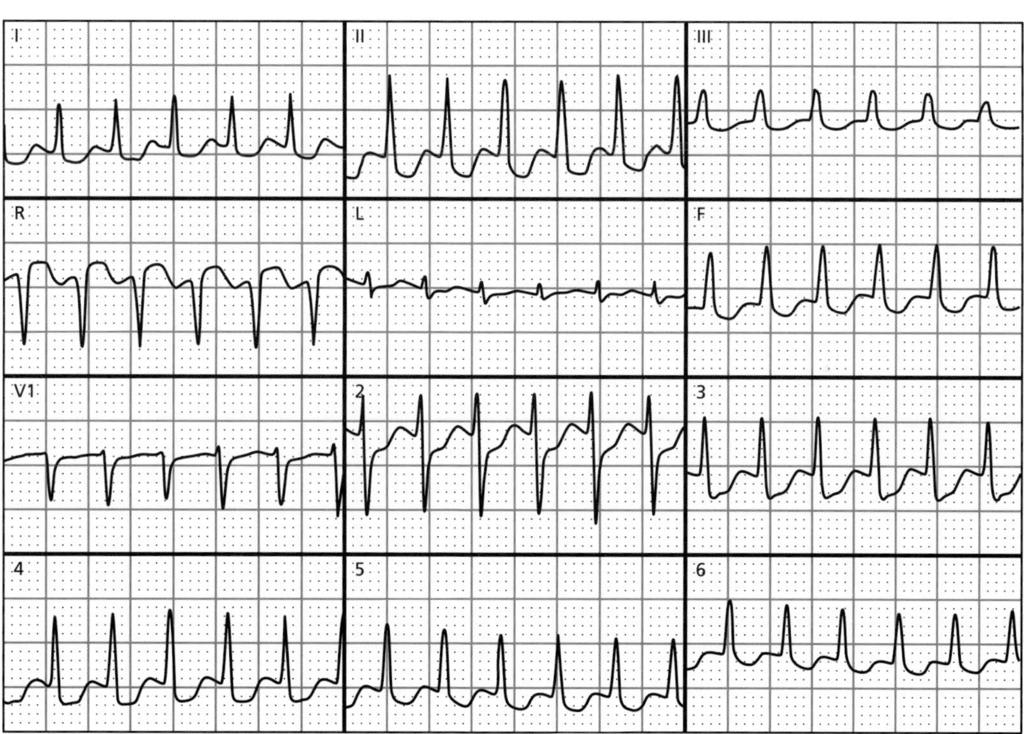

5.10.

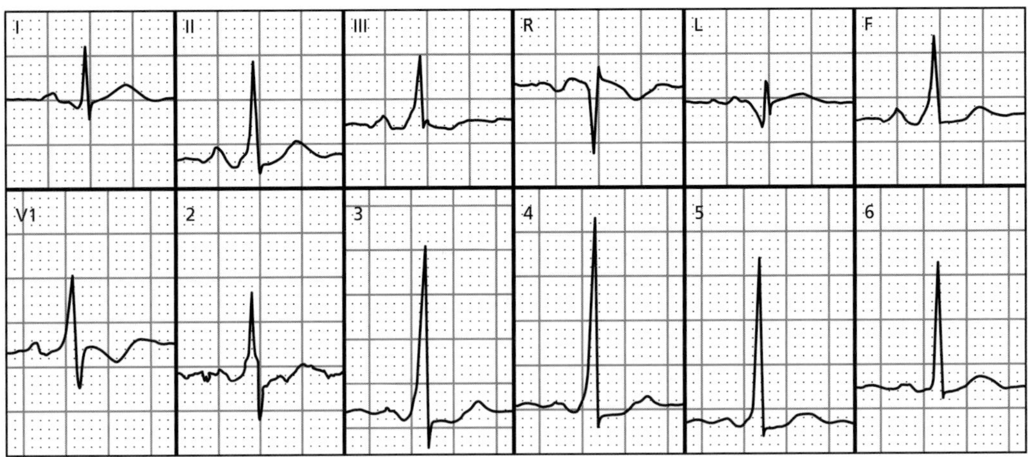

5.11.

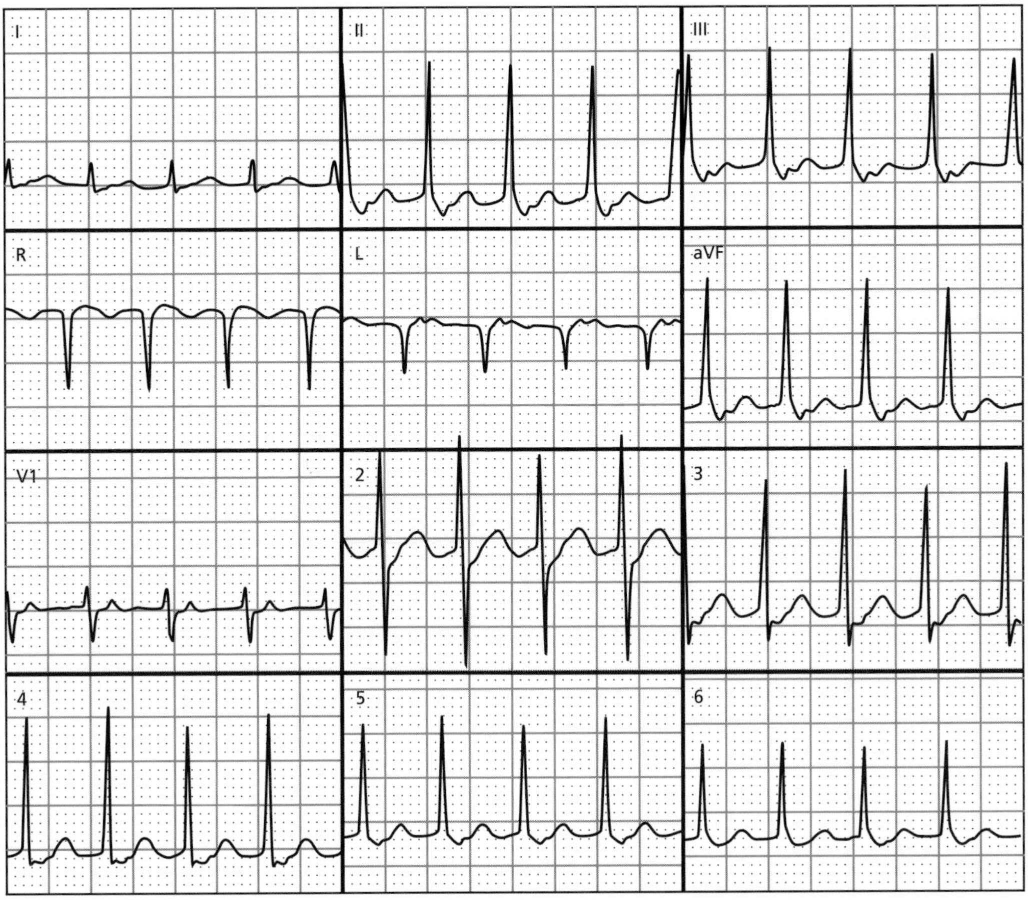

5.12.

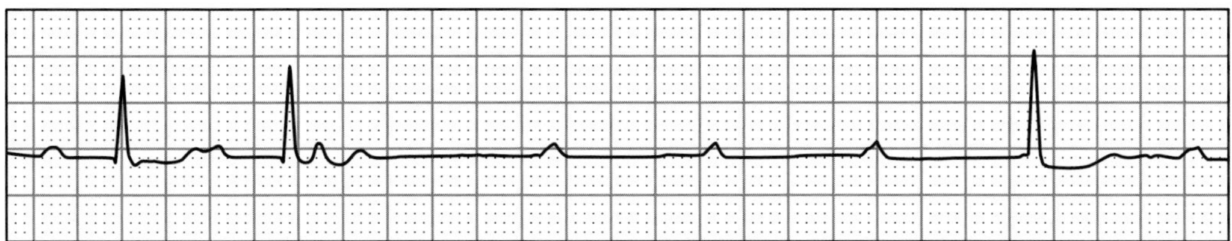

5.13.

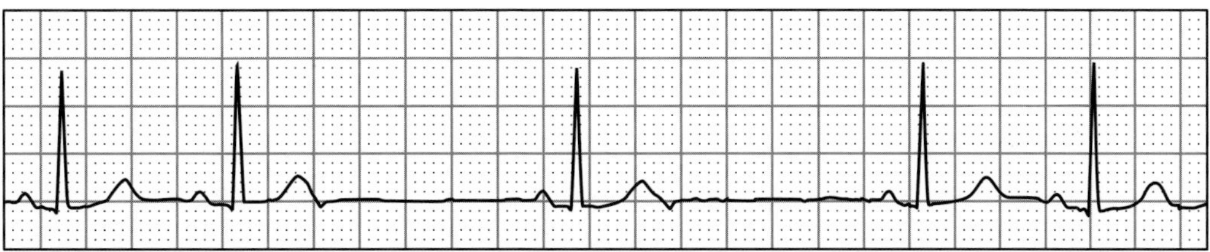

5.14.

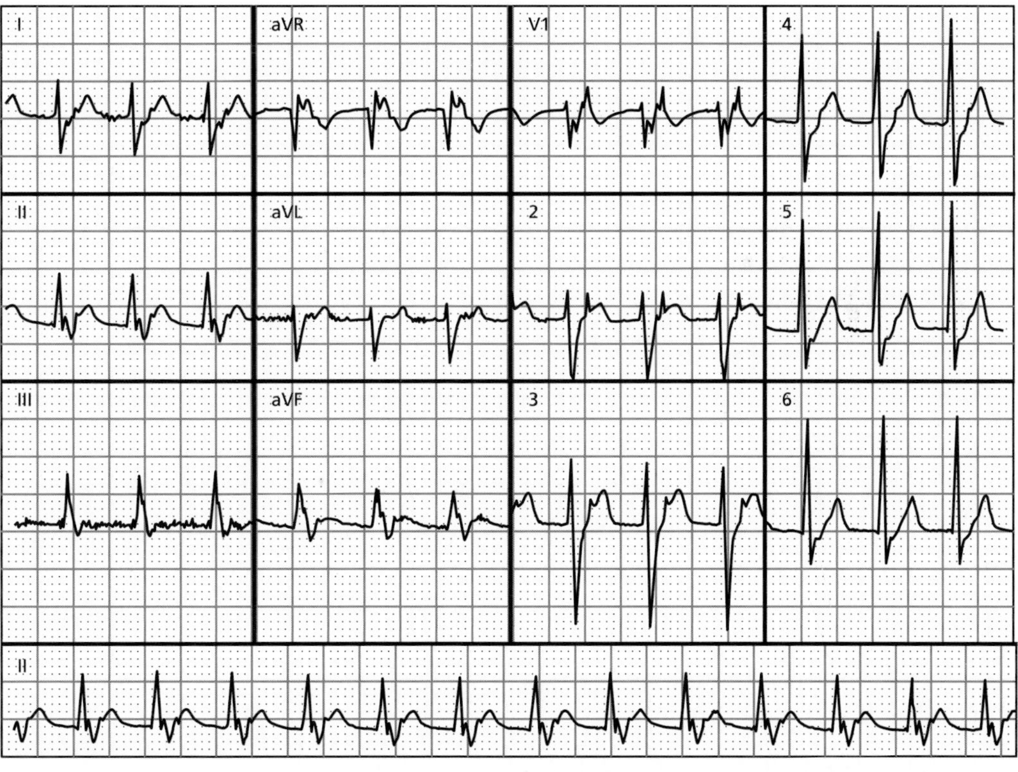

5.15.

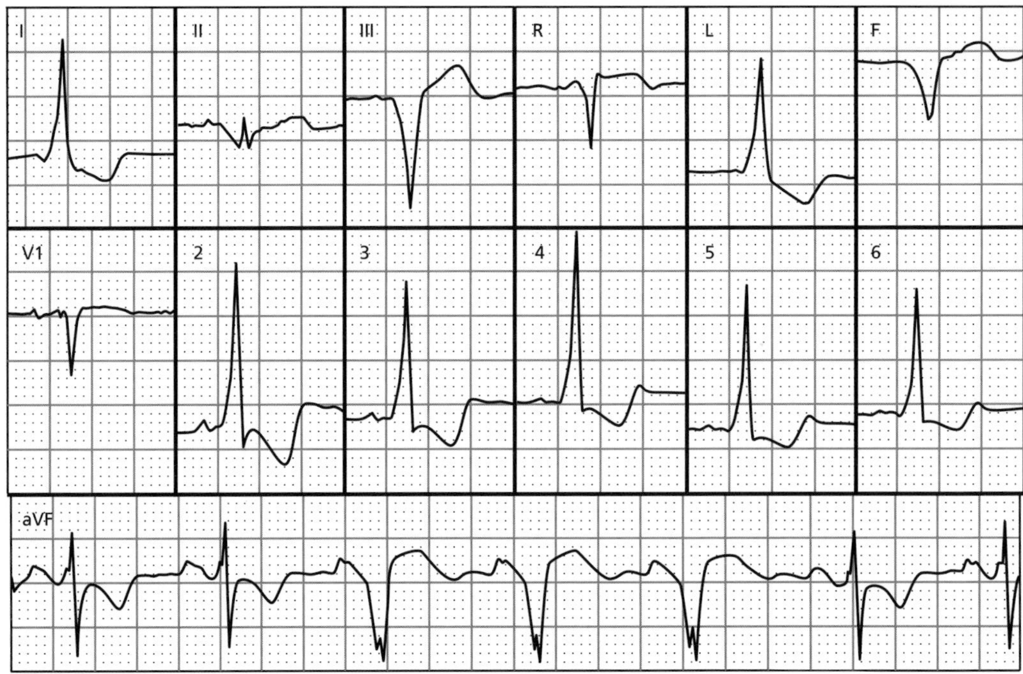

5.16.

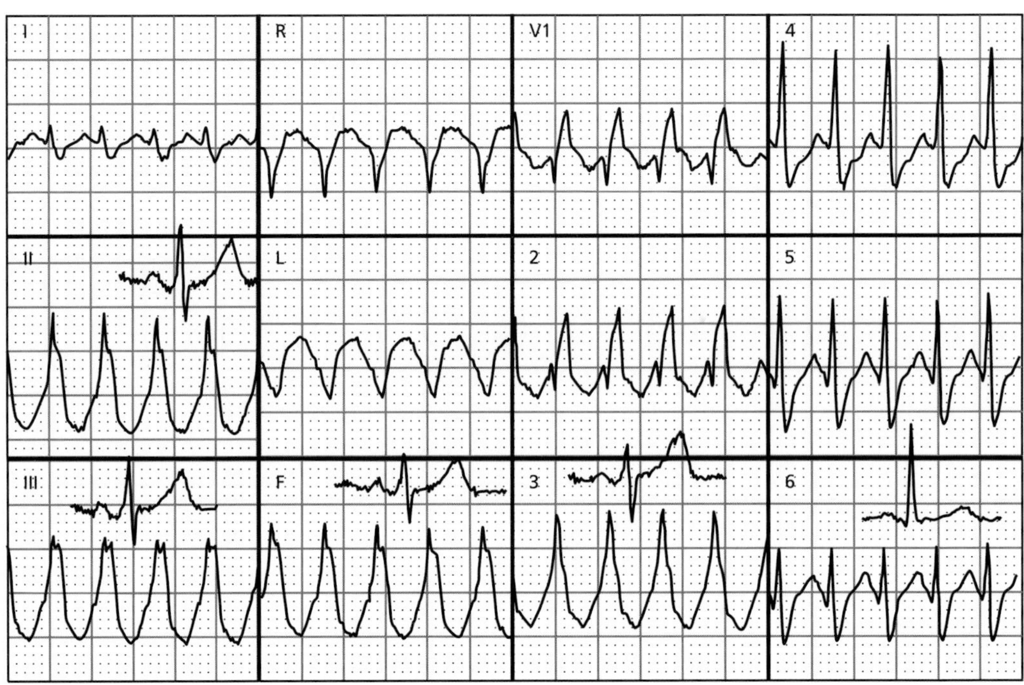

5.17.

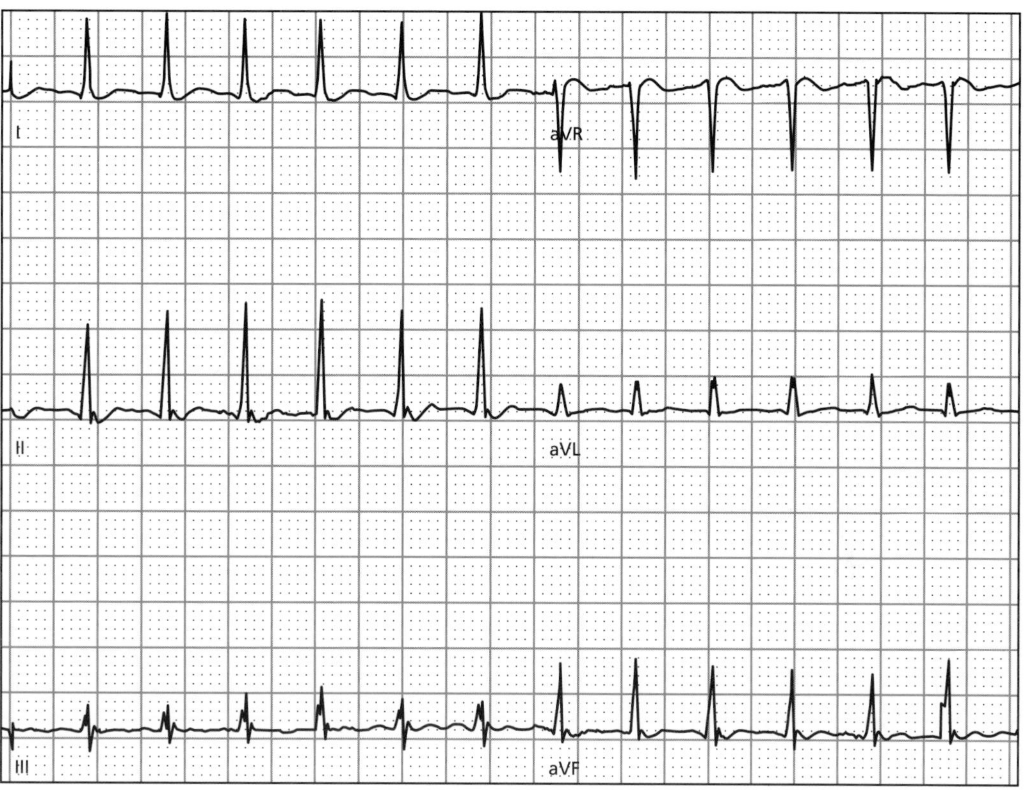

5.18.

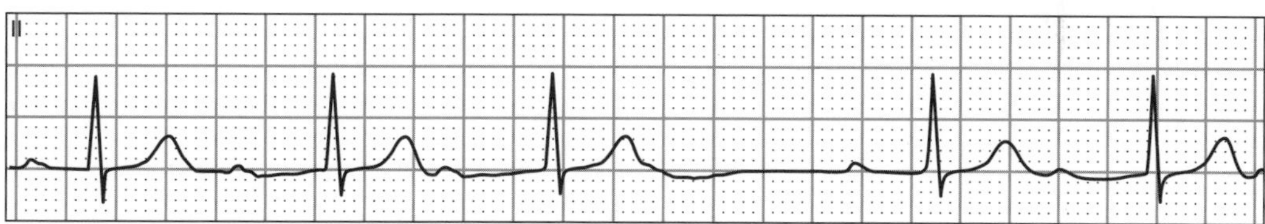

5.19.

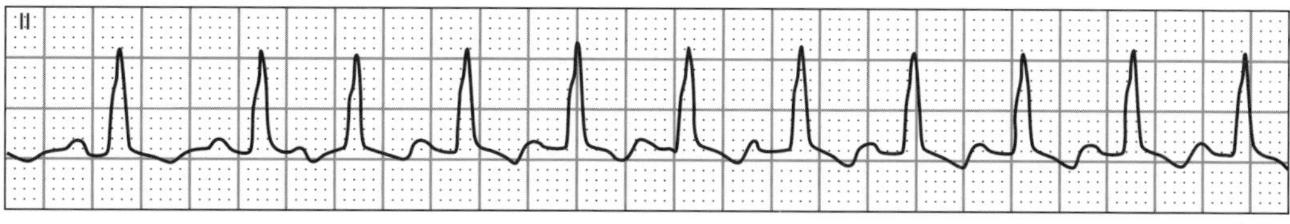

5.20.

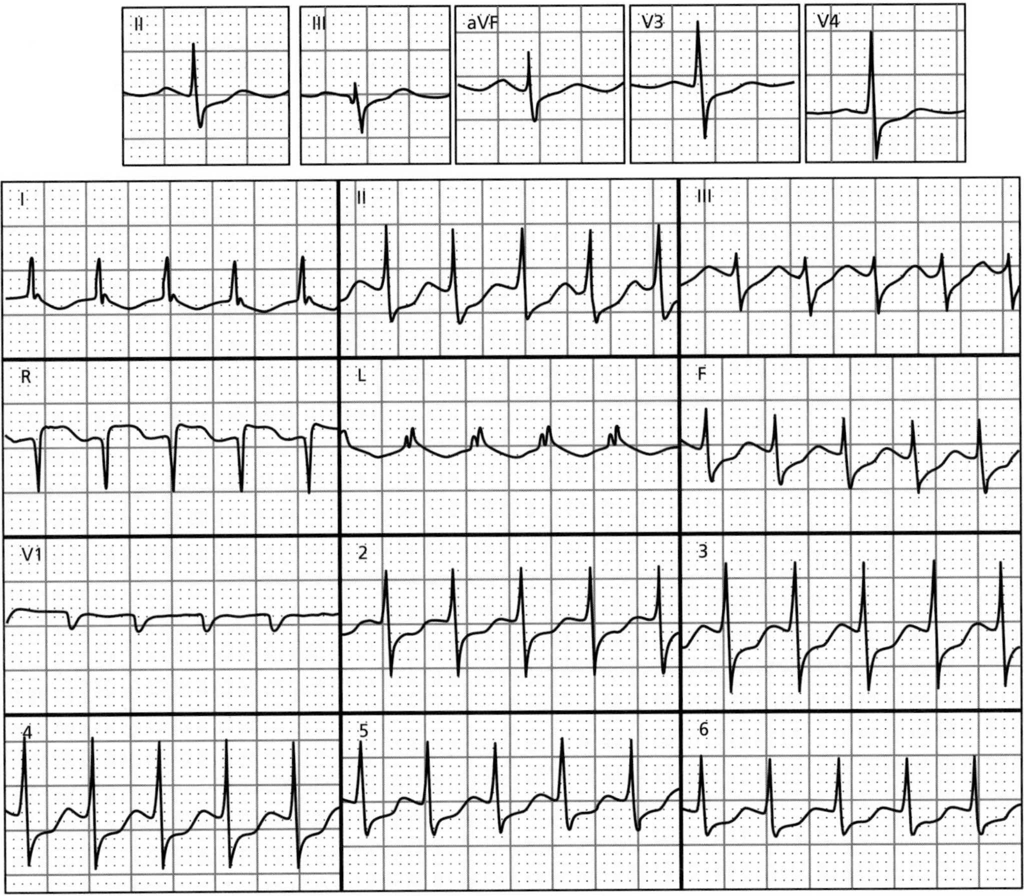

5.21.

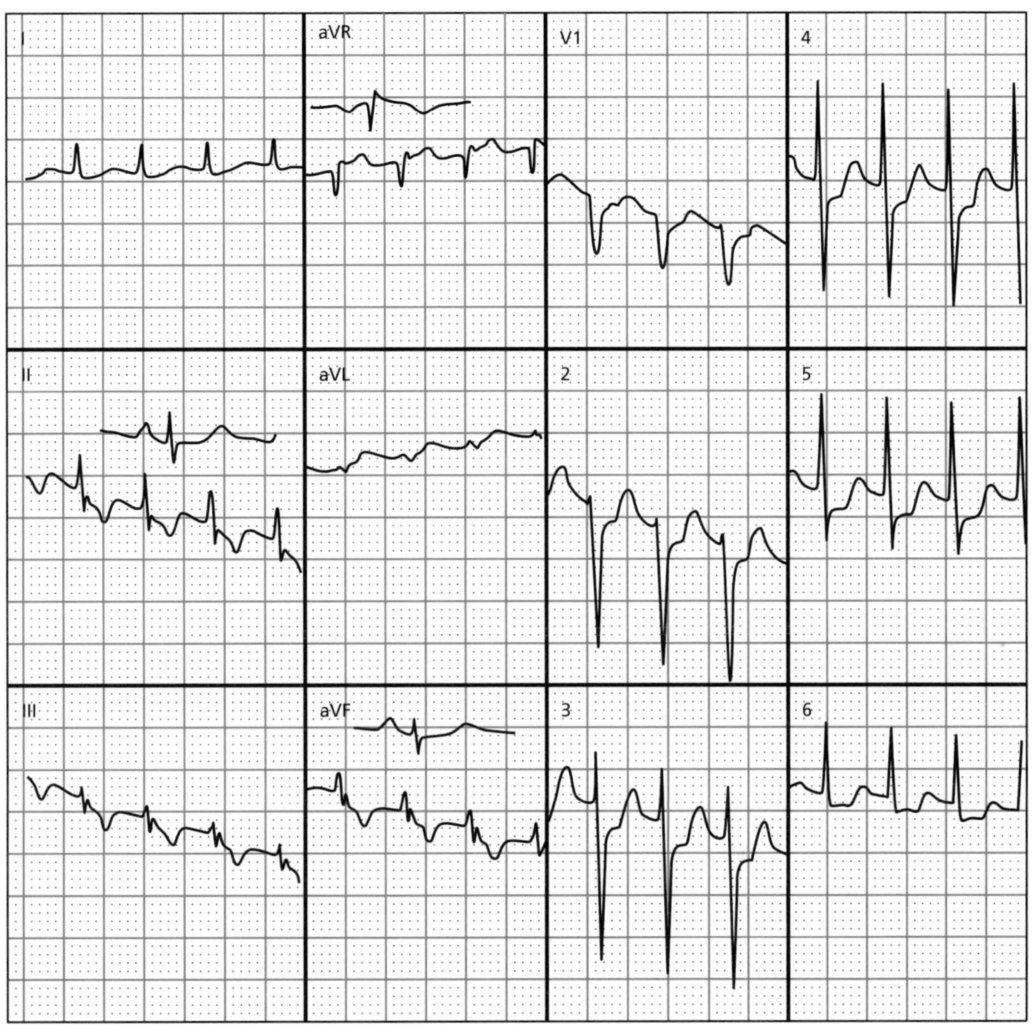

5.22.

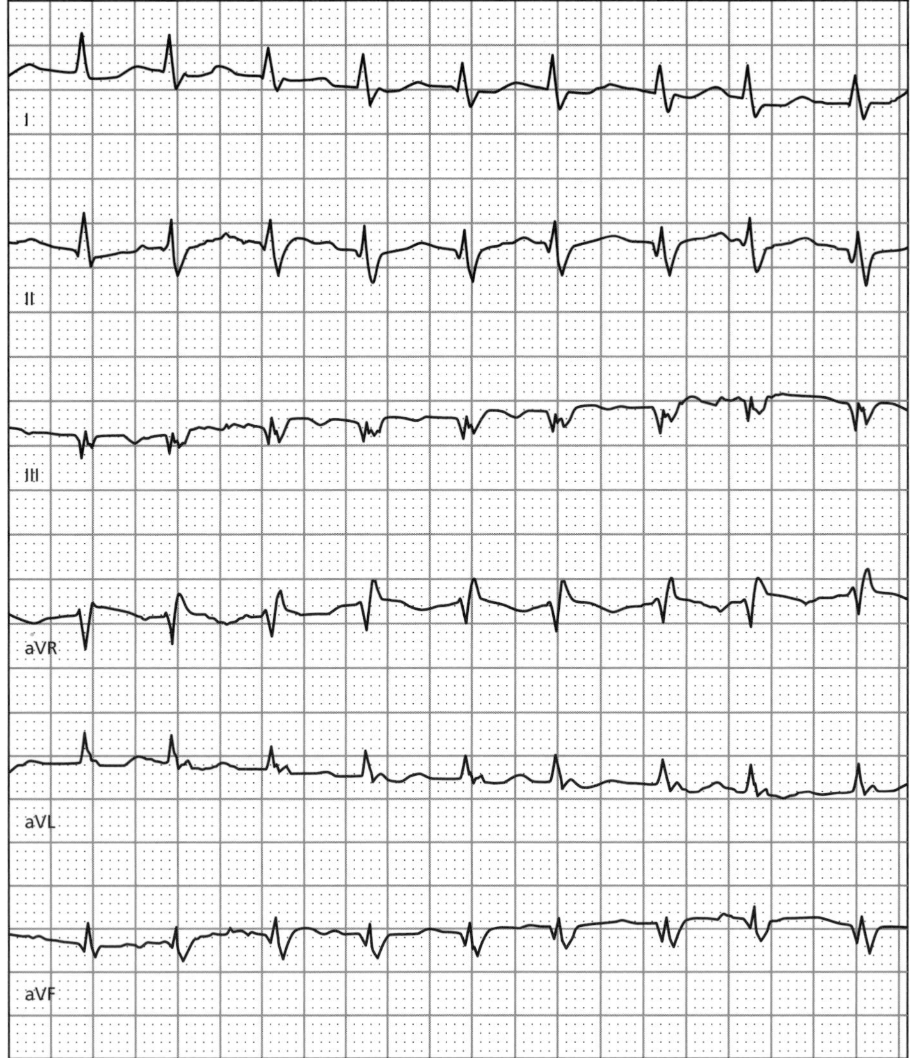

5.23.

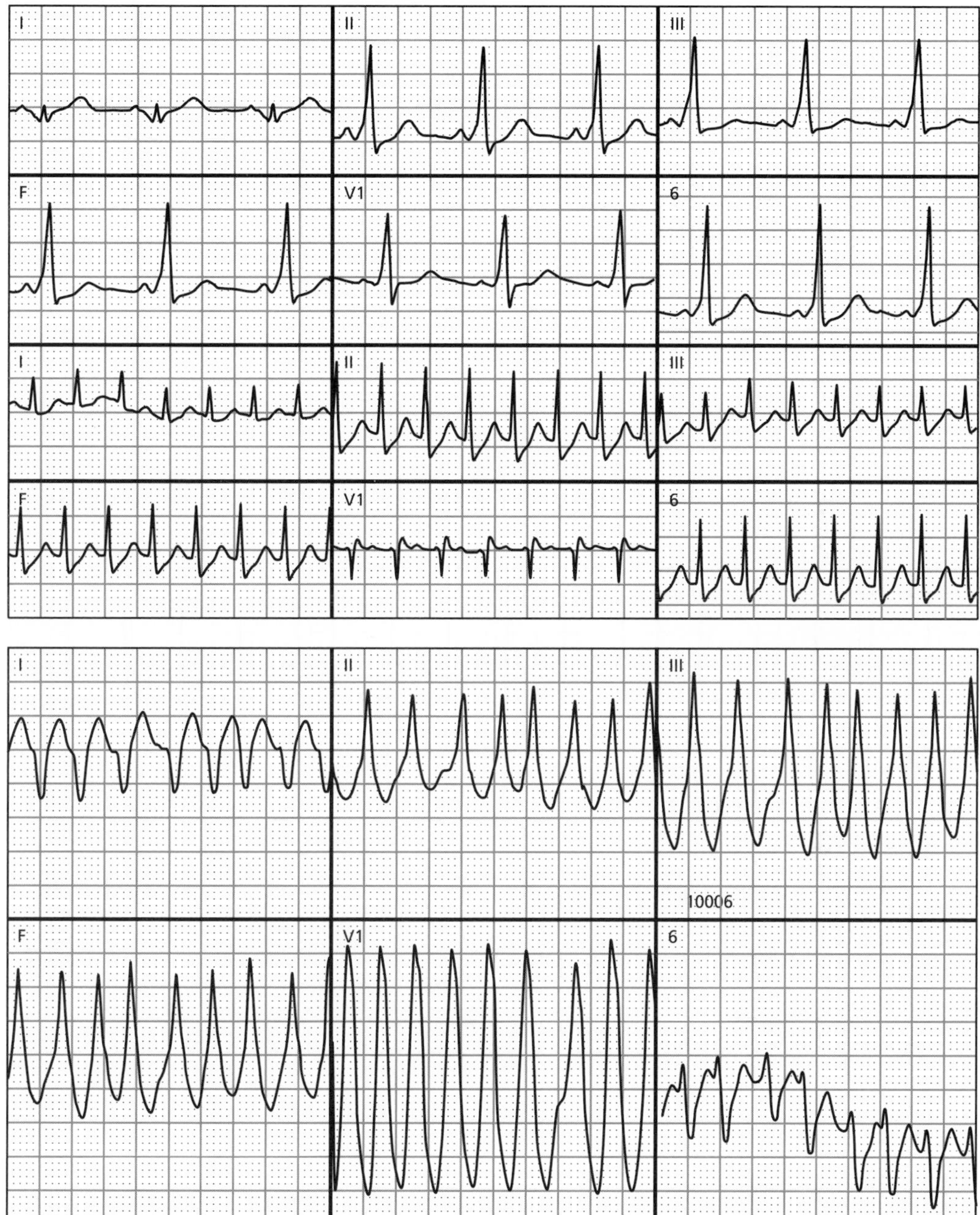

5.24.

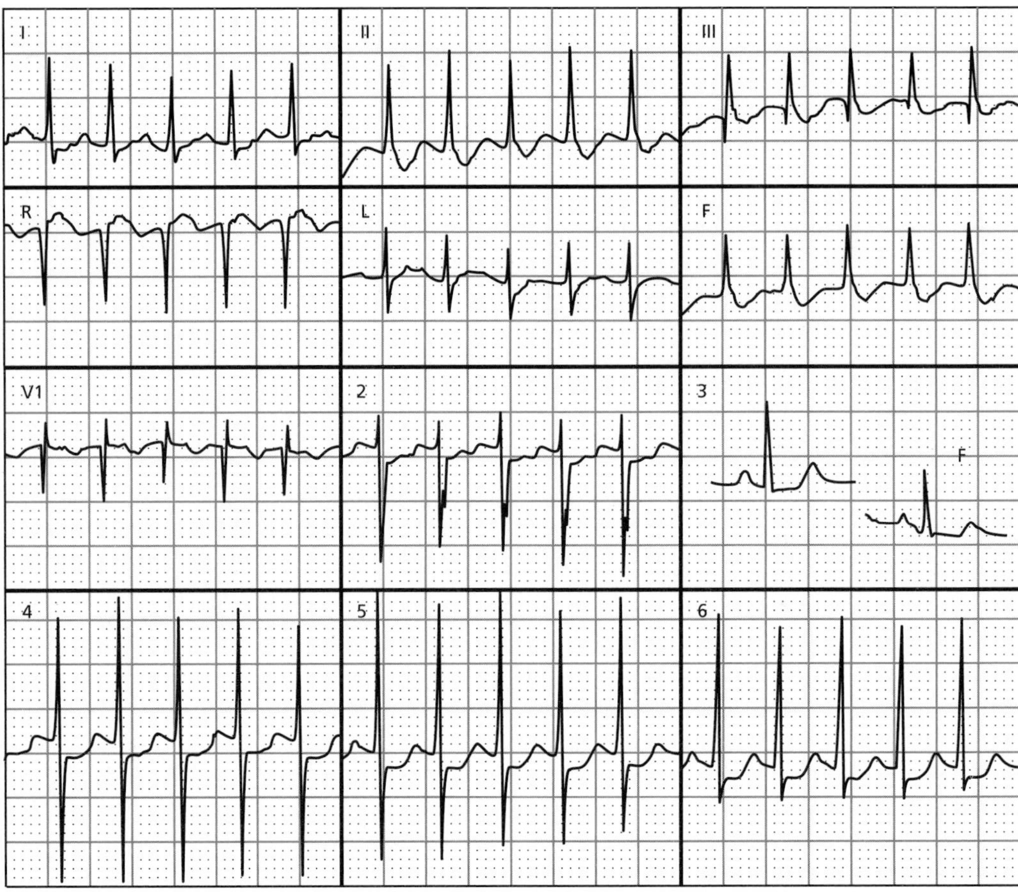

5.25.

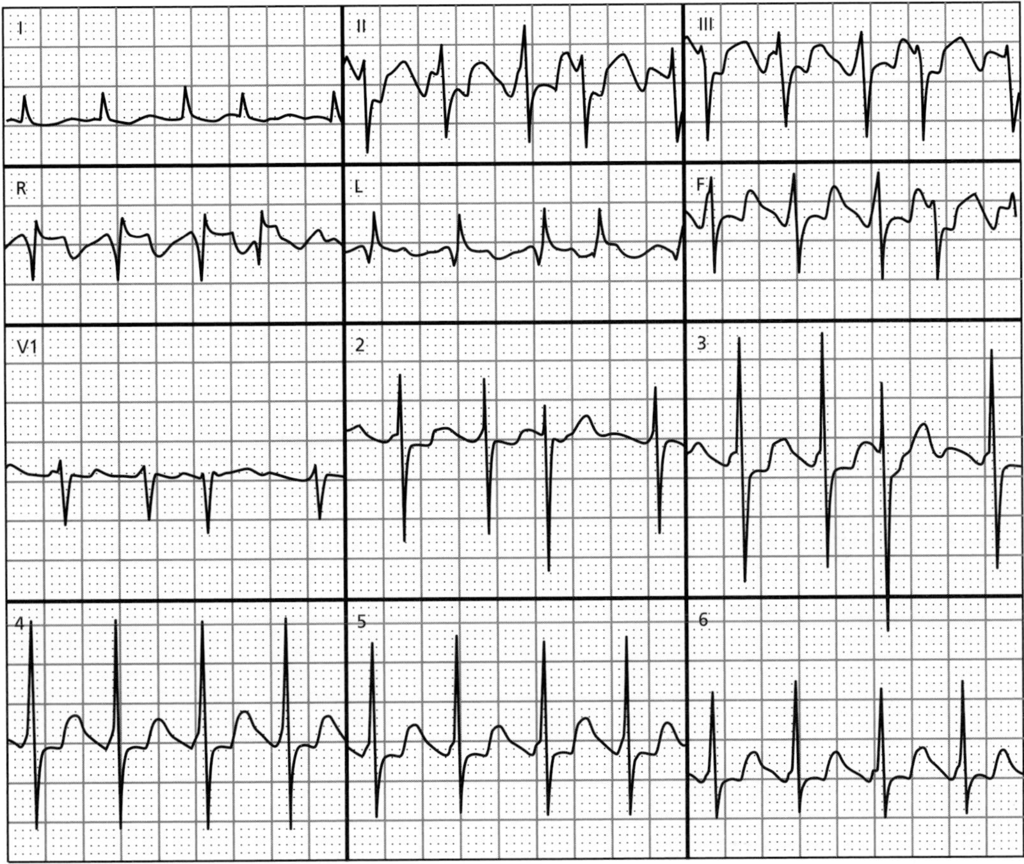

5.26.

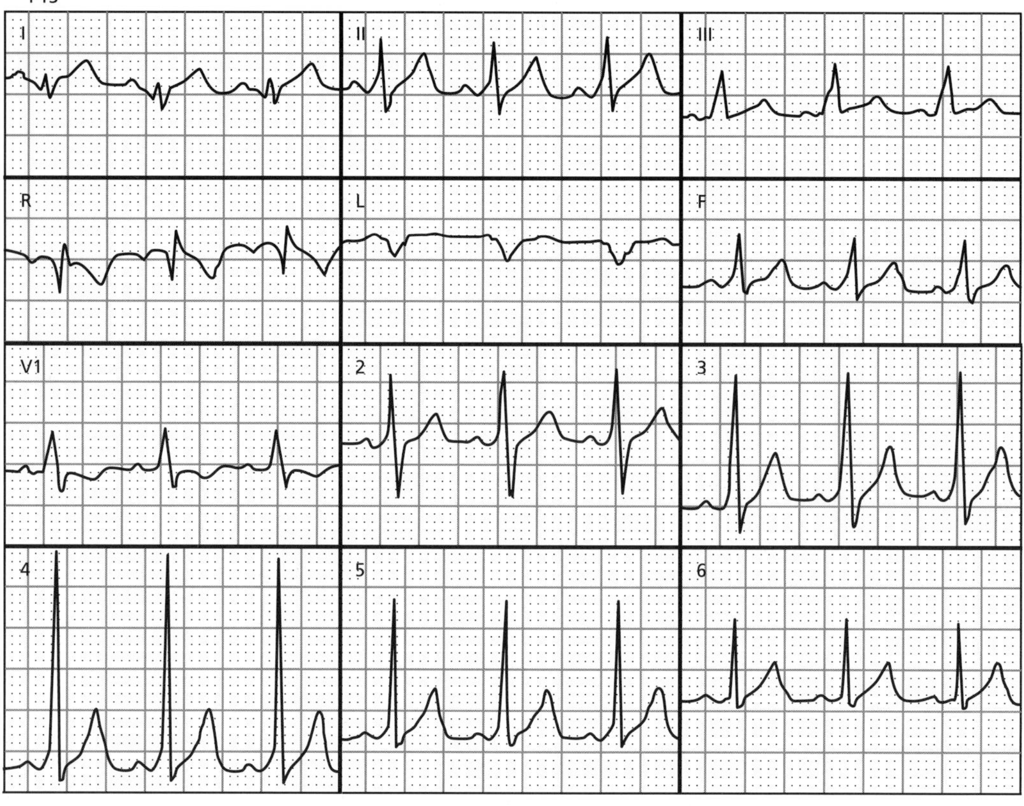

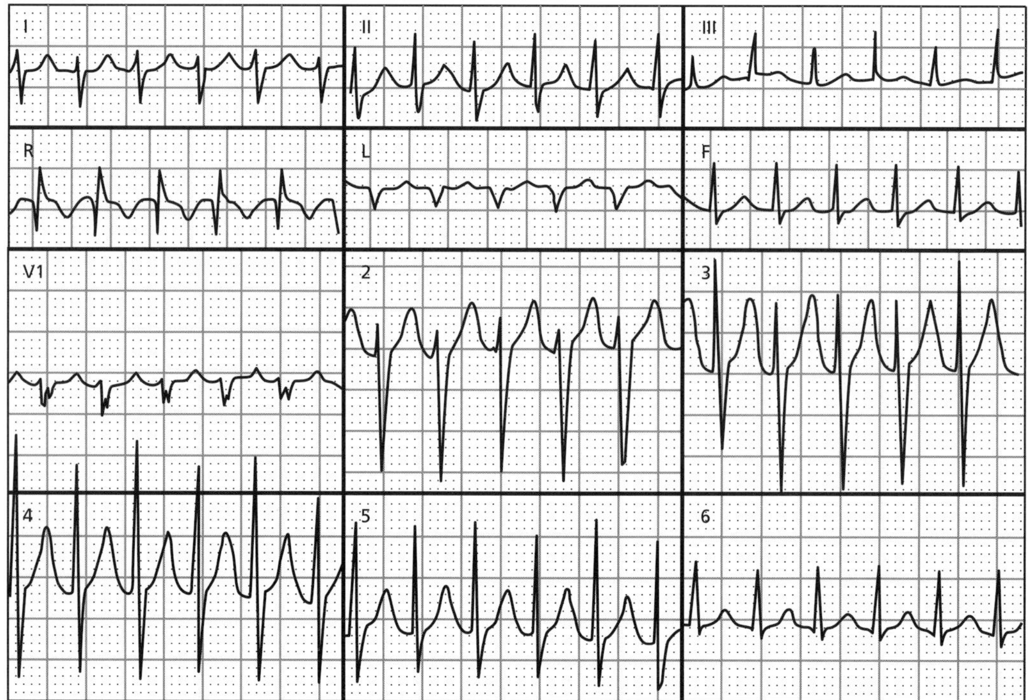

5.27.

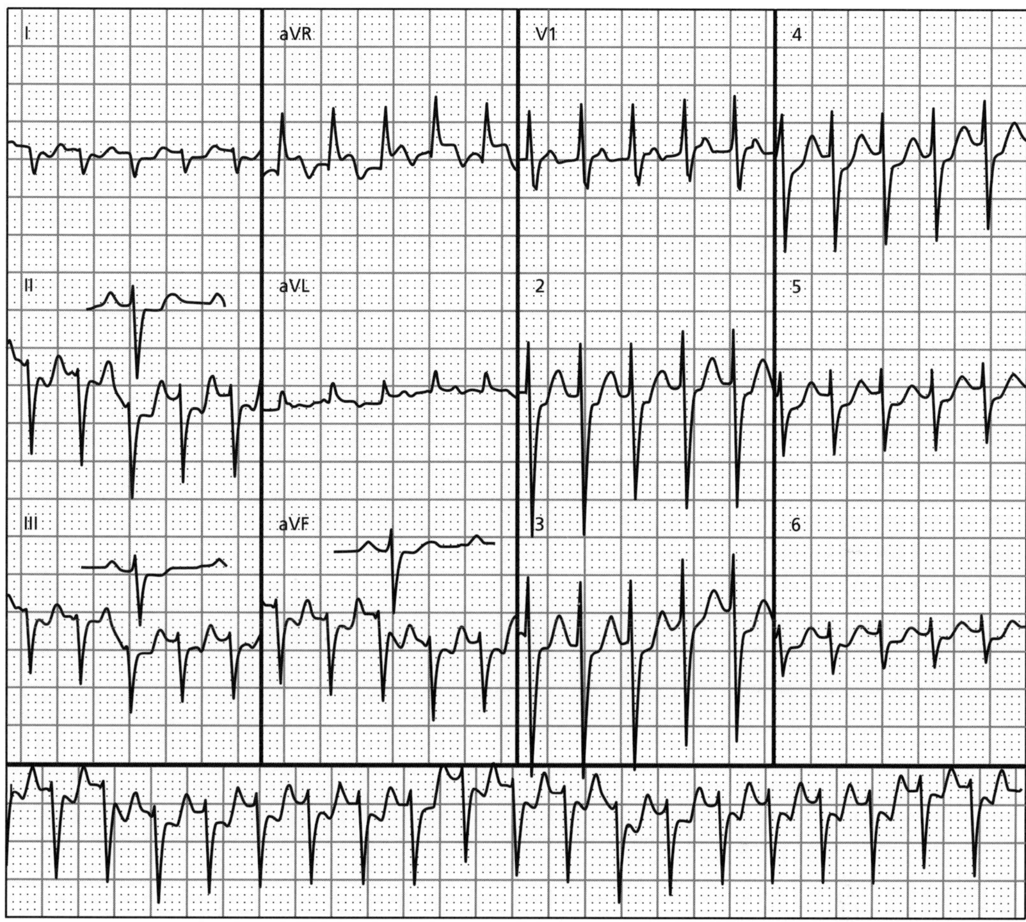

5.28.

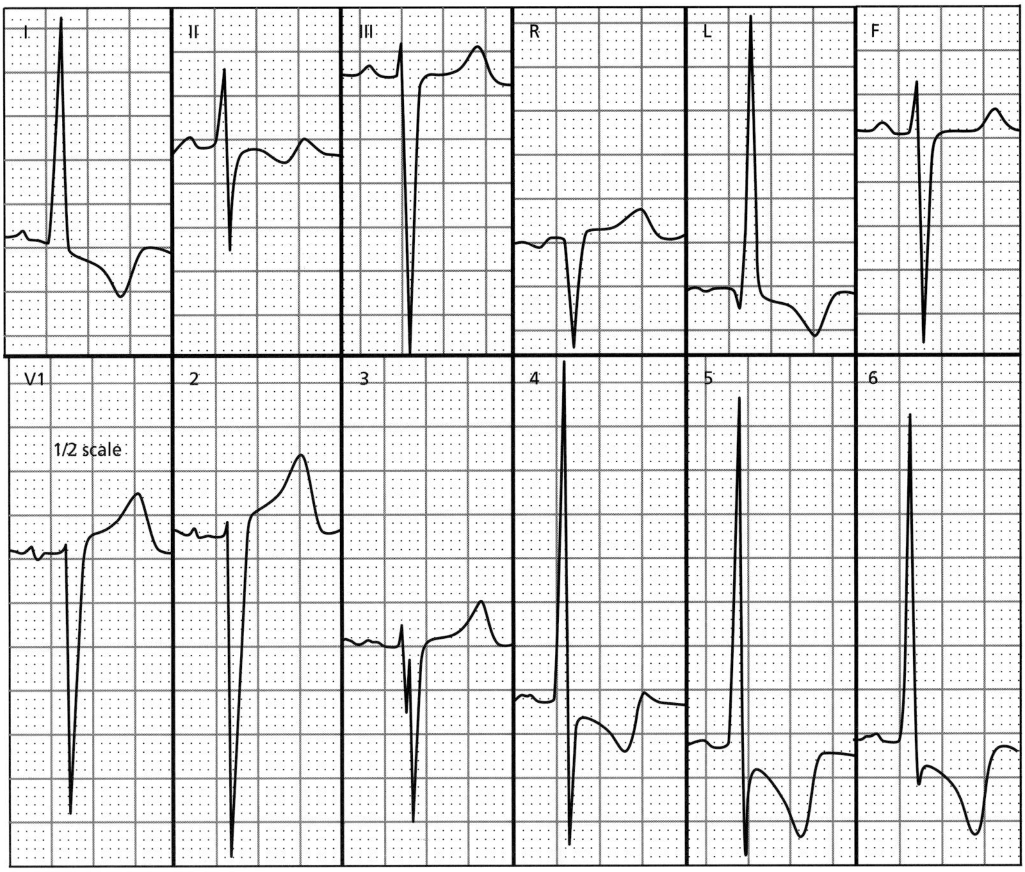

I II III R L F

V1 2 3 4 5 6

1/2 scale

5.29.

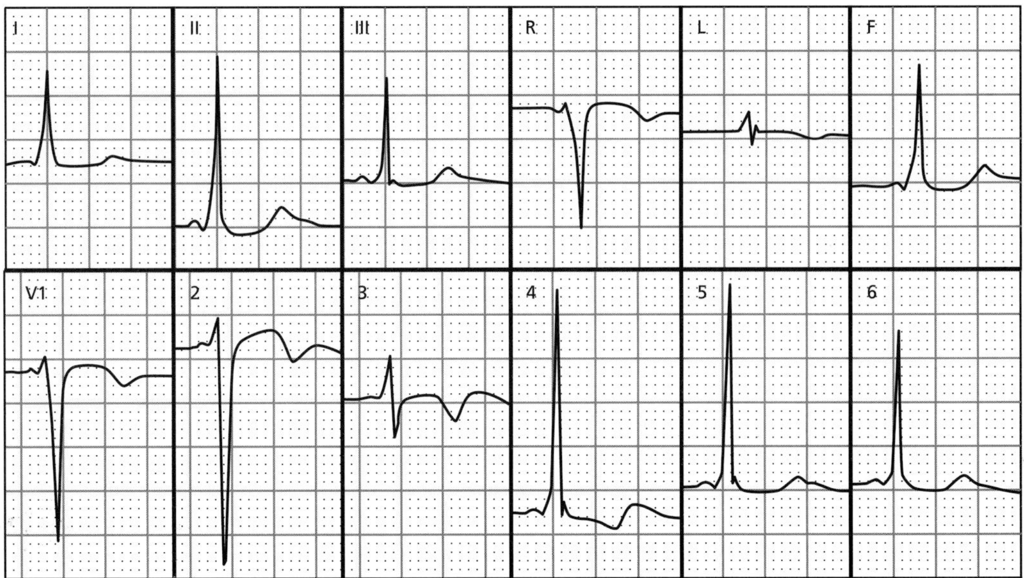

5.30.

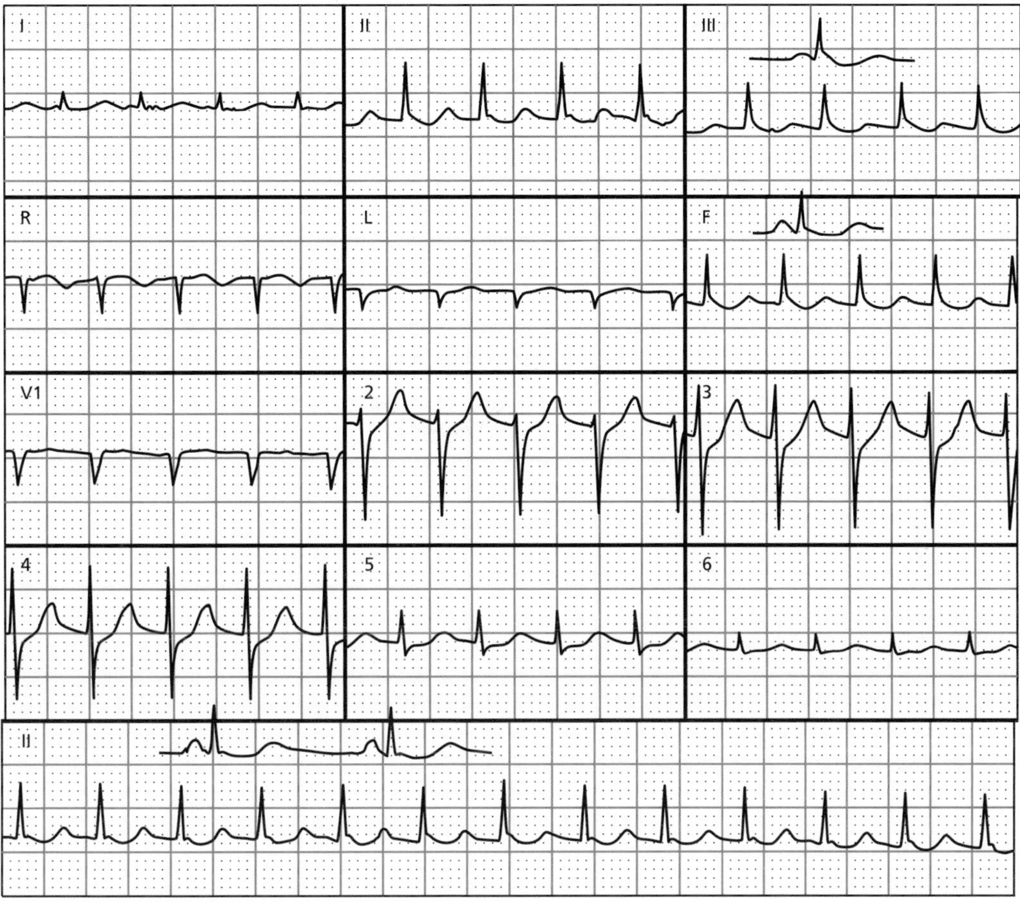

5.31.

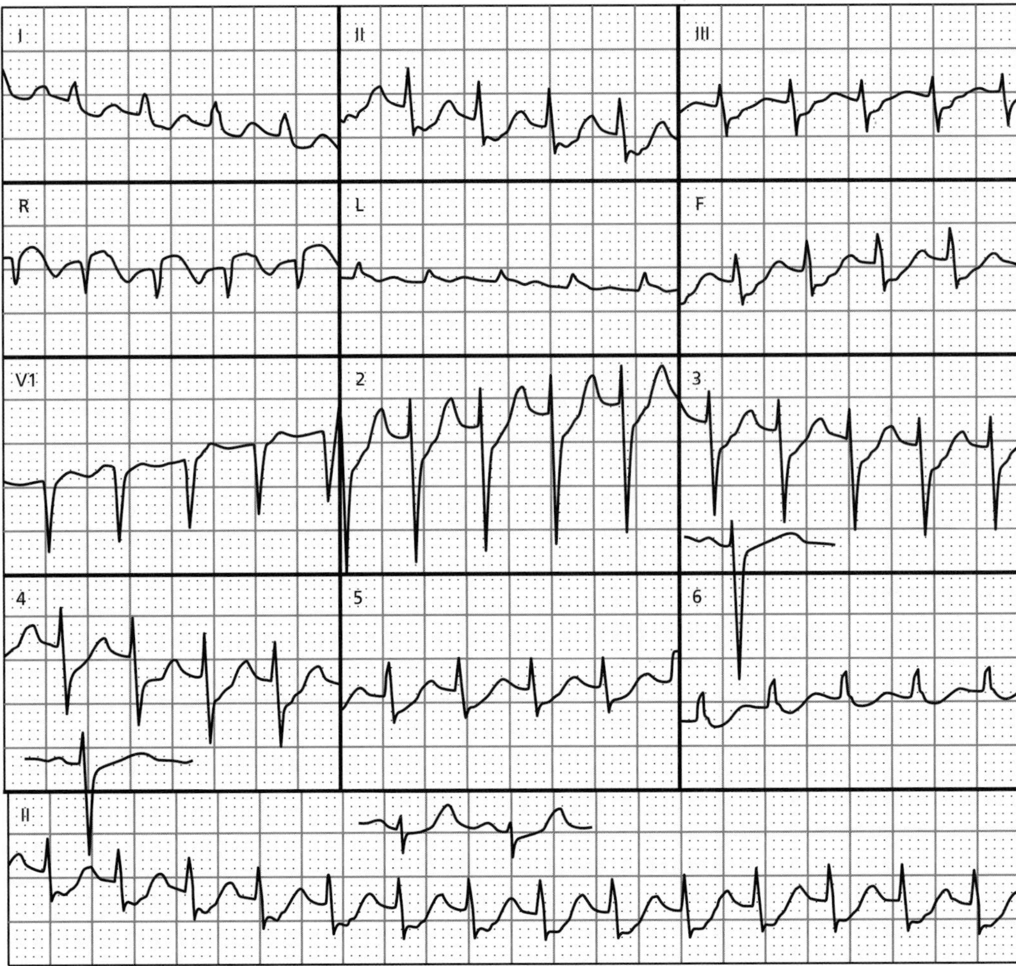

5.32.

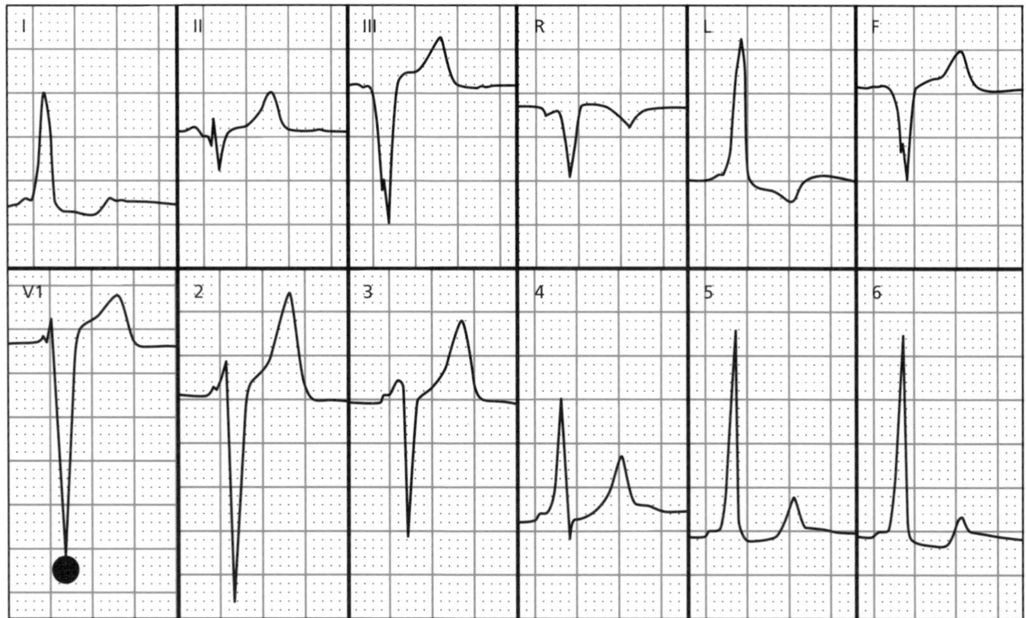

5.33.

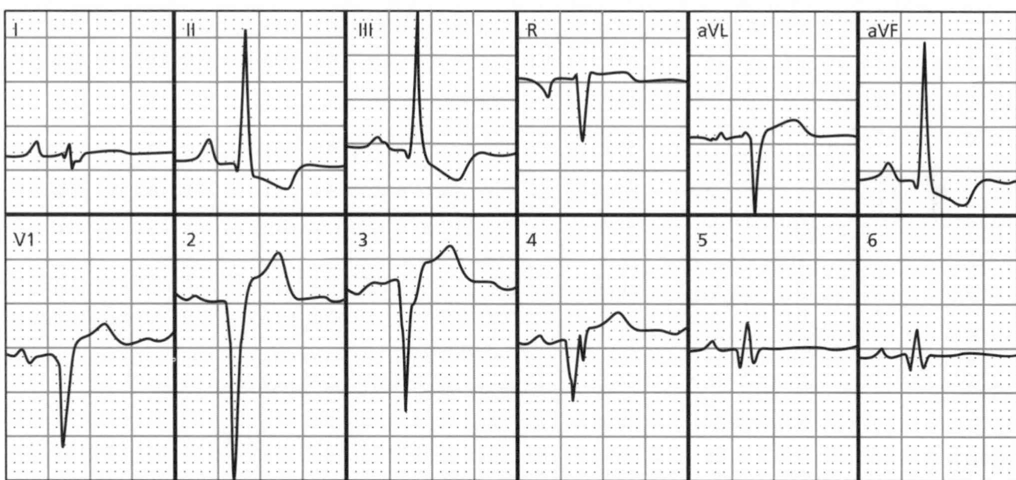

5.34.

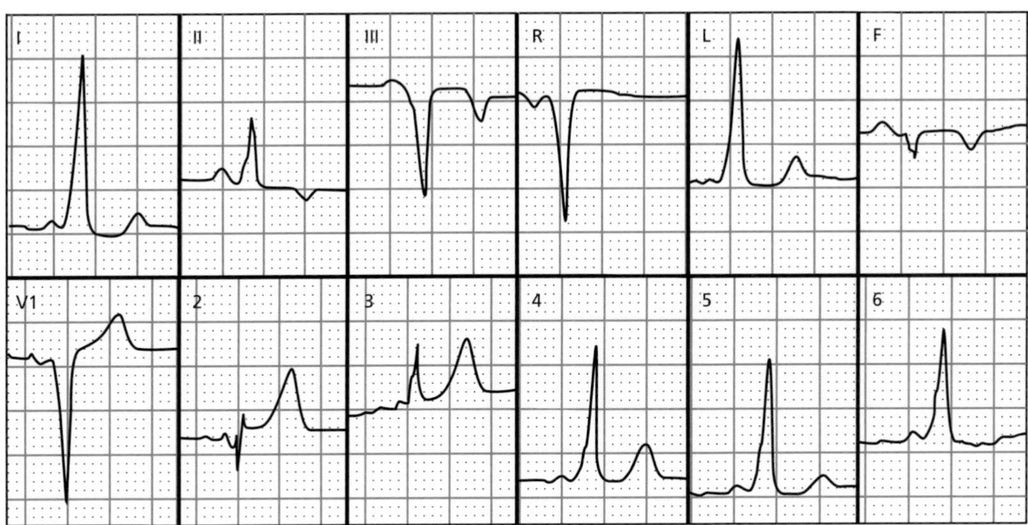

5.35.

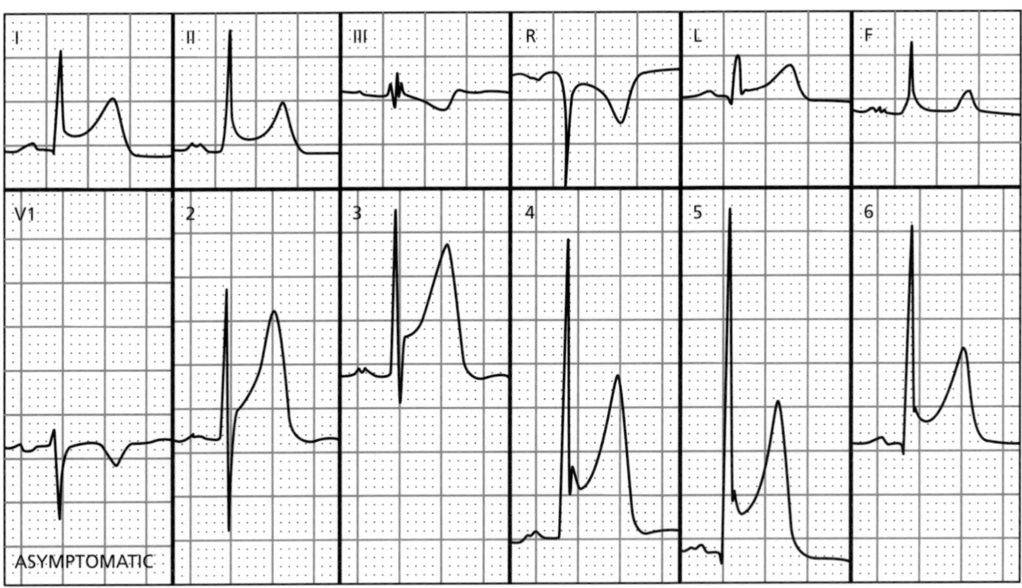

5.36.

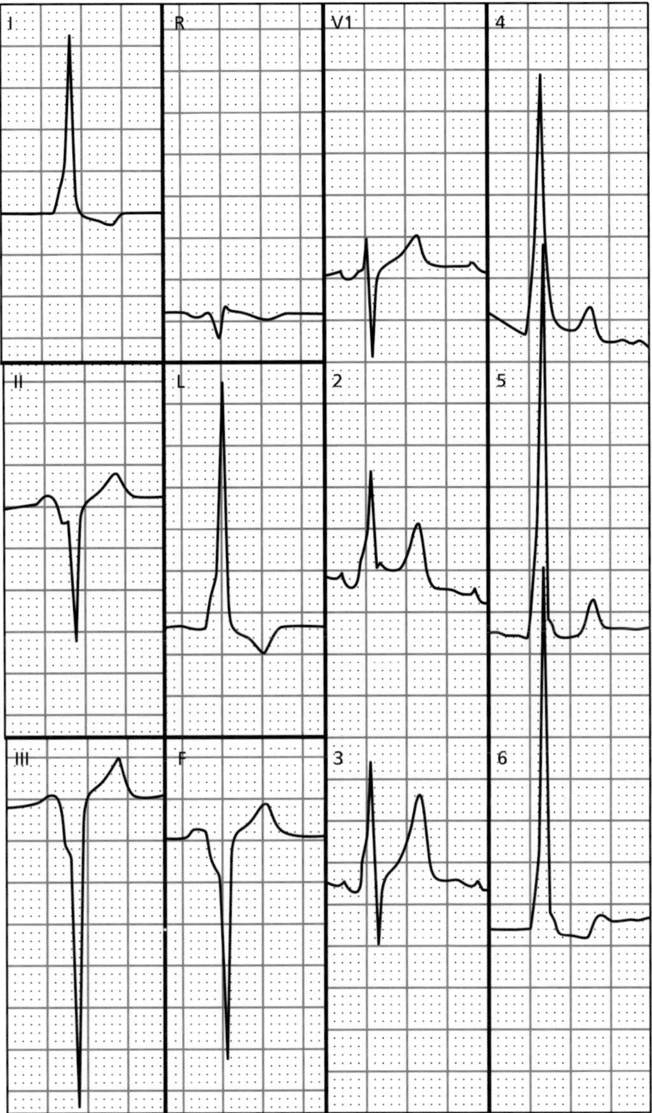

5.37.

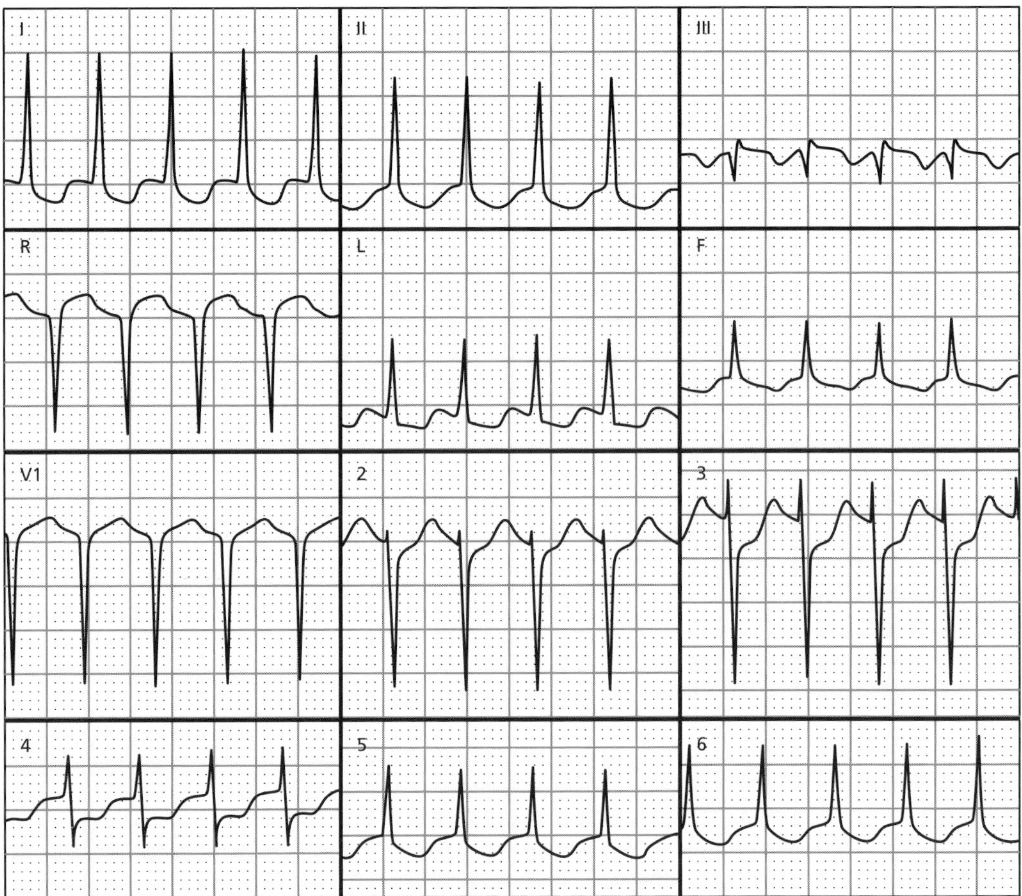

5.38.

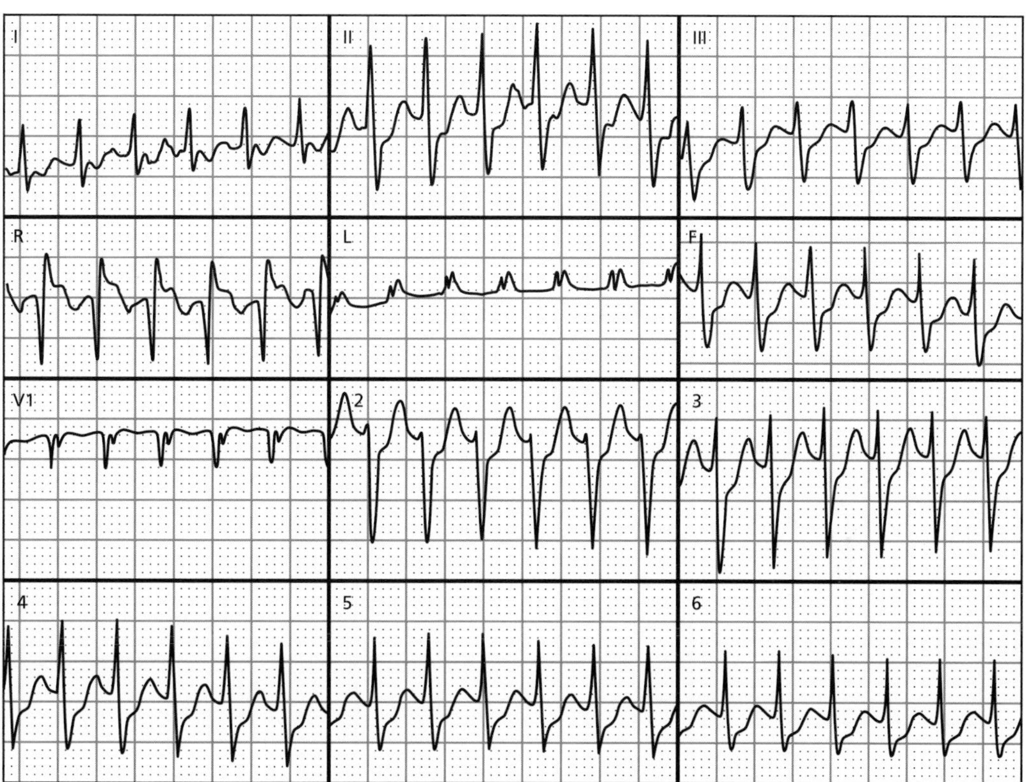

5.39.

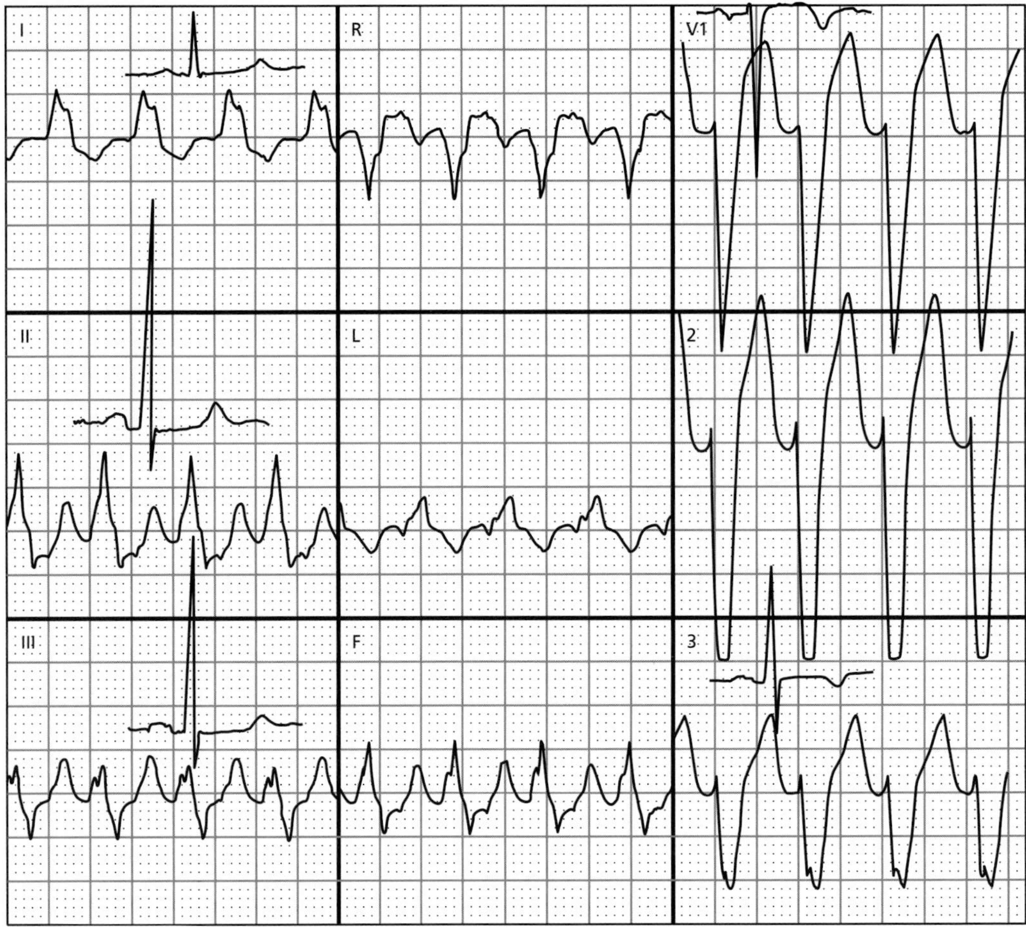

CHAPTER 13

Junctional arrhythmias

The atrioventricular junction is generally understood to include the atrial free wall and septum adjacent to the annuli of the atrioventricular valves ('atrial floor'), the atrioventricular node, and the penetrating portion of the bundle of His. This area contains both myocardium and conduction structures capable of generating extrasystolic beats and rhythms.

Impulses originating in the atrioventricular junction generally depolarize the atria in an inferior to superior or *retrograde* direction, resulting in P waves that are inverted in the inferior leads. Although P wave polarity is not a particularly accurate indicator of origin, inverted P waves are typically described as 'junctional.' Junctional P waves may precede, coincide with, or follow the QRS complex, and because these impulses usually conduct normally to the ventricular myocardium, the QRS complexes are typically narrow. *No wide-QRS tachycardia should be labeled 'junctional' without clear evidence of aberrant ventricular conduction or pre-existing bundle branch block.*

Premature junctional complexes and junctional rhythm

Examples of *premature junctional complexes* (PJCs) and *junctional rhythm* (JR) are shown in Figure 13.1. It should be noted that in most of the examples P waves are absent. Junctional tachycardia (>100 beats/minute) is the exception in adults (Figure 13.2); the usual junctional rate is in the 40 beats-per-minute range.

The sinus node maintains control of the cardiac rhythm because it has the fastest inherent rate, atrial pacemakers have a slower inherent rate, junctional pacemakers are slower yet, and the ventricular pacemakers are slowest of all. Therefore as pacing sites shift distally away from the sinoatrial node, the rate of impulse formation typically slows. Occasionally, however, subsidiary pacemakers defeat expectations and form impulses at a rate equal to or greater than the sinus rate. In the case of junctional sites, the result is called an *accelerated junctional rhythm* if the rate is below 100 per minute.

Accelerated junctional rhythm can coexist with sinus rhythm: the sinus node drives the atria and the junctional pacemaker drives the ventricles at a similar rate. The competing pacemakers are temporarily protected from each other by their nearly identical rates, resulting in *isorhythmic atrioventricular dissociation*. Such cases of dissociation are usually of short duration; as soon as the rate of one pacemaking focus exceeds the rate of the other, the faster will take control of both the upper and lower cardiac chambers.

Very rarely, sinus tachycardia coexists with junctional tachycardia, an example of *double tachycardia* (Figure 13.3).

Junctional escape rhythm

If sinus impulse generation fails or sinus impulses are blocked, the conduction system contains many other latent pacemaking sites capable of 'rescue' beating. The most proximal of these pacemakers, located in the atria, have relatively fast rates of impulse formation, whereas more distal sites have slower rates. Interruption of sinus rhythm permits the slower subsidiary sites to gain control, a phenomenon known as *escape* (Figure 13.4).

Because they emerge in response to slowing or block of sinus impulses, *escape beats are always late in relationship to sinus beats* or, to put it in other terms, although escape beats are ectopic, *they are never premature*. The interval from the last conducted beat to the escape beat is called the *escape interval*. In many cases the escape interval will be

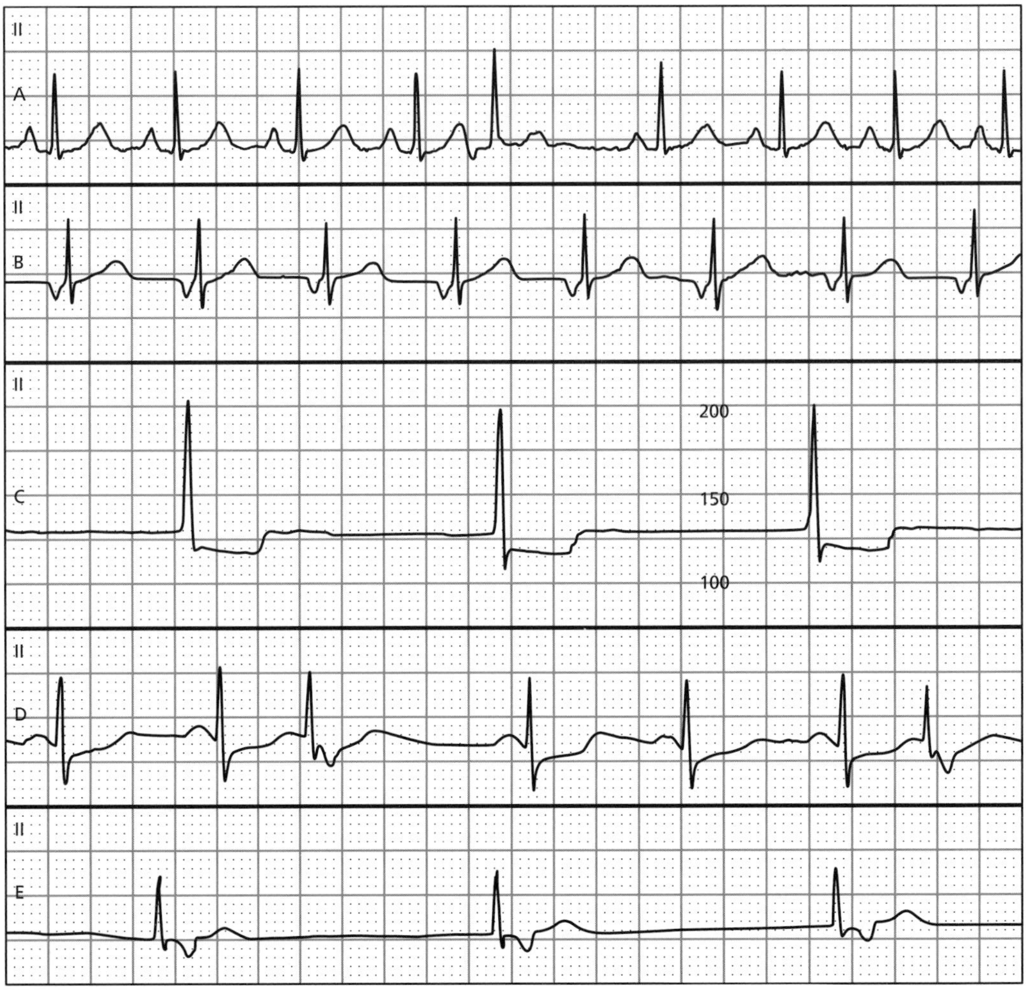

Figure 13.1 Premature junctional extrasystoles (A, D), accelerated junctional rhythm (B), a more typical junctional rhythm (C) in which P waves are missing, and rhythm likely originating in the bundle of His (E).

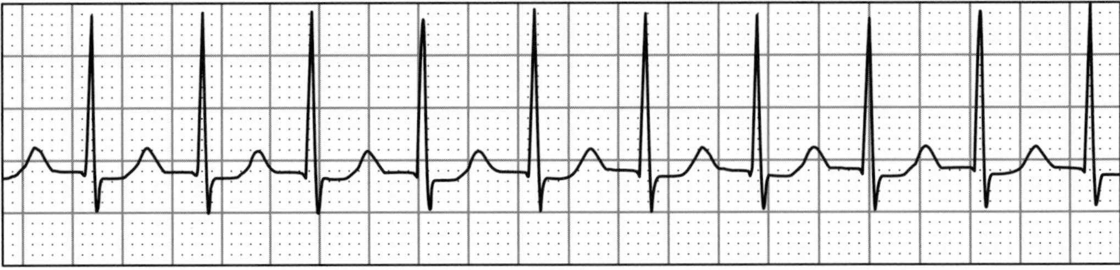

Figure 13.2 Junctional tachycardia.

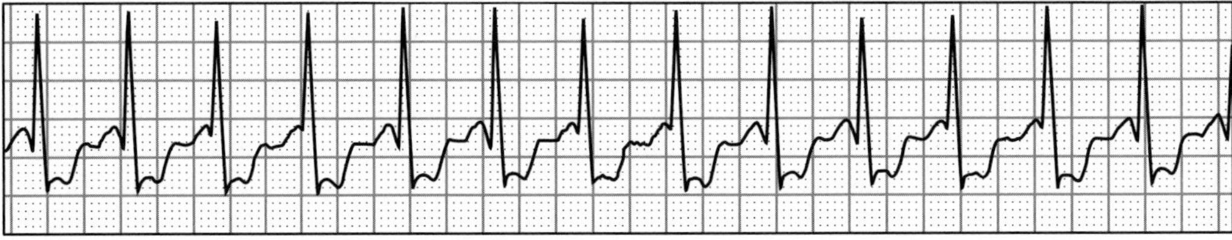

Figure 13.3 Double tachycardia: sinus tachycardia dissociated from junctional tachycardia.

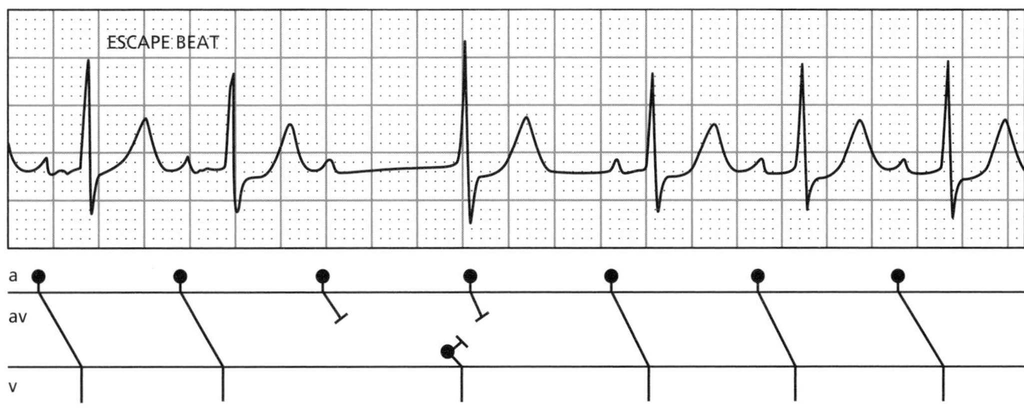

Figure 13.4 A junctional escape beat emerges in the setting of second-degree AV block.

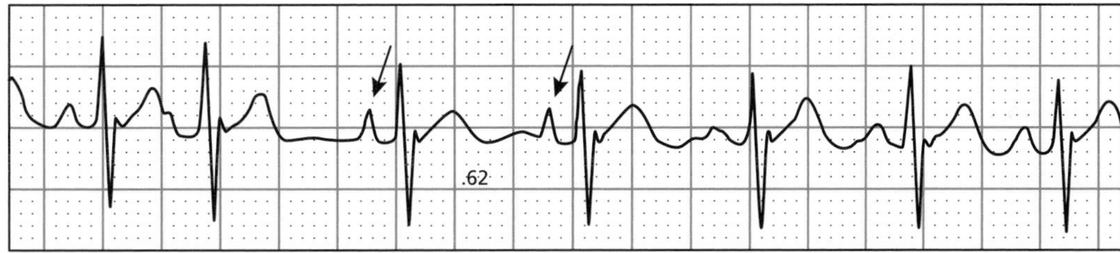

Figure 13.5 Two atrial escape beats (*arrows*) emerge during the pause caused by a premature atrial complex (PAC). The interval from the PAC to the first atrial escape beat is longer than the sinus cycle length, an example of hysteresis.

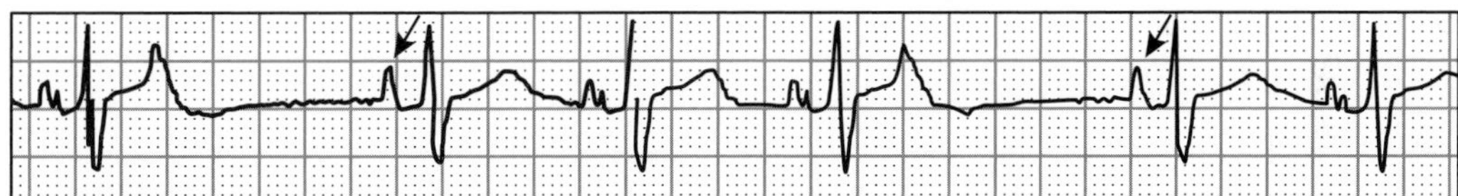

Figure 13.6 Atrial escape beats (*arrows*) following nonconducted atrial extrasystoles.

longer than the basic sinus rate, a phenomenon known as *hysteresis* (from the Greek word meaning 'late'; Figures 13.5 and 13.6).

Escape beats may arise from the atria, the junction, or the ventricles, and may be single or sequential. Sequential escape beats form an *escape rhythm*.

Escape-capture bigeminy

There are a number of circumstances in which conducted sinus beats ('capture' beats) alternate with (usually) junctional escape beats, forming a class of rhythms collectively called *escape-capture bigeminy* (Figures 13.7 to 13.9). The term 'capture' implies (1) capture of the atria or ventricles by a *sinus* impulse, or (2) capture of the atria or ventricles by an *electronic* pacemaker.

Concealed junctional extrasystoles

A junctional extrasystole that fails to conduct to either the atria or the ventricles depolarizes a segment of the conduction path but produces no deflection to signal its presence. The extrasystolic impulse will, however, produce conduction delay or block of the subsequent sinus impulse, producing a picture superficially consistent with atrioventricular block. *Concealed junctional extrasystoles* should be suspected if any one of the following is observed: (1) unexpected prolongation or

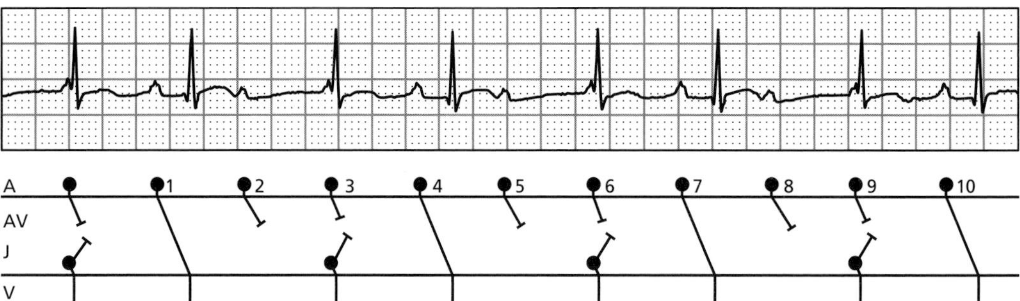

Figure 13.7 Escape-capture bigeminy in the setting of second-degree, type I AV block. The impulse from the junctional escape focus enters the AV node simultaneously with every third sinus impulse (3,6,9), preventing its conduction.

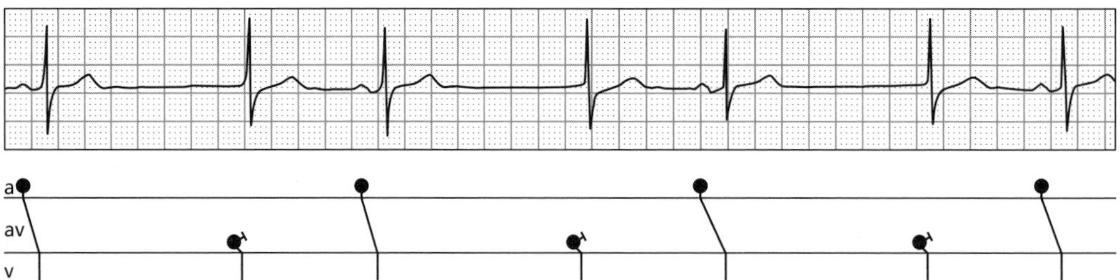

Figure 13.8 Escape-capture bigeminy due to extreme sinus bradycardia.

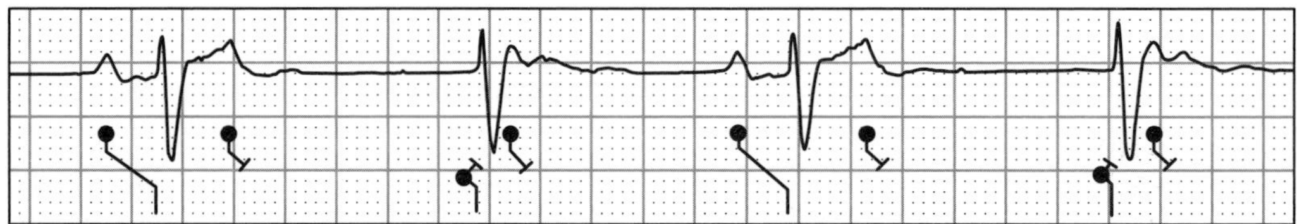

Figure 13.9 Escape-capture bigeminy due to nonconducted PACs. Each escape beat interferes with conduction of the following sinus beat.

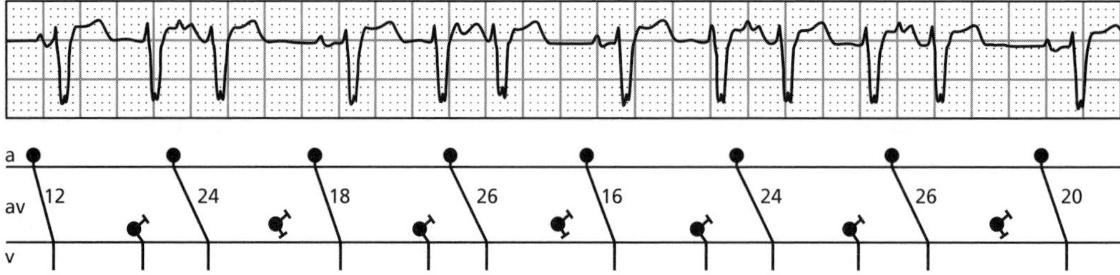

Figure 13.10 Concealed extrasystoles.

variability of PR intervals, (2) apparent type I and type II second-degree atrioventricular block noted on the same tracing, (3) apparent type II second-degree AV block with QRS complexes of normal duration, (4) manifest junctional extrasystoles elsewhere in the tracing, and/or (5) reciprocal beats.

Application of these diagnostic criteria is illustrated in Figure 13.10, in which four *manifest* junctional extrasystoles are noted (the second, fifth, eighth and tenth QRS complexes). Unexplained variability of the PR intervals signals the presence of three additional *concealed* extrasystoles (laddergram).

14

CHAPTER 14
Ventricular arrhythmias

Ventricular arrhythmias arise from sites distal to the bundle of His. Three basic mechanisms are thought to account for ventricular rhythms: (1) enhanced automaticity, (2) re-entry, and (3) triggered activity. In the case of *enhanced automaticity*, single or multiple excitable foci spontaneously form and discharge impulses. During *re-entry*, the impulse enters a circuit fulfilling the criteria for re-entry. The re-entry circuit may consist of *anatomically* separate pathways with different conduction properties, or disparate conduction properties in contiguous strands of myocardial fibers (*anisotropy*) may provide a *functional* basis for re-entry. If the circuit is very small, it is described as *micro re-entry*; if it consists of larger structures such as the fascicles of the bundle branches, it is referred to as *macro re-entry*. *Early after-depolarization*, a spontaneous depolarization that occurs during phase II of the action potential, is now widely believed to be a substrate of polymorphic ventricular tachycardia.

Premature ventricular complexes

Premature ventricular complexes (PVCs) may occur singly or in groups, and typically result in QRS complexes that are (1) early in relation to sinus beats, (2) abnormally wide (≥ 120 msec), and (3) of different morphology and axis. When every other beat is a ventricular extrasystole, *ventricular bigeminy* (Figure 14.1) is diagnosed; when every third beat is a ventricular extrasystole the rhythm is known as *ventricular trigeminy*.

Ventricular extrasystoles that fall between two conducted sinus beats are called *interpolated* PVCs and those that exhibit two or more morphologies are known as *multiform* PVCs (Figure 14.2) and are generally assumed to arise from different sites in the ventricle. Ventricular extrasystoles falling in pairs are called *couplets*, and those falling in runs of several beats, *salvos* (Figure 14.3). More than three ventricular beats in a row (assuming

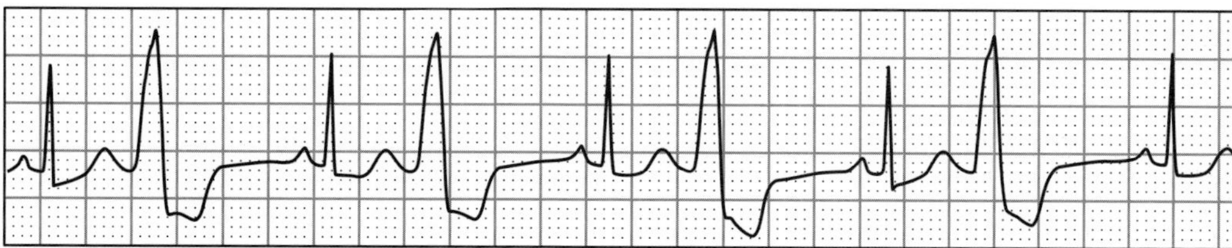

Figure 14.1 Ventricular bigeminy.

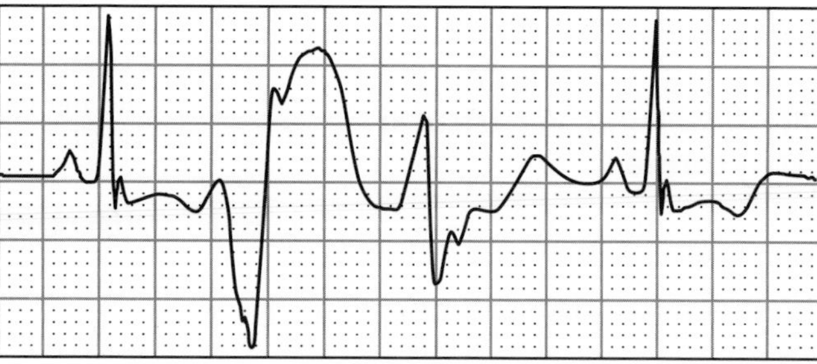

Figure 14.2 Multiform ventricular complexes.

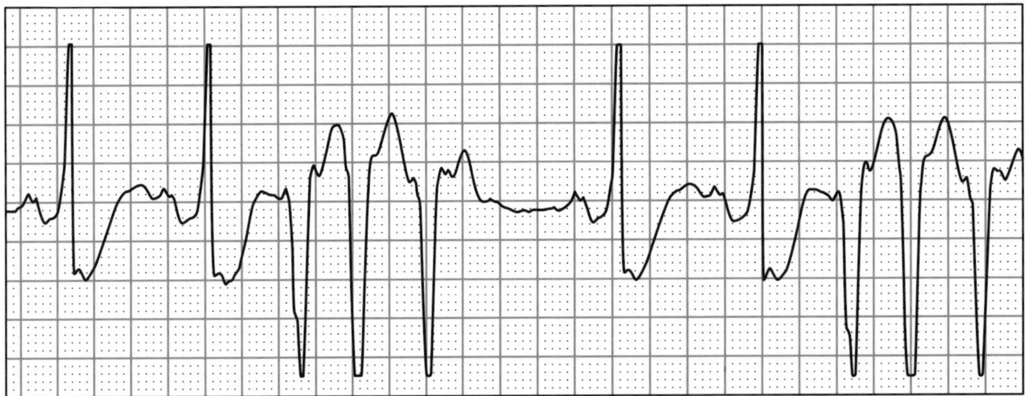

Figure 14.3 Salvos of ventricular beats.

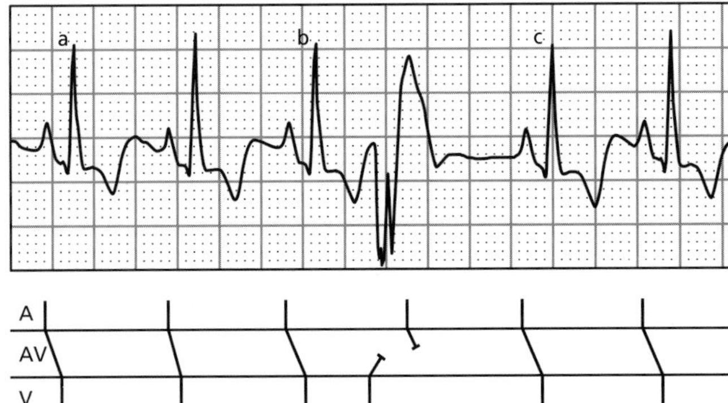

Figure 14.4 The interval containing the ventricular ectopic beat equals two sinus cycles: ab = bc.

a rate greater than 100 per minute) is *ventricular tachycardia.*

Ventricular extrasystoles usually prevent conduction of the following sinus impulse owing to concealed penetration into the distal AV nodal tissue (Figure 14.4). Therefore the interval containing the PVC is equal in length to two sinus cycles, the so-called 'compensatory pause.'

Any sudden change in cycle length (R–R interval) tends to precipitate ventricular ectopy, and ectopic ventricular beats tend to be self-perpetuating, a phenomenon so frequently noted that it has been named *the rule of bigeminy.*

Monomorphic ventricular tachycardia

Wide-QRS tachycardias are divided into four basic groups: (1) ventricular tachycardia, (2) supraventricular tachycardia with pre-existing bundle branch block, (3) supraventricular tachycardia with acceleration-dependent aberrant conduction, and (4) pre-excitation syndromes with antegrade conduction over an accessory pathway.

Ventricular tachycardia (VT) is defined as three or more ventricular beats in succession at a rate greater than 100 per minute. Short bursts of ventricular tachycardia are sometimes called *salvos.* Ventricular tachycardia is classified as *sustained* or *nonsustained*, and as *monomorphic* or *polymorphic.* Nonsustained VT is defined as VT lasting less than 30 seconds without producing hemodynamic collapse if induced in the EP lab, or lasting less than 15 seconds if it occurs spontaneously. *Monomorphic* VT refers to tachycardia that exhibits only one QRS morphology (Figure 14.5). Polymorphic VT exhibits multiple morphologies.

Differential diagnosis of wide-QRS tachycardia

Although the differential diagnosis of wide-QRS tachycardia is important given the therapeutic and

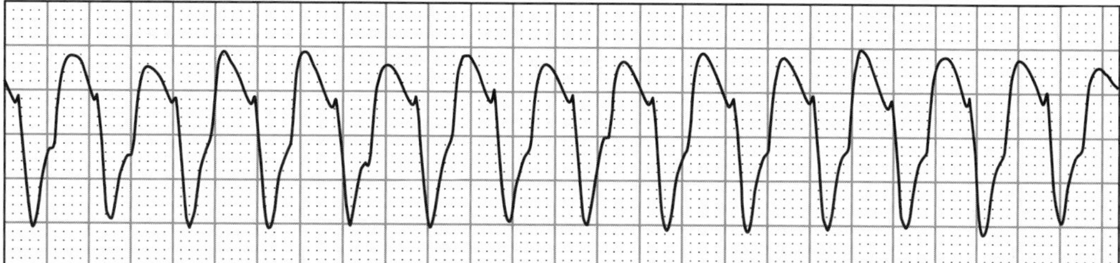

Figure 14.5 Monomorphic ventricular tachycardia.

prognostic implications, the issue of immediate clinical importance is the patient's hemodynamic status. Any tachycardia that provokes hemodynamic collapse should be cardioverted immediately. The common notion that ventricular tachycardia can be differentiated from other wide-QRS tachycardias merely on the basis of the patient's hemodynamic response is one of the most pernicious of electrocardiography's old wives' tales. Some patients can tolerate ventricular tachycardia, particularly if the rate is less than 170, whereas supraventricular tachycardia is capable of producing sudden collapse in some otherwise healthy individuals.

The width of the QRS complex is a frequently cited criterion for the diagnosis of ventricular tachycardia. While it is true that QRS duration of more than 140 msec (0.14 sec) is highly suggestive of VT and that a QRS width of less than 120 msec (0.12 sec) favors a supraventricular origin, the findings are not specific. As a general rule, the cell-to-cell impulse transmission that occurs during ventricular tachycardia is slower than transmission over the His–Purkinje network. Therefore the QRS complexes of VT are typically wide and slurred, whereas QRS complexes that result from transmission through the normal conduction system are typically narrower and more crisply inscribed.

The width of the QRS complex is directly related to where ventricular depolarization begins: if near the septum or fascicle, the QRS complex will be narrower because right and left ventricular depolarization will be more nearly simultaneous, i.e. more nearly like normal. However, if depolarization begins from the ventricular free wall, the QRS complex will be wider because depolarization is occurring sequentially as the impulse travels through the more slowly conducting ventricular myocardium. Following this logic, *if QRS complexes are wider during sinus rhythm than during tachycardia, the tachycardia is likely to originate from the ventricular septum.*

Accessory pathways that insert into the septum will follow this same basic principle: a septal point of insertion will cause a more normal sequence of ventricular depolarization, resulting in a narrower QRS complex. Conversely, if the point of insertion is in the lateral free wall, an eccentric sequence of depolarization occurs, resulting in a wider QRS complex during pre-excited tachycardia.

Since QRS complexes with bundle branch block morphology are abnormally wide to begin with, a wide-complex tachycardia with right bundle branch block morphology is more likely to be ventricular if the QRS complexes are equal to or greater than 140 msec in duration, and with left bundle branch block morphology, more likely to be ventricular if the QRS complexes are equal to or greater than 160 msec.

Axis deviation favors a diagnosis of VT, particularly if the axis deviates more than 40 degrees from its value during sinus rhythm. However, the literature on ventricular tachycardia uses a somewhat different terminology to describe axis deviation, so a brief description of that terminology is in order.

If ventricular tachycardia originates at or near the base of the ventricle, the mean QRS axis will be directed inferiorly, resulting in positive QRS complexes in inferior leads (Figure 14.6). Ventricular tachycardia with positive complexes in the inferior leads (II, III and aVF) is therefore said to exhibit *inferior axis.*

If ventricular tachycardia originates at or near the apex of the ventricle, the mean QRS axis will be directed superiorly, resulting in negative QRS complexes in inferior leads (Figure 14.7).

If ventricular tachycardia originates in the left posterior ventricular wall, the wave of depolarization will be directed anteriorly in the horizontal

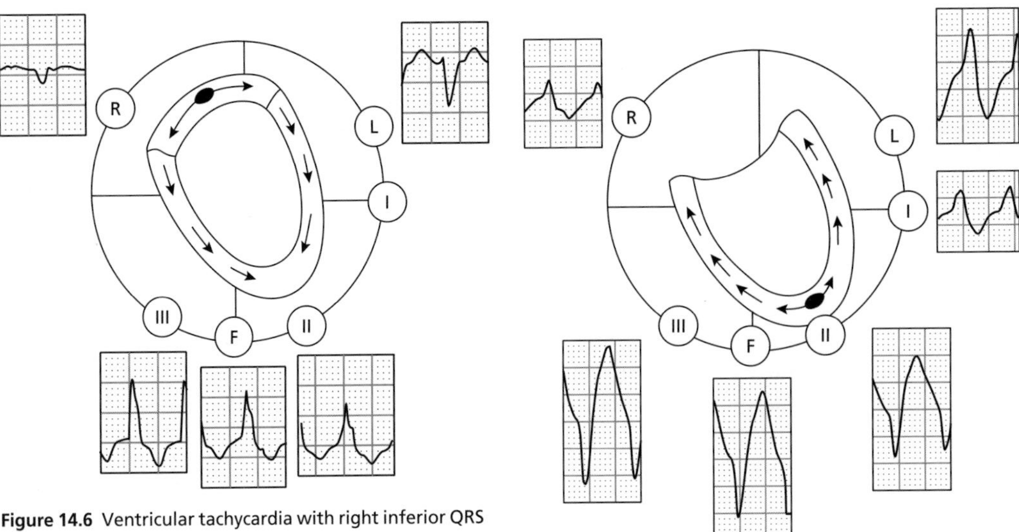

Figure 14.6 Ventricular tachycardia with right inferior QRS axis: the origin is at the base of the ventricular cone.

Figure 14.7 Ventricular tachycardia with left superior axis: the origin is at the apex of the ventricular cone.

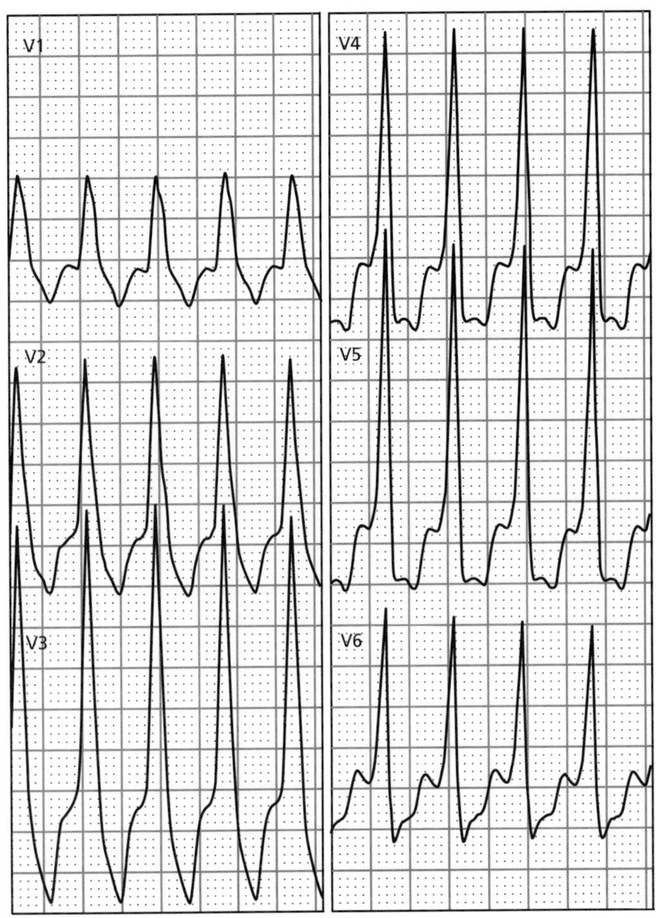

Figure 14.8 Positive precordial concordance (V1–V6): the tachycardia originates in the posterior ventricular wall.

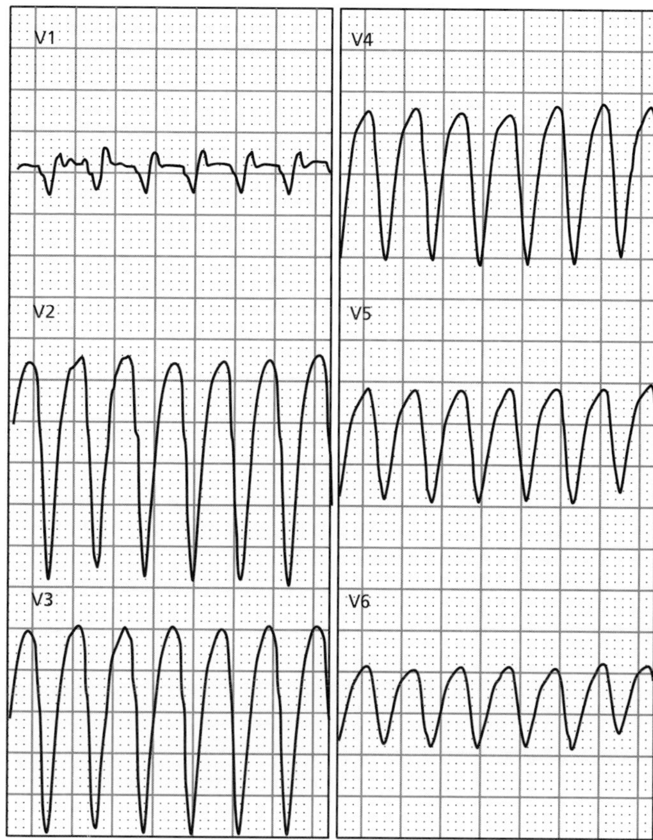

Figure 14.9 Negative precordial concordance (V1–V6).

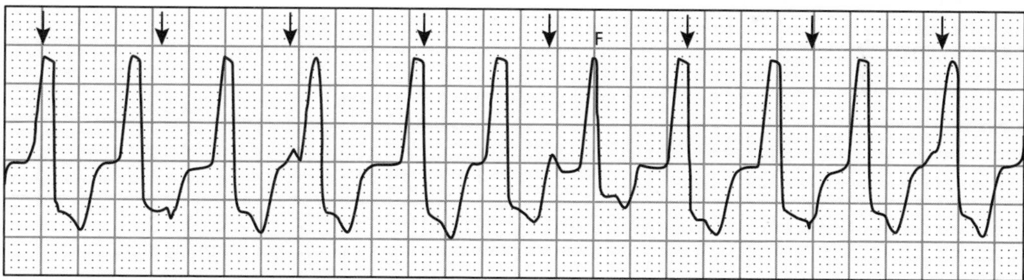

Figure 14.10 Dissociated sinus P waves (*arrows*) with partial capture producing a fusion beat (F).

plane, resulting in *positive concordance* and uniformly positive QRS complexes in the precordial leads (Figure 14.8). Positive concordance is strongly suggestive of VT, but may also occur during antidromic tachycardia with antegrade conduction over a left posterior accessory pathway.

Negative concordance – uniformly negative QRS complexes in the precordial leads (Figure 14.9) – is highly suggestive of VT originating in the apical area of the left ventricle. In this case, negative QRS complexes are inscribed because depolarization is moving away from the positive pole of the precordial leads.

All investigators agree that the presence of *atrioventricular dissociation* argues strongly for VT (Figure 14.10.), but strictly speaking, atrioventricular dissociation merely excludes an atrial origin. Unfortunately for diagnostic accuracy, ventricular tachycardia with atrial entrainment is common, and very fast VT can completely mask atrial activity,

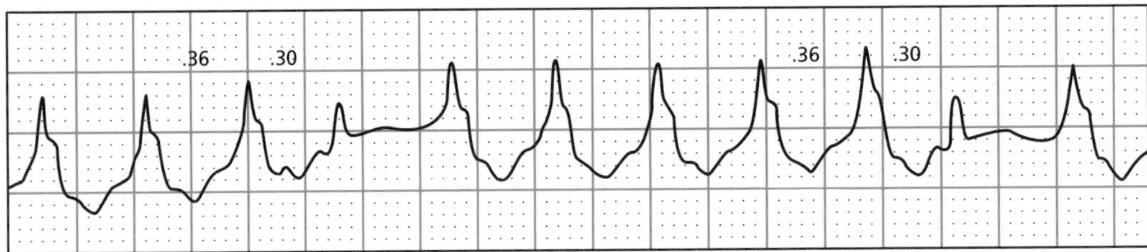

Figure 14.11 Intermittent ventricular capture by sinus beats shortens the R–R interval from 0.36 to 0.30 sec and normalizes the QRS complex.

making dissociation impossible to recognize. Atrioventricular dissociation may be present in 20% of proven ventricular tachycardias.

Ventricular fusion beats are highly suggestive of VT. Ventricular fusion occurs when an appropriately timed sinus impulse and a ventricular ectopic impulse share in ventricular activation, resulting in a hybrid QRS complex (*F* in Figure 14.10). However, fusion beats are not commonly seen during VT. If an extrasystole occurs from the contralateral ventricle during VT, it may also alter the morphology of the QRS and may be mistaken for a fusion beat.

Sinus capture beats during VT are shown in Figure 14.11. Intermittent capture of the ventricles by sinus impulses causes the QRS complex to normalize, and shortens the R–R interval of the tachycardia. Partial capture will result in a fusion beat. Because sinus rhythm must persist during VT for capture beating to occur and atrioventricular dissociation cannot be complete, capture beats are uncommon.

The *morphology of the QRS complex* during wide-QRS tachycardia is often invoked to distinguish between supraventricular and ventricular tachycardias.

Ventricular tachycardia has traditionally been divided into two broad categories based on the QRS morphology in lead V1. Predominantly positive complexes in V1 are regarded as exhibiting *right bundle branch block morphology* and are thought to represent tachycardia originating from the left ventricle, whereas predominantly negative complexes in V1 are considered to exhibit *left bundle branch block morphology* and are thought to represent tachycardia originating from the right ventricle. Subsequent investigation has lent qualified support to this thesis. Ventricular tachycardia with right bundle branch block morphology nearly always arises in the left ventricle; VT with left bundle branch block morphology indicates a right ventricular or septal origin. An algorithm for localizing a VT focus based on frontal plane axis and precordial progression is shown in Figure 14.12. Various types of right bundle branch block morphology and their correlations are shown in Figure 14.13. Monophasic or biphasic QRS complexes with right bundle branch block morphology in V1 are suggestive of VT.

Ventricular ectopy with left bundle branch block morphology is shown in Figure 14.14. Particular note is drawn to the *r wave* in lead V1, which is

MORPHOLOGY	*if* LBBB morphology, *then*: **septum**		*if* RBBB morphology, *then*: **free wall**	
AXIS	*if* superior axis, *then*: **inferior septum**	*if* inferior axis, *then*: **superior septum**	*if* superior axis, *then*: **inferior free wall**	*if* inferior axis, *then*: **superior free wall**
R WAVES	*if* progression, *then*: **infero-basal septum**	*if* none/late, *then*: **infero-apical septum**	*if* reverse/late, *then*: **infero-lateral free wall**	*if* abrupt loss, *then*: **antero-apical free wall**

Figure 14.12 Algorithm for locating ectopic ventricular foci.

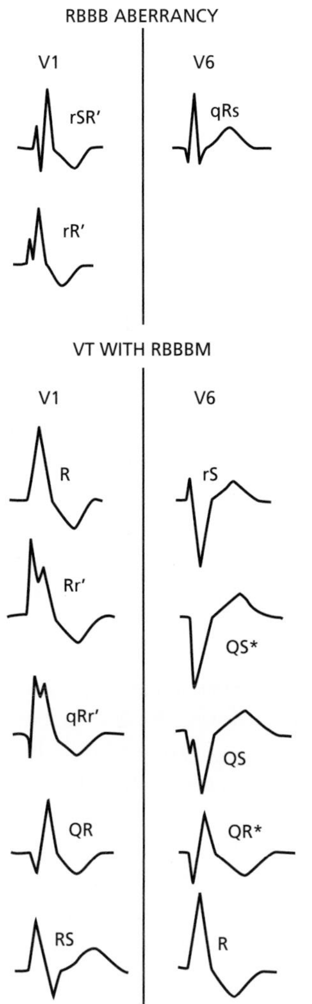

Figure 14.13 QRS morphologies in VT. Complexes marked * are typical of VT with left bundle branch block morphology in V6.

wider than expected in a true left bundle branch block pattern. Four morphologic criteria, the *Kindwall criteria,* are shown in Figure 14.14. These left bundle branch block morphology criteria, which have been demonstrated to have high predictive accuracy, are (1) an *initial R wave greater than 30 msec* (0.03 sec) in leads V1 or V2, (2) the presence of a *Q wave in lead V6*, (3) a duration *greater than 60 msec* (0.06 sec) *from the beginning of the QRS complex to the nadir of the S wave* in leads V1 or V2, and (4) *notching of the downstroke of the S wave* in leads V1 or V2.

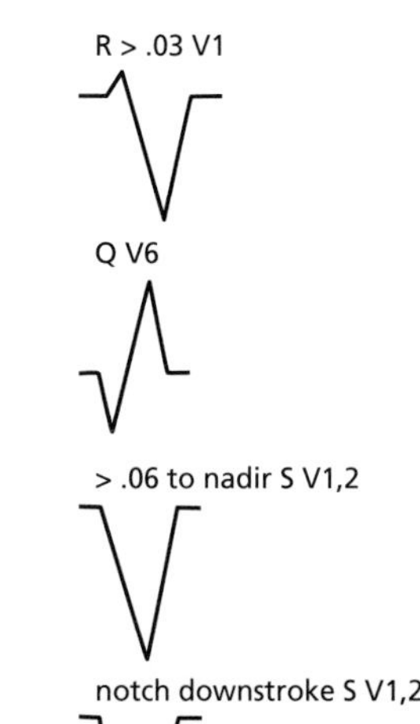

Figure 14.14 The Kindwall criteria illustrated.

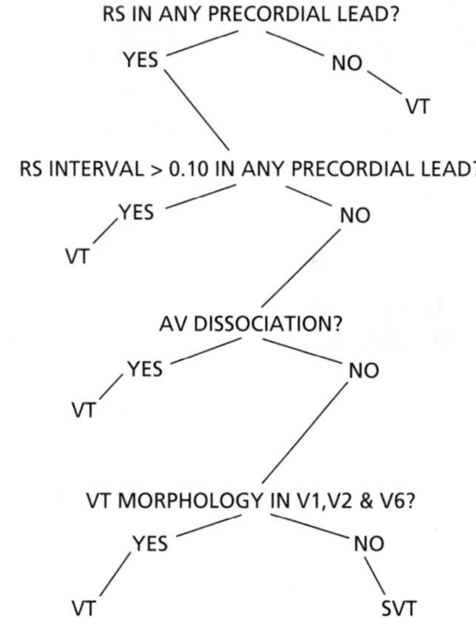

Figure 14.15 The Brugada algorithm.

The Brugada algorithm is a four-step approach to the diagnosis of VT based in part on the QRS morphology in the precordial leads (Figure 14.15). If there is *no RS complex* in any of the precordial leads, a diagnosis of VT is automatically made. If RS complexes are seen, an *RS duration greater than 100 msec* (0.10 sec) indicates that the rhythm is VT (Figure 14.16). If the RS interval is less than 100

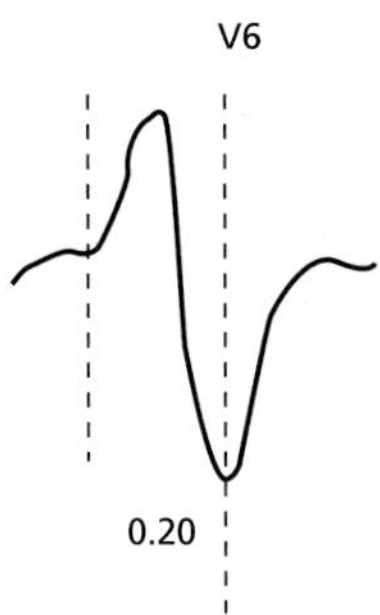

Figure 14.16 The RS duration is measured from the beginning of the QRS complex to the nadir of the S wave.

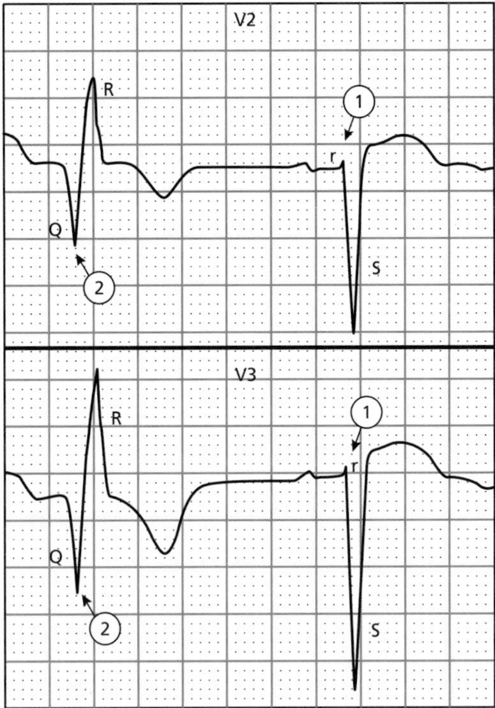

Figure 14.17 Ventricular premature beats unmasking a previous infarction.

msec, evidence of *atrioventricular dissociation* is sought. If AV dissociation exists, the rhythm is VT. If no atrioventricular dissociation is seen, the usual *criteria for morphology in V1 and V6* (discussed above) are applied.

The presence of Q waves in ventricular beats is shown in Figure 14.17. Asynchronous myocardial depolarization can unmask Q waves that do not appear in normally conducted beats. To be diagnostically significant, Q waves should be accompanied by a strong positive component (QR, 2 in Figure 14.17). The presence of Q waves during ventricular tachycardia points to re-entry in or around a scar from previous infarction as the probable mechanism of the arrhythmia. A wide complex tachycardia in the presence of a previous history of myocardial infarction is likely to be VT.

Arrhythmogenic right ventricular dysplasia

Arrhythmogenic right ventricular dysplasia (ARVD) is a cardiomyopathy characterized by extensive replacement of the right ventricular free wall myocardium by adipose tissue, sometimes with complete absence of the muscular layer (Uhl's anomaly). The syndrome is almost three times more common in men. The typical presentation consists of a young to middle-aged male with palpitations, syncope, heart failure, and ventricular tachycardia with left bundle branch block morphology. It may result in sudden cardiac death. The QRS axis during tachycardia usually ranges from +60 to +140 degrees, but may vary from one episode of tachycardia to the next. The baseline electrocardiogram often exhibits *QRS prolongation* (> 110 msec) *in the right precordial leads* (V1–V3) accompanied by *T wave inversion. Epsilon waves,* small postexcitation waves seen following the QRS complex in V1–V3, are visible in about 30% of subjects. On signal-averaged electrocardiograms, the right precordial QRS duration ranges from 180 to 290 msec, with postexcitation waves extending to 360 msec.

Right ventricular outflow tract tachycardia

Ventricular tachycardia originating from the *right ventricular outflow tract* (RVOT) is more common in females, usually nonsustained, and is rarely associated with sudden cardiac death. The tachycardia typically exhibits left bundle branch block morphology with inferior (normal to rightward) axis (Figure 14.18). It is often triggered by exercise. There is generally a good therapeutic response to calcium channel blockers or β-blockers. Ablation of the offending focus could be considered if medical management fails.

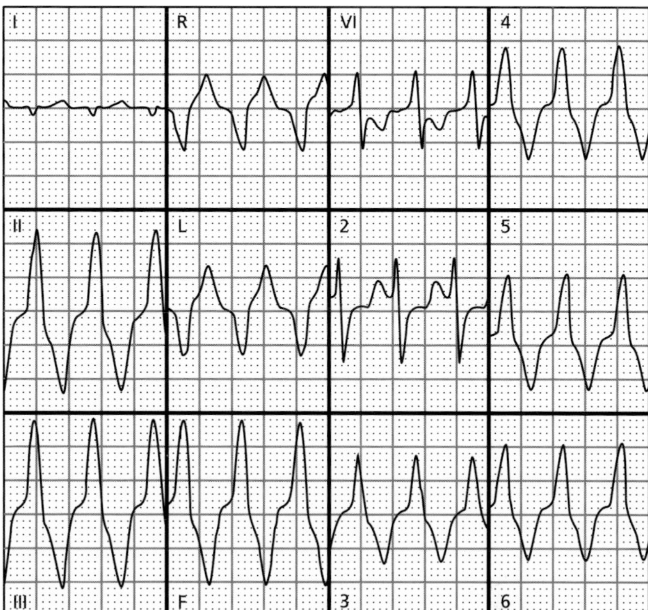

Figure 14.18 Right ventricular outflow tract tachycardia.

Bundle branch re-entry and fascicular ventricular tachycardia

The bundle branches can serve as the anatomical substrate for re-entry. In these cases, antegrade conduction usually occurs over the right bundle branch (Figure 14.19). Because depolarization begins in the right ventricle, the ECG shows left bundle branch block morphology. If the circuit is reversed, antegrade conduction will occur over the left bundle and the VT will exhibit right bundle branch block morphology. Ventricular tachycardias in patients without structural heart disease are commonly classified as *idiopathic ventricular tachycardia*.

The fascicles of the left bundle branch can also serve as the re-entry circuit for ventricular tachycardia. In the majority of cases (> 90%), antegrade conduction occurs over the left posterior fascicle (Figure 14.20).

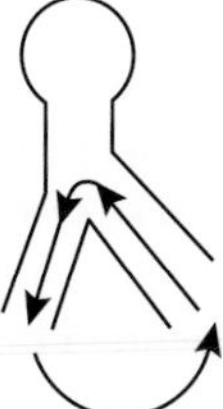

Figure 14.19 Bundle branch block re-entry with antegrade conduction through the right bundle branch.

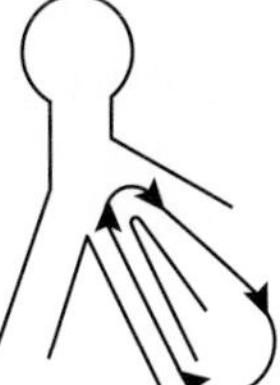

Figure 14.20 Fascicular re-entry with antegrade conduction through the left posterior fascicle.

Because ventricular depolarization begins in the left ventricle, the VT will exhibit right bundle branch block morphology, and because the left anterior fascicle is used for retrograde conduction, superior axis is recorded (Figure 14.21). If the circuit is reversed, VT with right bundle branch block and left posterior fascicular block morphology (inferior axis) will be observed. Unlike VT that originates from scar tissue, VT that utilizes the conduction structures as part of the re-entry circuit tends to produce narrower and more sharply inscribed QRS complexes (note lead aVL in Figure 14.21).

Fascicular tachycardia is more common in men. Since there is rarely evidence of structural heart disease, the baseline ECG tends to be normal. Patients typically present with complaints of palpitations, dizziness, and syncope induced by exercise or emotional distress.

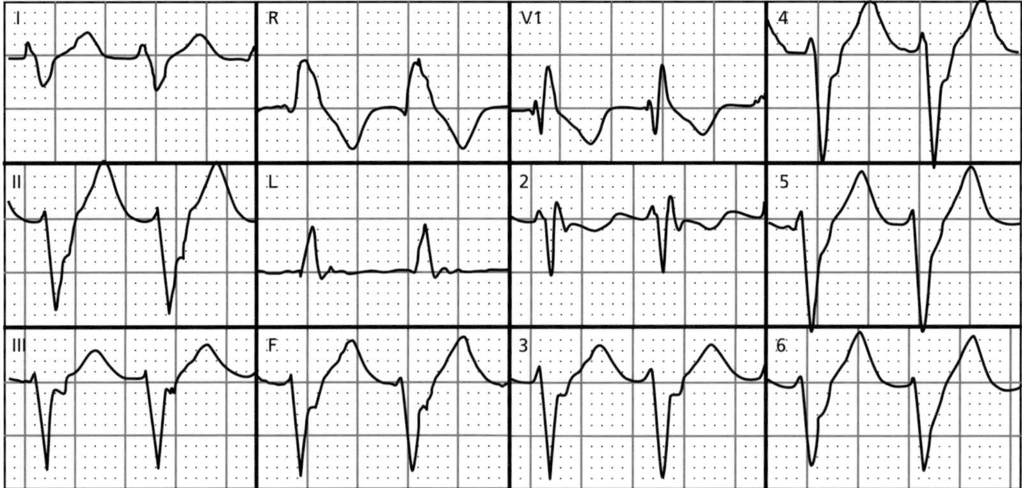

Figure 14.21 Fascicular tachycardia with antegrade conduction through the left posterior fascicle.

Bidirectional ventricular tachycardia

Bidirectional ventricular tachycardia, an unusual form of VT, typically exhibits right bundle branch block morphology in the precordial leads with alternating right and left axis deviation manifest in the limb leads (Figure 14.22). The arrhythmia is particularly associated with digitalis toxicity, but has also been documented in cases of Andersen–Tawil syndrome, a rare condition characterized by QT interval prolongation and periodic paralysis, as well as in *catecholaminergic polymorphic ventricular tachycardia* (CPVT), in which syncope due to VT is induced by emotional stress or exercise. Catecholaminergic VT is a suspected factor in drowning deaths among competent swimmers. The onset occurs in infancy or childhood and the resting ECG is typically normal. Males show a slight preponderance. The arrhythmia responds to β-blockers.

Polymorphic ventricular tachycardia

Polymorphic ventricular tachycardia, universally known by its French appellative, *torsade de pointes* (TDP), is characterized by changing morphology and QRS vector that results in the distinctive 'twisting' appearance (Figure 14.23). Several subsets of polymorphic VT are recognized based on: (1) *normal versus prolonged QT intervals*, (2) *pause-dependent versus non pause-dependent* initiation of tachycardia, and (3) *stress-related versus non stress-related* initiation of tachycardia.

Strictly speaking, *torsade de pointes* should be reserved for those cases of polymorphic VT in which QT interval prolongation is a feature. Polymorphic VT may also be encountered in subjects with ischemia and/or infarction, hypokalemia and hypomagnesemia. In these cases, bradycardia and/or sudden changes in R–R intervals (heart rate) are often the triggers that initiate VT. At least fifty drugs, including antiarrhythmics and antibiotics, have been implicated in the induction of polymorphic VT. Various substrates of polymorphic VT are discussed in the following chapter on channelopathies.

Accelerated idioventricular rhythm

Accelerated idioventricular rhythm (AIVR) arises from an automatic focus with a rate that usually ranges from 45 to 100 beats per minute, and almost invariably occurs owing to slowing of the sinus pacemaker. Atrioventricular dissociation is common but generally of short duration. Occasionally ventricular impulses conduct in a retrograde direction, entraining the atria. Owing to the slow rate, fusion between ventricular and sinus impulses is usually observed (Figure 14.24). The rhythm is almost always transient, typically alternating with periods of sinus rhythm. Aside from the loss of 'atrial kick' that occurs during atrioventricular

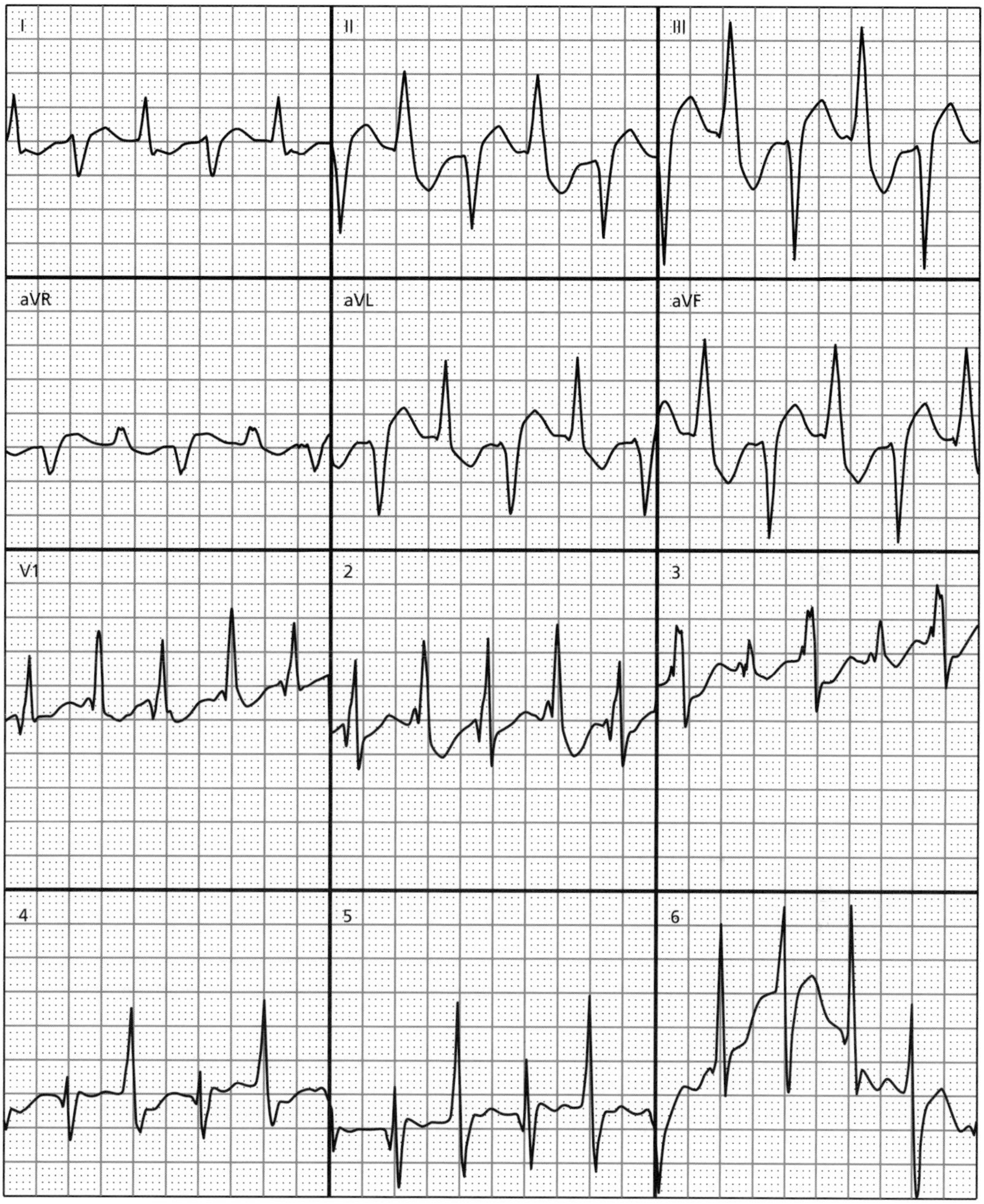

Figure 14.22 Bidirectional ventricular tachycardia.

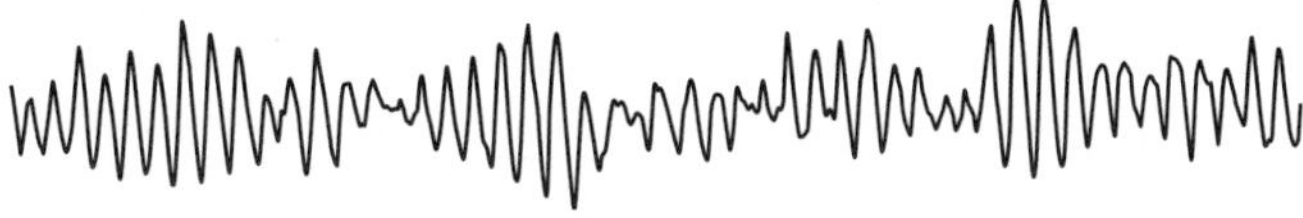

Figure 14.23 Polymorphic ventricular tachycardia: torsade de pointes.

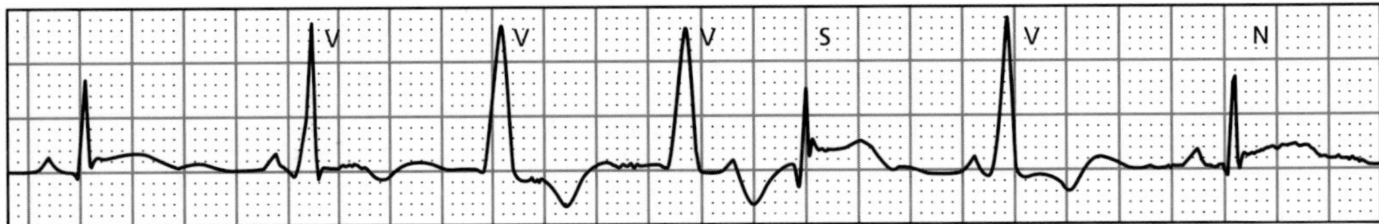

Figure 14.24 Accelerated idioventricular rhythm. The second QRS complex is a fusion beat, the fifth QRS complex is a sinus capture beat.

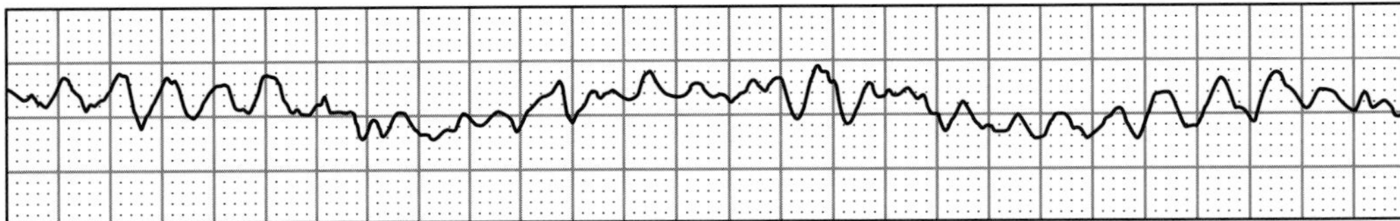

Figure 14.25 Ventricular fibrillation.

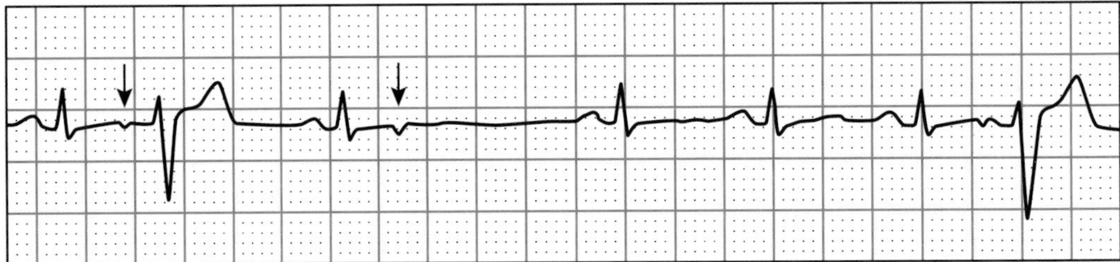

Figure 14.26 PACs masquerading as PVCs.

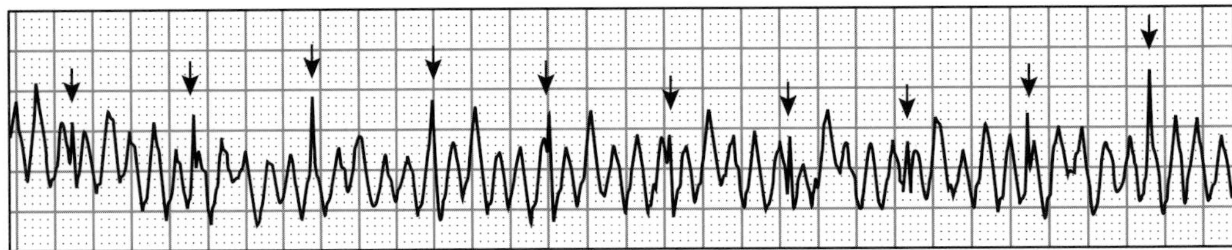

Figure 14.27 Artifact masquerading as ventricular fibrillation: the subject's native R waves are indicated (*arrows*).

dissociation, AIVR rarely has hemodynamic consequences that merit intervention, and attempts to suppress AIVR are therefore generally not required.

Ventricular fibrillation

Ventricular fibrillation (VF) is characterized by a low-amplitude, undulating baseline without discrete P–QRS–T waves (Figure 14.25). Defibrillation is the only effective treatment and takes priority over other interventions since the probability of successful defibrillation decreases dramatically over time even if properly done cardiopulmonary resuscitation is performed. Uncorrected VF leads rapidly to ventricular asystole, a total absence of ventricular activity.

Diagnostic pitfalls

Often the simplest diagnostic clues are overlooked. The rhythm in Figure 14.26, read as 'PVCs,' is, on closer examination, sinus rhythm with PACs (*arrows*) aberrantly conducted. There is even a pause due to nonconduction of a PAC!

Artifact produced by regular, repetitive movement, sometimes called 'toothbrush tachycardia,' can result in wide, regular deflections that are sometimes mistaken for VT. The section of tracing shown in Figure 14.27, obtained from a subject with a history of syncope, is part of a longer record interpreted as ventricular fibrillation. On closer inspection the tracing is obviously artifact; the native R waves are indicated by arrows.

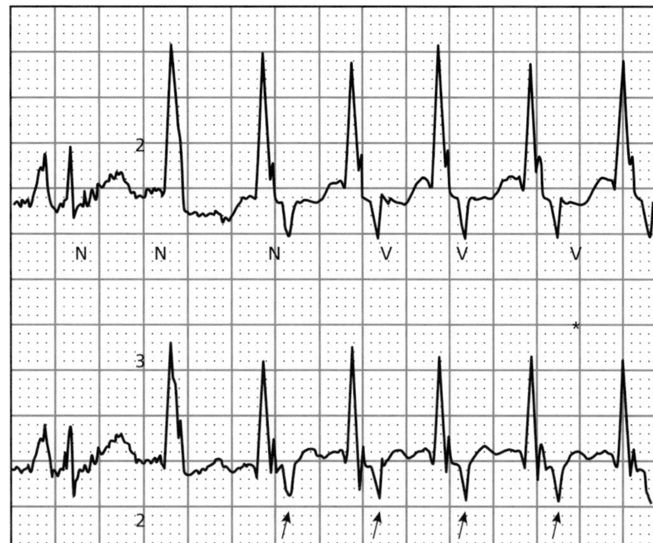

Figure 14.28 Ventriculoatrial conduction (1:1).

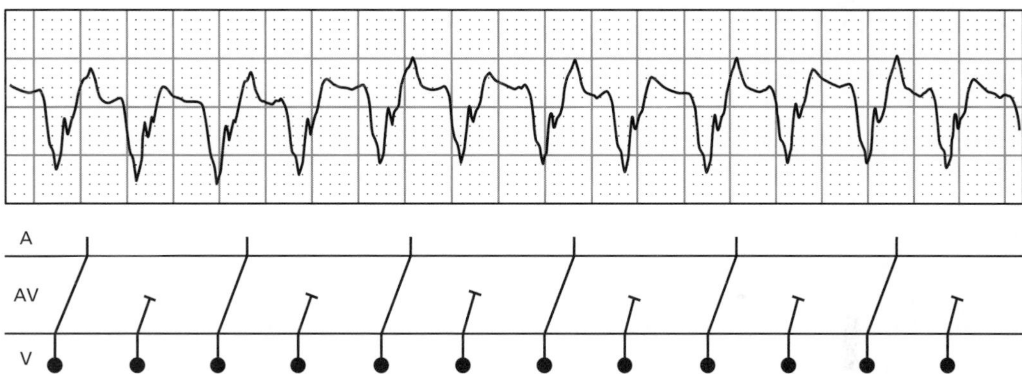

Figure 14.29 Ventriculoatrial conduction (2:1).

Ventriculoatrial conduction

Ventriculoatrial conduction – retrograde conduction from the ventricles to the atria – has been touched upon already in the context of echo beats (*reciprocal beats*) and atrioventricular re-entrant tachycardia, in which the atria form an obligatory part of the re-entrant circuit. Ventriculoatrial conduction is also common during ventricular tachycardia.

The brief segment of tracing shown in Figure 14.28, recorded from leads II and III, illustrates 1:1 ventriculoatrial conduction that begins following the second ventricular QRS complex. In this case, deeply inverted P waves (*arrows*) follow each QRS complex, indicating atrial entrainment by the ventricular rhythm. In the case shown in Figure 14.29, ventricular impulses are conducted to the atria in a 2:1 ratio during VT.

In the next example (Figure 14.30), type I (Wenckebach) second-degree ventriculoatrial block with a 3:2 conduction ratio is noted during VT. As these cases illustrate, the faster pacemaker, whatever its origin, tends to usurp control of cardiac rhythm overall. As a result, complex forms of ventriculoatrial conduction are often encountered during junctional and ventricular tachycardia.

Parasystole

Under normal circumstances, no potential cardiac pacemaker has protection from any other. For this reason, the impulse generated by the inherently

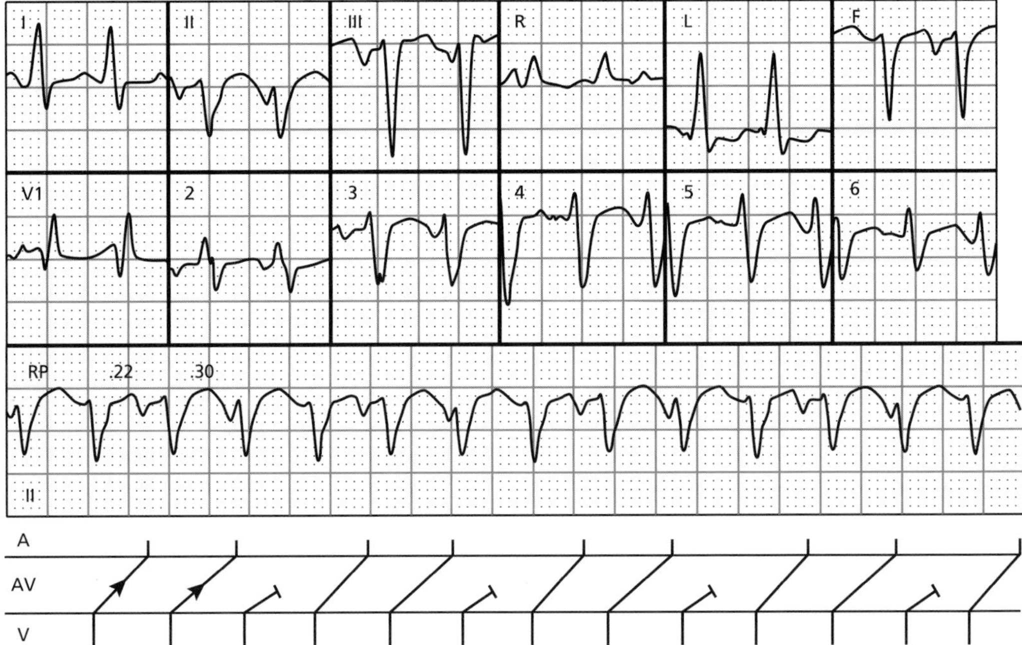

Figure 14.30 Ventriculoatrial conduction (3:2).

fastest pacemaker, the sinoatrial node, reaches and passively depolarizes all slower subsidiary sites before they spontaneously depolarize. The sinus node thereby maintains exclusive control of the cardiac rhythm because it has the fastest rate of spontaneous impulse formation and because the slower subsidiary pacemakers are vulnerable to being passively discharged and reset by successive sinus impulses.

Diseased segments of the conduction system can retain the capacity for spontaneous depolarization (impulse formation) while acquiring protection from passive discharge by the sinus impulse. Because the sinus impulse cannot 'enter' the ectopic focus to discharge and reset it, the ectopic focus is said to exhibit *entrance block*. Under these circumstances, the protected ectopic pacemaker coexists with the sinus pacemaker and competes with it for control of the cardiac rhythm. The phenomenon of a protected ectopic pacemaker is called *parasystole*. Parasystolic pacemakers may be atrial, junctional, or ventricular.

The diagnostic criteria for parasystole include (1) variable coupling intervals, (2) interectopic intervals that are constant or have a common denominator, and (3) fusion beats. A *coupling interval* is the interval between a sinus beat and the following ectopic beat. An *interectopic interval* is the interval between consecutive ectopic beats, including any intervening sinus beats.

Figure 14.31 illustrates the differences between ordinary ventricular ectopy and ventricular parasystole. In the upper strip (A), ventricular bigeminy is seen. The coupling intervals between sinus beats and the following ventricular beats are always the same, i.e. the coupling intervals are constant. In the case of the ventricular parasystolic rhythm (B), the coupling intervals vary (0.64, 0.58, 0.48 and 0.38 second, respectively) but the interectopic intervals (*II*) remain the same (1.92 sec). The varying coupling intervals of a parasystolic rhythm reflect the fact that the parasystolic rhythm is independent (dissociated) from the sinus rhythm and is discharging at its own rate.

Figure 14.32 illustrates another example of ventricular parasystole. The basic interectopic interval (1.40–1.42 sec) and its multiples are indicated for ease of reference. This parasystolic focus is protected from both sinus and atrial or ventricular ectopic impulses. Parasystolic impulses that fall within the ventricular refractory period fail to depolarize the ventricles (*arrows*), resulting in pauses

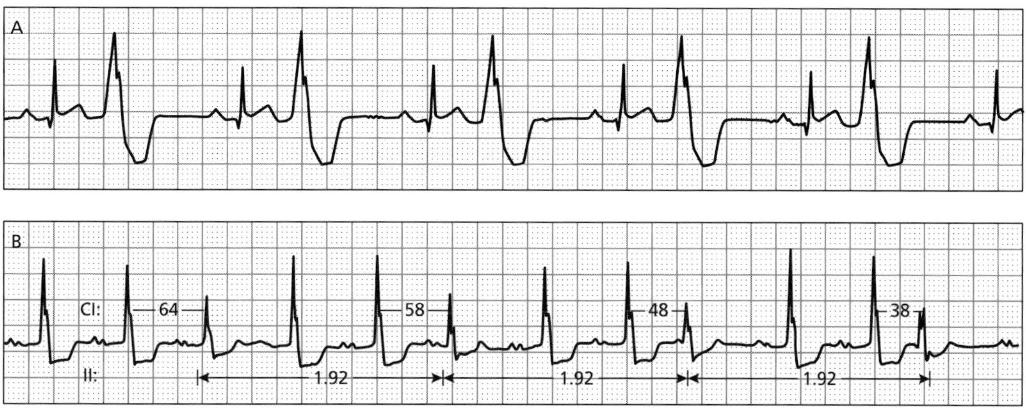

Figure 14.31 A: Ventricular bigeminy, B: Ventricular parasystole, CI: coupling interval, II: Interectopic interval.

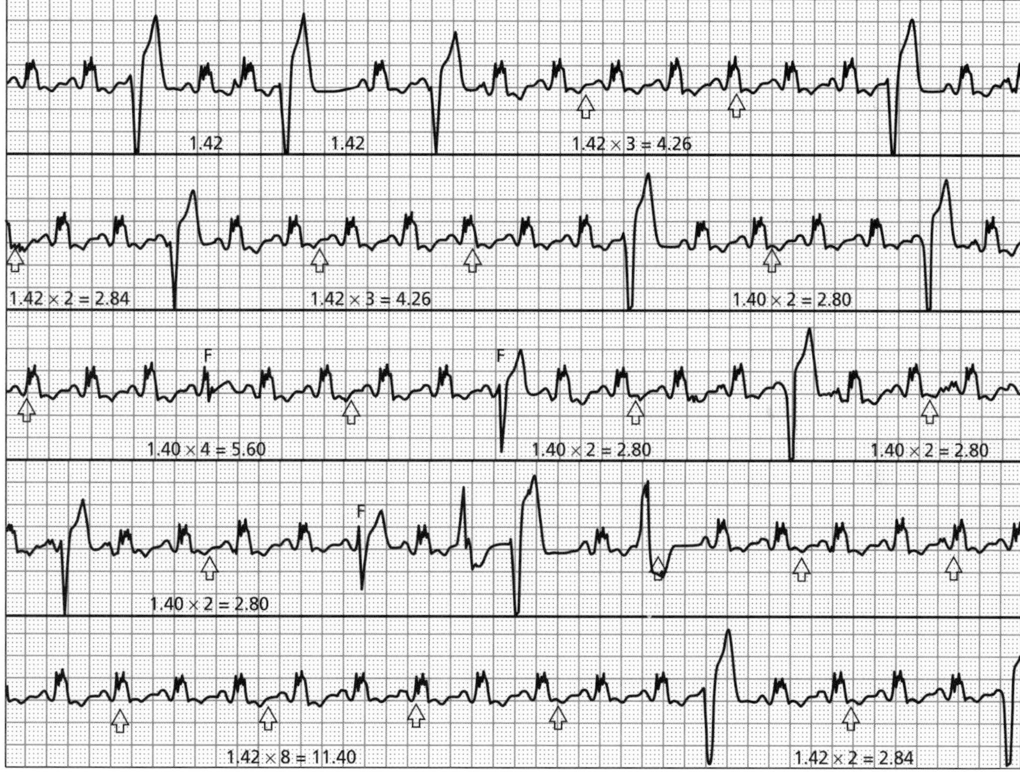

Figure 14.32 Ventricular parasystole.

between parasystolic complexes that are exact multiples of the basic parasystole cycle length. At several places, the sinus impulse and parasystolic impulse share in ventricular depolarization, resulting in fusion beats (*F*).

An example of atrial parasystole is shown in Figure 14.33. The manifest parasystolic beats are indicated by *arrows*; parasystolic impulses that fail to capture are marked by *empty circles*. In this case the parasystolic rhythm is accompanied by a degree of *exit block* (discussed in the next section): some parasystolic impulses that fall well outside the atrial refractory period fail to capture, implying that they could not exit from the parasystolic focus.

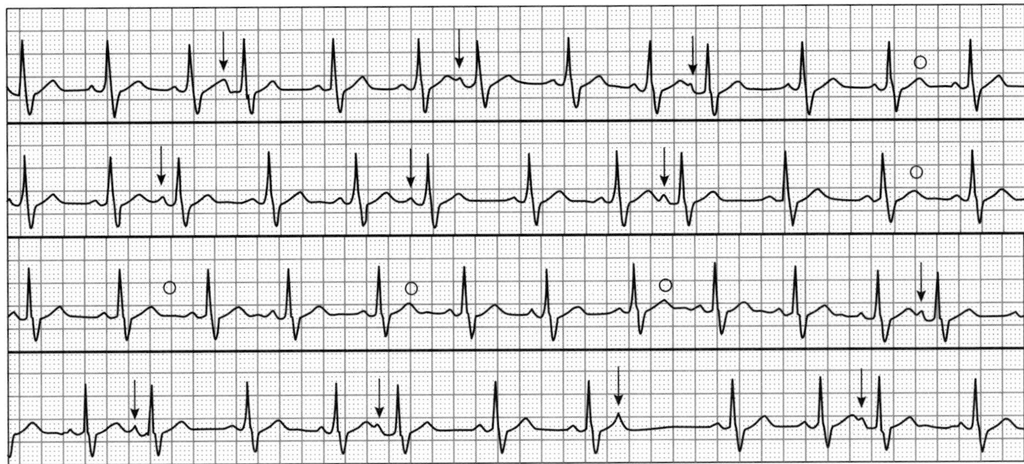

Figure 14.33 Atrial parasystole.

Parasystolic rhythms may be transient or persistent. Some have been documented to discharge consistently on tracings taken years apart. Ventricular parasystole tends to be benign; ventricular fibrillation precipitated by parasystole is exceedingly rare. Rapidly discharging parasystolic foci rarely manifest as ventricular tachycardia owing to the frequency of coexisting exit block from the parasystolic focus and competition from sinus rhythm. In some cases, only multiples of the basic parasystolic cycle length are ever seen. In those cases, the true cycle length, which will be the lowest common denominator of the observed cycle lengths, must be calculated.

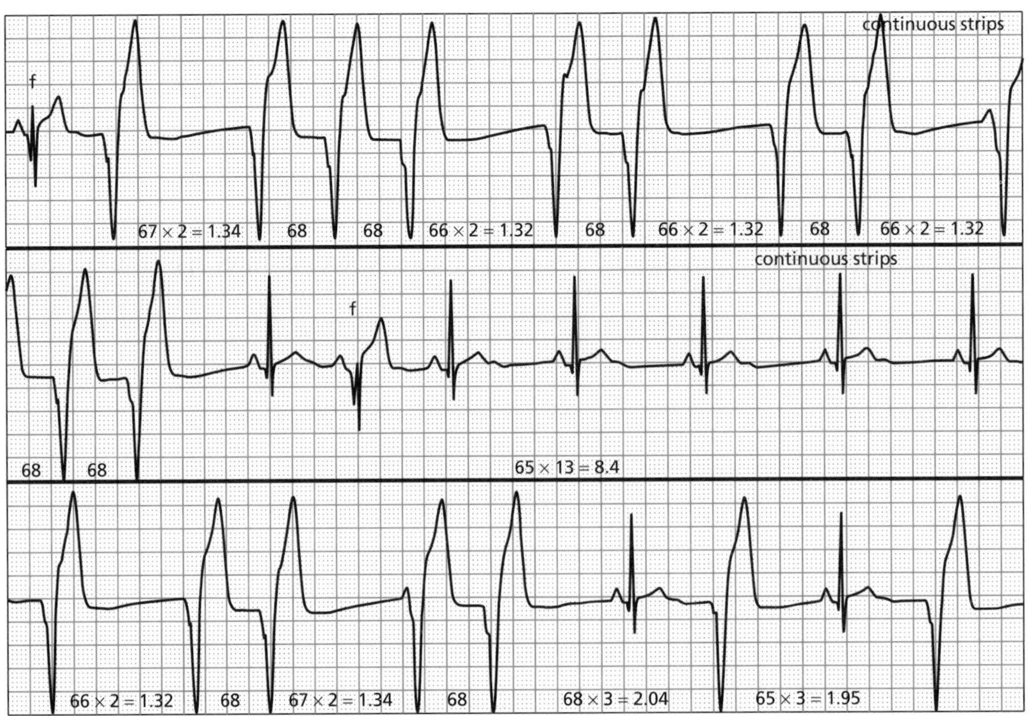

Figure 14.34 Ventricular exit block.

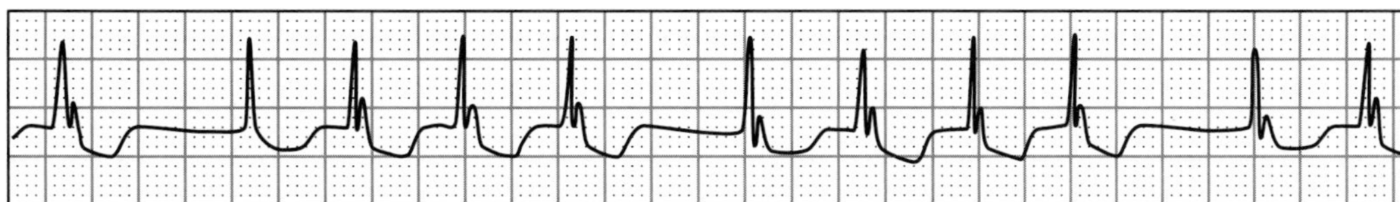

Figure 14.35 Junctional exit block (5:4).

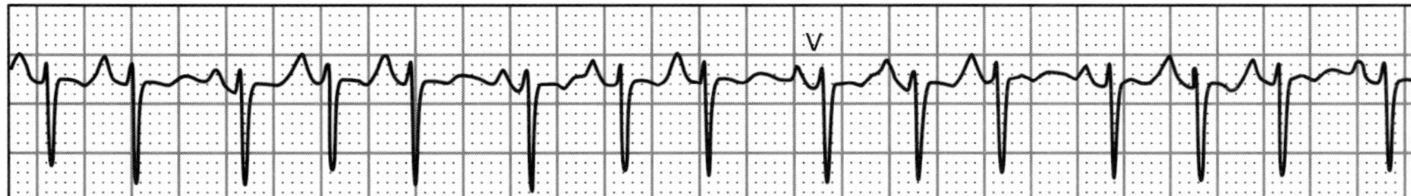

Figure 14.36 Atrial exit block (4:3).

Exit block

Spontaneous impulse formation, or automaticity, is an intrinsic property of cardiac tissue. Once generated, the impulse must successfully conduct to and depolarize atrial or ventricular myocardium to produce any deflection on the ECG. Impulse conduction can fail *within the specialized conduction pathway*, resulting in atrioventricular, fascicular or bundle branch block, or fail *between the impulse source and the contiguous myocardium*, a condition known as *exit block*. Exit blocks are recognized between the sinoatrial node and the contiguous atrial myocardium (sinoatrial block), between the pacing terminal of an electronic pacemaker and the contiguous myocardium, or between natural ectopic pacemakers and the contiguous cardiac tissue. Exit block may occur abruptly, without previous detectable conduction delay, or after increasing increments of conduction delay (Wenckebach periodicity).

Failure of atrial or ventricular complexes to appear when expected is the *sine qua non* of exit block. An example of exit block from a ventricular ectopic focus is shown in Figure 14.34. The R–R intervals of this accelerated ventricular rhythm range from 0.65 to 0.68 sec (88–92/minute). The interectopic intervals, including one of 8.4 sec, are multiples of this basic cycle length. During the longer pauses, sinus rhythm re-establishes control, resulting in the appearance of fusion beats (f). The fact that the sinus impulse does not passively discharge and reset the ventricular focus indicates that the ectopic focus is parasystolic.

Figure 14.35 is an example of junctional tachycardia, 125 per minute, in which QRS complexes appear in clusters separated by pauses. The observations that (1) cycle lengths (R–R intervals) tend to shorten and (2) the pauses are less than the sum of any two preceding cycle lengths argue for a Wenckebach exit block with a 5:4 conduction ratio distal to the junctional focus.

The P waves of the atrial tachycardia shown in Figure 14.36 consistently appear in clusters of three. Cluster beating, a tendency for the P–P intervals to shorten, and the presence of pauses that are less than the sum of any two preceding P–P intervals, are indicative of a 4:3 Wenckebach exit block from an ectopic atrial focus.

prolongation of the PR interval. Prolonged QT

assumed to occur. If a diagnosis of Brugada syn-

15

CHAPTER 15

The channelopathies

The *channelopathies* are a diverse constellation of diseases caused by mutations of genes that encode for ion channel proteins. They are now understood to include myotonic diseases, cystic fibrosis, and various cardiac syndromes resulting in arrhythmias and sudden death. Although representing defects in a number of genes, the channelopathies create a substrate for polymorphic ventricular tachycardia through a single basic mechanism: transmural dispersion of repolarization owing to electrical heterogeneity in the ventricular myocardium.

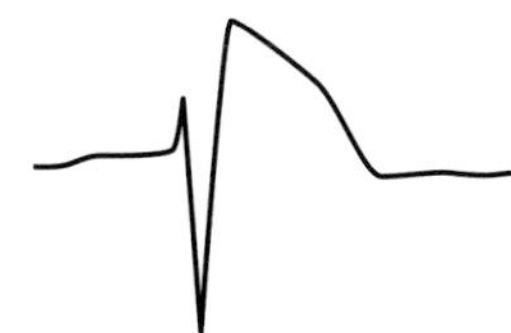

Figure 15.1 The Brugada syndrome: J point elevation with ST segment coving in lead V2.

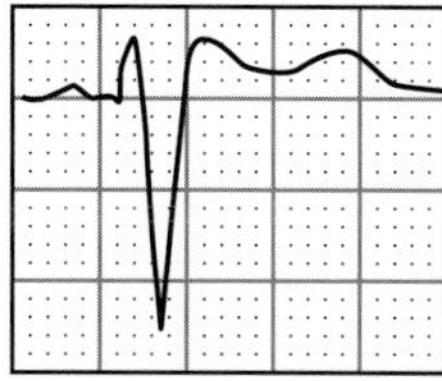

Figure 15.2 The Brugada syndrome: J point elevation with ST segment 'saddleback' deformity in lead V2.

Brugada syndrome

The *Brugada syndrome*, first identified in the Western medical literature in 1992, is due to a defect in the SCN5A gene on the short arm of chromosome 3 that results in a sodium channel defect. The mode of inheritance is autosomal dominant. The typical subject presents after a syncopal episode caused by polymorphic VT. The heart is structurally normal. Some 60% of subjects give a history of sudden cardiac death among family members. Although *de novo* gene mutations are assumed to occur, if a diagnosis of Brugada syndrome is made in one family member, the other members should be screened.

Previously known as *sudden unexpected nocturnal death syndrome* (SUNDS), Brugada syndrome occurs worldwide, but is particularly common in Southeast Asians (Filipinos, Japanese, Thais and Cambodians). Among affected populations it is a common cause of sudden death, exhibiting a strong male preponderance. Among Thais the disease occurs almost exclusively in males.

The baseline ECG may reveal *Brugada's sign*, J point elevation greater than 2 mm and ST segment coving in leads V1–V3 (Figure 15.1), which gives the QRS complex a right bundle branch block morphology. A second morphology, ST segment elevation with a 'saddleback' deformity in leads V1–V3, is a variant (Figure 15.2). The saddleback deformity can exist without J point or ST segment elevation. Around 10% of subjects experience paroxysmal atrial fibrillation, and around half exhibit prolongation of the PR interval. Prolonged QT intervals are not a notable feature of the syndrome. In these patients *VT is not induced by exercise.*

Unfortunately, the occurrence of Brugada's sign is not constant: the syndrome may be *concealed*, *intermittent*, or *permanent*. The sodium channel dysfunction is also temperature dependent in some subjects in whom polymorphic VT is more likely to occur during fever. In many, VT occurs at night during sleep owing to slowing of the heart rate. In subjects with concealed or intermittent ECG manifestations, the typical ST segment changes can often be provoked by administering procainamide, flecainide or ajmaline. The syndrome may be aggravated by numerous drugs, by high or low levels of serum potassium, and by hypercalcemia. Acquired forms

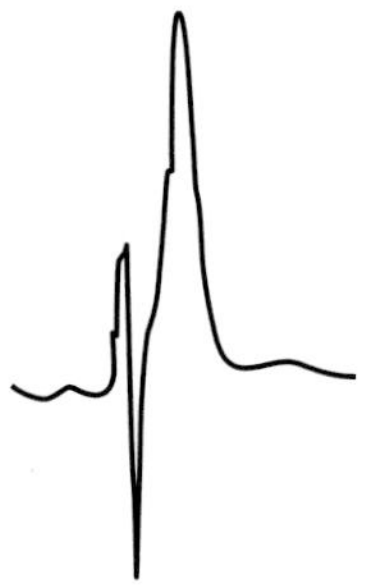

Figure 15.3 Short QT syndrome: the QT interval is short, and T waves tend to be tall and compressed.

exist, presumably caused by pharmacologic sodium channel modulation in susceptible subjects.

Even in persons with concealed or intermittent ECG manifestations of Brugada syndrome, the likelihood of sudden cardiac death (SCD) due to ventricular tachycardia is high. The treatment of choice is implantation of a cardioverter–defibrillator (ICD).

Short QT syndrome

First described in 2000, the *short QT syndrome* (SQTS) has been linked to defects in three different genes (KCNH2, KCNQ1 and KCNJ2). Subjects with SQTS exhibit a corrected QT interval of less than 300 msec (Figure 15.3). The severity of symptoms is quite variable. Atrial fibrillation and a family history of sudden death, often at an early age, are common. At present, implantation of a cardioverter–defibrillator is the only definitive treatment.

Genetically caused long QT syndromes

At present, eight genetically caused *long QT syndromes* (LQT) have been described. Such long QT syndromes are thought to affect approximately 1 in 7000 persons and are now recognized as an important cause of sudden cardiac death (SCD) in the young. Recurrent syncope and resuscitation from SCD are the hallmarks of high-risk patients. However, many patients with frequent self-terminating episodes of polymorphic VT are asymptomatic and unaware of their arrhythmias. Even patients without marked QT prolongation may experience syncope and cardiac arrest.

Long QT syndrome 1 (LQT1) is the most common variant, accounting for about 50% of reported cases. It is due to mutation of the KCNQ1 gene on chromosome 11, resulting in abnormally regulated potassium transport across the cell membrane. Two phenotypes are recognized: the *Romano–Ward syndrome*, in which QT prolongation occurs without deafness, and the *Jervell and Lange–Nielson syndrome*, in which QT prolongation is accompanied by deafness.

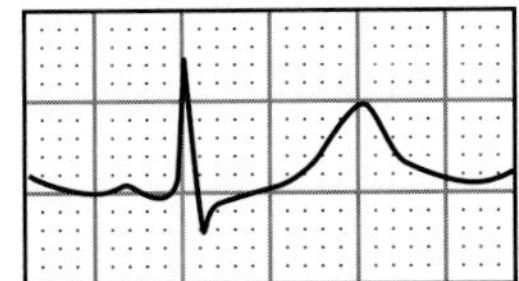

Figure 15.4 LQT1: broad-based T waves and QT prolongation.

Subjects with LQT1 often develop torsade de pointes tachycardia in response to sympathetic stimulation, particularly during exercise (running, swimming) and heightened emotional states (fright, anger). Premature systoles may provoke torsade owing to sudden changes in cycle length (R–R intervals). In LQT1, T waves tend to be *broad based* (Figure 15.4) and the QT interval prolonged beyond 440 msec. It should be noted, however, that up to 15% of subjects with symptomatic LQT syndrome exhibit normal QT intervals, at least intermittently, and that prolongation of the QT interval may occur as a normal variant, during myocardial ischemia, or in response to electrolyte imbalances, particularly hypokalemia. Because sympathetic stimulation is a trigger for polymorphic VT in patients with LQT1, β-blockers may prove effective in suppressing VT.

Long QT syndrome 2 (LQT2) is the second most common variant, accounting for about 40% of cases. It is due to mutation of the KCNH2 gene located on chromosome 7, and results in abnormally regulated potassium transport. Subjects with LQT2 syndrome may exhibit bifid or notched T waves in addition to prolonged QT intervals (Figure 15.5) and experience torsade de pointes tachycardia in response to sympathetic stimuli.

Long QT syndrome 3 (LQT3) is a rare variant due to mutation of the SCN5A gene located on chromosome 3. It is characterized by late-appearing T waves and QT prolongation (Figure 15.6) and represents a mutation of the same sodium channel that

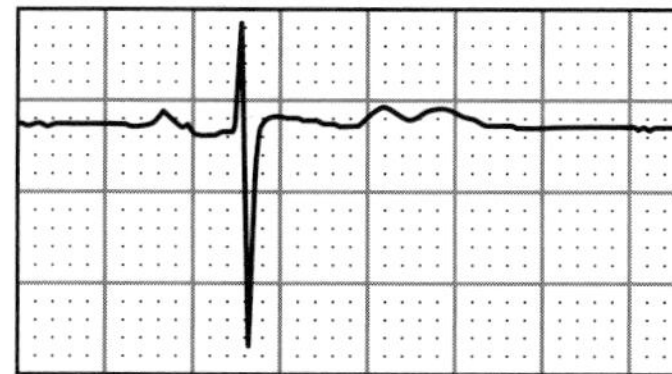

Figure 15.5 LQT2: bifid ('double-humped') T waves and QT prolongation.

causes Brugada syndrome. LQT3, however, represents a 'gain of function' defect, Brugada syndrome a 'loss of function' defect.

Bradycardia accentuates the effect of the defective gene, accounting for the tendency of polymorphic VT to occur during sleep in subjects with LQT3. In these subjects, β-blockers are contraindicated. The QT interval may be shortened, increasing the heart rate.

Long QT syndrome 4 (LQT4), caused by a mutation in gene ANK2 on chromosome 4, has not been linked to any particular T wave abnormality.

Long QT 5 (LQT5), resulting from a mutation of gene KCNE1 on chromosome 21, results in a broad-based T wave.

Long QT 6 (LQT6), due to a mutation of gene KCNE2 on chromosome 21, produces a bifid T wave.

Long QT 7 (LQT7), due to a mutation of gene KCNJ2, results in disordered cardiac and skeletal muscle excitability, the *Andersen–Tawil syndrome* (ATS). Notched or bifid T waves and QT prolongation accompany dysmorphic features and periodic paralysis. These patients experience bidirectional VT as well as torsade de pointes, but are usually unaware of the arrhythmias. Those who are symptomatic may benefit from ICD implantation.

Long QT 8 (LQT8), related to a defect of gene CACNA1C, occurs in the setting of *Timothy syndrome*, an extremely rare disorder characterized by malignant ventricular arrhythmias, atrioventricular block, immune deficiency, cardiac, facial and hand abnormalities (syndactyly) and autism. Death due to polymorphic VT or infection is common, frequently occurring in infancy.

In addition to altered T wave morphology, several other manifestations of long QT syndromes are known to predispose to ventricular arrhythmias. Among them are *T wave alternans*, a beat-to-beat change in T wave polarity (Figure 15.7) that is regarded as a clear signal of electrical instability.

Any situation in which R–R intervals change abruptly can trigger polymorphic VT (Figure 15.8); premature beats followed by pauses, bradycardia and atrioventricular block are particularly well-known offenders. Any sudden change in cycle length is likely to accentuate inhomogeneous ventricular repolarization, an important precondition for polymorphic VT.

Subjects with long QT syndromes are particularly likely to experience exacerbation of VT if exposed to medications that prolong repolarization. Particular care must be exercised when prescribing to these patients (see below under *Acquired long QT syndrome*).

Acquired long QT syndrome

Drug-related prolongation of the QT interval accounts for the majority of cases of *acquired long QT syndrome*. Over sixty medications, as well as illicit substances such as cocaine, are known or suspected to cause torsade de pointes tachycardia. Medications that do not directly prolong the QT interval may contribute indirectly by increasing the serum levels of other drugs as a side effect.

Three broad classes of drugs account for most of the offending agents.

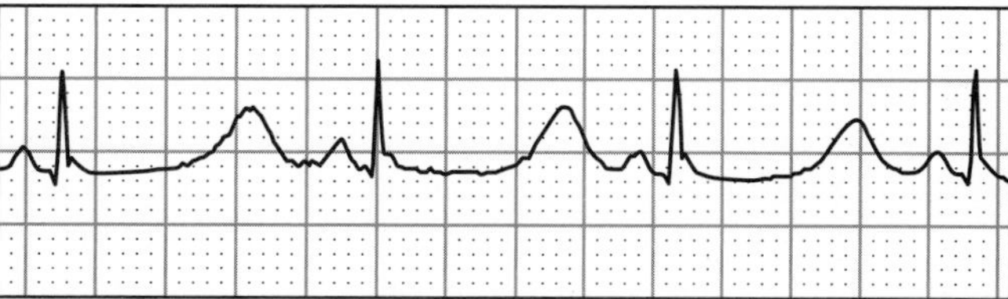

Figure 15.6 LQT3: late-appearing T wave and QT prolongation in lead II.

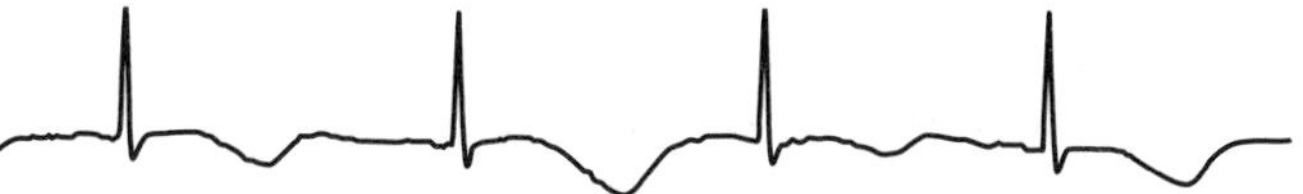

Figure 15.7 T wave alternans in long QT syndrome.

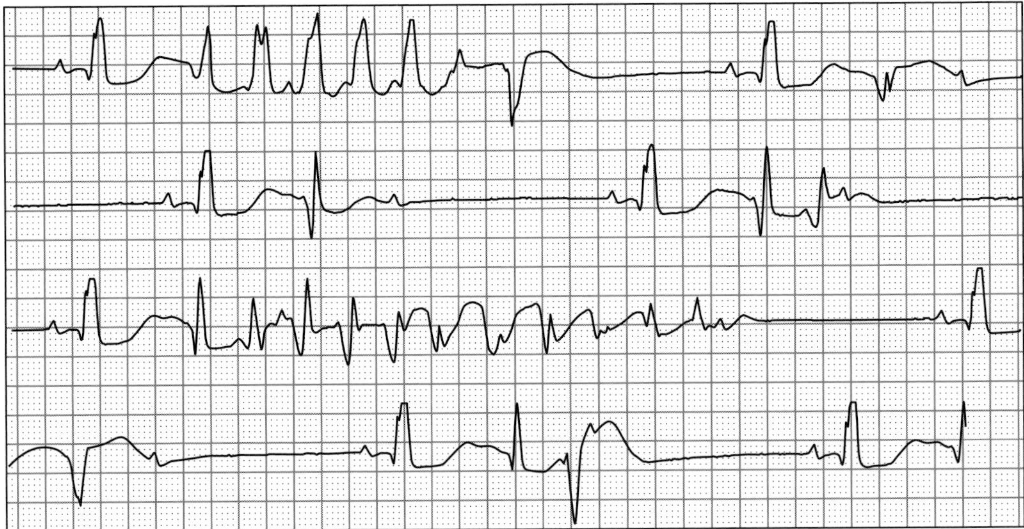

Figure 15.8 Prolongation of the QT interval and sudden cycle length changes precipitate bursts of polymorphic VT (lead V1).

Antiarrhythmics: such as amiodarone, disopyramide, dofetilide, ibutilide, procainamide, quinidine and sotalol.

Psychotropics: such as amitriptyline, chlorpromazine, haloperidol, mesoridazine, thioridazine and pimozide.

Antibiotics: such as chloroquine, clarithromycin, erythromycin, halofantrine, pentamidine and sparfloxacin.

These categories are offered as a general guide and are by no means inclusive. Agents which affect gastrointestinal motility, bronchodilators, muscle relaxants and other medications that act on cell membranes may prolong the QT interval.

Electrolyte imbalance, particularly hypokalemia and hypomagnesemia, is a second important cause of QT interval prolongation. Other factors such as female gender, renal failure, and use of diuretics may contribute to QT prolongation.

Infusion of magnesium sulfate is the treatment of choice for polymorphic VT. Offending medications must be identified and discontinued.

Catecholaminergic polymorphic ventricular tachycardia

Catecholaminergic polymorphic ventricular tachycardia (CPVT), an important cause of syncope and sudden cardiac death in children and adolescents with otherwise normal hearts, is caused by as many as four identified mutations of genes located on chromosome 1, the cardiac ryanodine receptor gene (RyR2), ankyrin-B mutations, calstabin 2, and CASQ2. All are involved in calcium ion exchange within the sarcoplasmic reticulum.

The baseline ECG is typically normal. Polymorphic VT and/or bidirectional VT are induced by exercise or emotional stress, with the frequency and complexity of ventricular ectopy increasing as the heart rate increases. During exercise, atrial fibrillation may precede ventricular arrhythmias.

CPVT can be induced by isoproterenol infusion. The use of volatile anesthetics or succinylcholine may result in malignant hyperthermia in carriers of the RyR1 mutation in skeletal muscle, but those complications have not been reported in carriers of RyR2 mutations or subjects with CPVT. Substantial protection from CPVT can be achieved with β-blockers, and intravenous propranolol is used for acute management of tachycardia. A combination of β-blockers and implantation of a cardioverter–defibrillator provides the greatest degree of protection from sudden cardiac death.

CHAPTER 16

Electronic pacing

Regardless of its particular functional parameters, an electronic pacemaker consists of three basic elements: (1) a power source, (2) electronic circuitry that determines the pacemaker's functional parameters, and (3) leads that connect the pacemaker to the cardiac tissues. Pacemakers can be internal or external, temporary or permanent, and may include anti-tachycardia features such as defibrillation and/or overdrive pacemaking.

Pacemaker leads consist of (1) coaxial metal wires, (2) a connector pin that joins the lead wire to the pacemaker, and (3) one or more distal electrodes that both sense intrinsic ('native') cardiac electrical events and deliver the artificially generated impulse to cardiac tissues. *Unipolar leads* consist of a single-tip electrode at the end of the pacing wire, with the metallic outer skin ('the can') of the pacemaker serving to complete the circuit. The pacemaker artifact ('spike') generated by a unipolar pacemaker is typically large. *Bipolar leads* consist of a tip electrode and a neighboring ring electrode located near the tip of the lead. The tip electrode is used for sensing and pacing and the ring electrode is used to complete the electrical circuit. The pacer artifact produced by a bipolar pacemaker is typically small and may even be hard to see on a monitor set at normal gain.

An *endocardial* lead refers to a lead that has been placed transvenously. The leads are generally placed in the apex of the right ventricle and the atrial lead is placed in the right atrial appendage. Placement is confirmed by chest radiography and by the appearance of characteristic left bundle branch block morphology on the ECG.

Basic functional parameters

Regardless of the sophistication of their electronics, all pacemakers have two basic functional parameters: *sensing* and *pacing*.

Sensing or *sensitivity* refers to the pacemaker's ability to detect the patient's intrinsic (native) impulses. Detection of an intrinsic impulse suppresses the pacemaker's impulse formation, a response known as *inhibition*. Inhibition prevents the pacemaker from competing with the heart's intrinsic beats. The *sensing threshold* is the smallest atrial or ventricular complex amplitude that can be detected by the pacemaker. Sensitivity is measured in millivolts (mV).

The sensitivity of an implanted pacemaker can be adjusted ('reprogrammed') electronically. External pacemakers have a dial that can be set to adjust the pacemaker's sensitivity to the patient's beats. A sensitivity of 4 millivolts (4 mV) means that the pacemaker will detect any intrinsic complex equal to or greater than 4 mV. *Increasing the sensitivity* means that the setting in millivolts must be *decreased*. In other words, with the sensitivity set at 3 mV, the pacemaker will now detect a smaller complex, i.e. be more sensitive. At a sensitivity of 20 mV, complexes must exceed 20 mV in order to be detected. Because in most subjects intrinsic cardiac activity falls well short of that value, the pacemaker will not sense the patient's own beats and will fire *asynchronously*, ignoring the patient's intrinsic beats. The nominal sensitivity for detecting P waves is 1 millivolt, and for R waves it is 2–4 millivolts. The pacemaker lead senses the electrogram from a particular vantage point; if the vector of the electrogram changes, the resulting complex may fall within the null plane of that lead and prove too small to be detected.

The basic *pacing rate* or beats per minute (BPM) is the number of impulses per minute the pacemaker will produce in the absence of intrinsic cardiac beats (pure pacing). The impulse-to-impulse interval is measured in milliseconds and can be calculated by dividing the base rate into 60,000. For example, a base rate of 80 per minute results in an impulse-to-impulse interval of 750 msec. The base rate is dialed in on external pacemakers and electronically programmed into permanent implantable pacemakers. *Output*, which refers to the amount of energy the pacemaker generates with each impulse, is measured in milliamperes (mA). Output is increased until atrial or ventricular depolarization results from the pacer stimulus ('capture'). The smallest amount of current necessary to achieve and sustain capture is the *pacing threshold*. Lower pacing thresholds prolong the pacemaker's battery life. A pacemaker that supplies a stimulus when no intrinsic complexes are sensed is said to be in *demand mode*.

The generic pacemaker code

A universally recognized five-letter code is used to describe pacemaker functions. The first letter of the code indicates the chamber paced, the second indicates the chamber sensed, and the third, the response to sensed impulses. The fourth letter indicates programmable functions, and the fifth, anti-arrhythmic functions. The code is summarized below:

I	II	III	IV	V
A	A	T	P	P
V	V	I	M	S
D	D	D	C	D
O	O	O	O	O

In this system *A* stands for *atrium*, *V* for *ventricle*, *D* for *dual* (both atrium and ventricle or both triggers and inhibits), *T* for *triggers* pacing, *I* for *inhibits* pacing, *O* for *none*, *P* in position IV for *programmable* rate/output, *M* for *multiprogrammability* (rate, output, sensitivity), *C* for *communicating* functions, *P* in position V for *pacing* as an anti-arrhythmic function, and *S* for *shock*, another anti-arrhythmic function.

Thus a pacemaker classed as an *AAI* paces the *atria*, senses the *atria*, and if a native P wave is sensed the pacemaker is *inhibited* from firing. A *VAT* classification describes a pacemaker that senses *atrial* activity which then *triggers* a *ventricular* paced beat in response. A *VVI* pacemaker senses the *ventricle*, paces the *ventricle*, but is *inhibited* from firing if a native QRS complex is sensed. A *DDD* pacemaker program paces *both* the atria and ventricles, senses *both* the atria and ventricles, is *both* inhibited by native P waves or QRS complexes and triggered to pace in their absence.

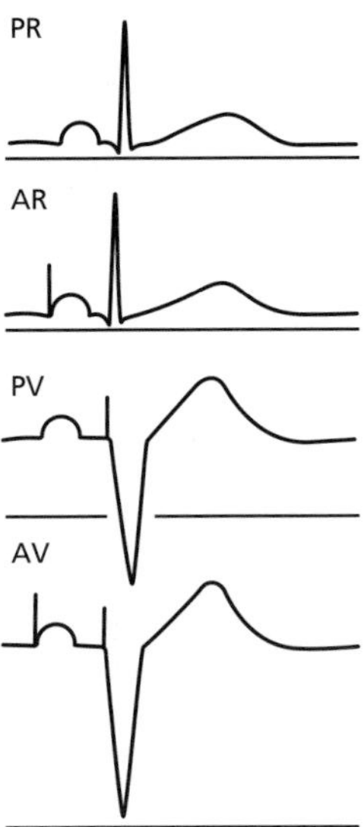

Figure 16.1 The four states of DDD pacing.

DDD pacemakers present several complexities related to the sophistication of the device. There are four states of DDD pacemaker function, which are represented in Figure 16.1. In DDD terminology, *P* stands for an *intrinsic atrial event* (a native P wave), *R* stands for an *intrinsic ventricular event* (a native QRS complex), *A* stands for a *paced atrial event*, and *V* for a *paced ventricular event*. For example, an *AR* state would indicate that a *paced* atrial beat is conducted to produce a *native* QRS complex while an *AV* state would indicate that a *paced* atrial beat was followed after an appropriate interval by a *paced* ventricular beat, the latter state implying that the atrial impulse could not be conducted to the ventricles.

Pacemaker intervals

Remembering a simple basic principle helps to clarify the subject of pacemaker intervals: pacemakers are designed to mimic the behavior of the cardiac conduction system. A pacemaker, like the conduction system, has *refractory periods*, time intervals when the pacemaker's sensing mechanism becomes unresponsive. As in the normally functioning conduction pathway, intrinsic activity will reset the pacemaker, a response known as *inhibition*.

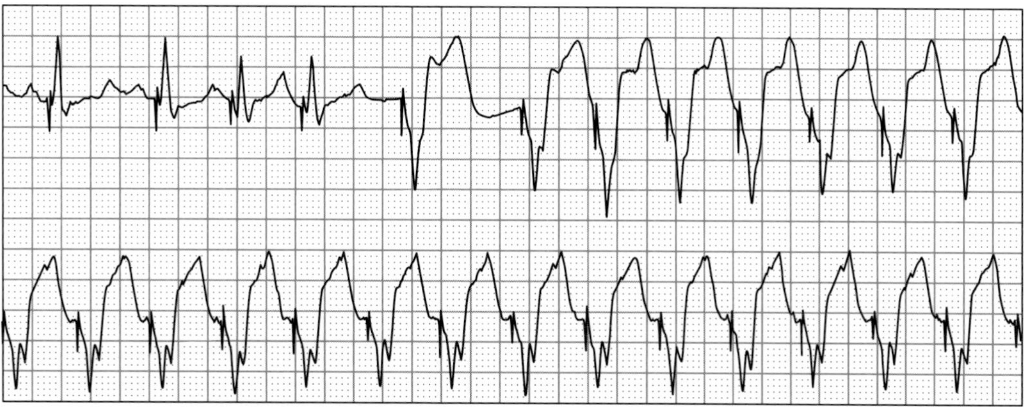

Figure 16.2 Pacemaker-mediated tachycardia: each retrograde P wave is sensed by the pacemaker and triggers a ventricular paced beat.

A normally functioning pacemaker may sense its own output. Such abnormal sensing is known as *cross-talk*. Cross-talk is prevented in dual chambered (DDD) pacemakers by a *blanking period*, a brief ventricular refractory period that is initiated by a paced atrial event. This blinding of the ventricular channel prevents the atrial stimulus from resetting the ventricular pacing interval.

The *atrial refractory period* (ARP) consists of two components: the *atrioventricular interval* (AVI), the pacemaking equivalent of the PR interval, and the postventricular atrial refractory period. The atrioventricular interval permits ventricular filling by the atrial contraction and should be carefully programmed to optimize cardiac output.

The *postventricular atrial refractory period* (PVARP) prevents the atrial channel from sensing retrograde conduction of ventricular impulses. The PVARP is initiated by the release of a ventricular stimulus and its duration is programmable. In a dual-chamber pacemaker, a retrograde P wave can be sensed, triggering a paced QRS complex in response. If the paced ventricular impulse is again conducted in a retrograde manner to the atria, yet another paced QRS complex would be triggered, and so on, producing a *pacemaker-mediated* ('endless loop') *tachycardia* (Figure 16.2). The length of the PVARP is programmed to prevent this kind of feedback. The PVARP can also prevent the atrial channel from responding to very early atrial extrasystoles.

The intervals used in DDD pacing are shown diagrammatically in Figure 16.3.

The *ventricular refractory period* (VRP) prevents the ventricular channel from sensing the T wave and being inhibited (reset) by it (Figure 16.4). A short ventricular refractory period, the *ventricular blanking period* (*B* in Figure 16.3), coincides with the atrial pacemaker spike in DDD pacing. This blinds the ventricular channel to the atrial pacemaker spike, preventing ventricular inhibition by atrial channel output (cross-talk).

Most pacemakers also have an *upper rate protection circuit* that prevents the ventricular channel from responding to very rapid atrial rates. In the event that rapid atrial impulses are sensed, the pacemaker will revert to a 2:1 pacing ratio or a Wenckebach pattern of response that protects the ventricle from entrainment by atrial tachyarrhythmias. The highest rate at which the ventricular channel will track atrial activity is the *maximal tracking rate*.

A native atrial or ventricular beat will normally reset the corresponding channel, thereby inhibiting pacemaker discharge. Pacemaker inhibition by native beats prevents the pacemaker from competing with native beats and rhythms. The sensed native beat initiates an *escape interval*. If *hysteresis* is programmed in, the escape interval may exceed the length of the normal pacemaker cycle. An escape interval longer than a basic pacing cycle functions to permit resumption

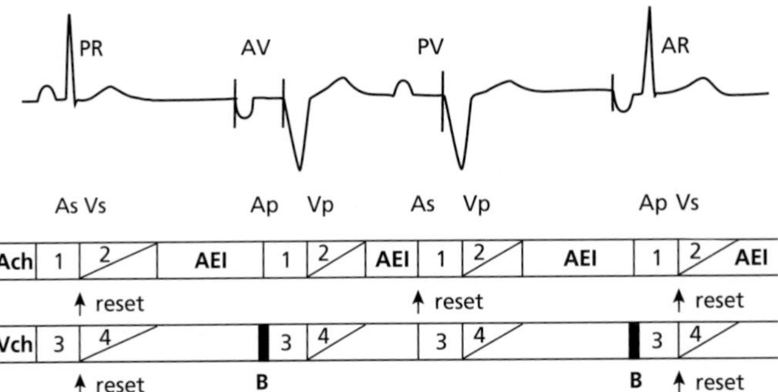

Figure 16.3 DDD pacemaking intervals, Ach: atrial channel, AEI: atrial escape interval, Ap: atrium paced, As: atrium sensed, B: blanking period, Vch: ventricular channel, Vp: ventricle paced, Vs: ventricle sensed, 1: atrial refractory period, 2: postventricular atrial refractory period, 3: AV interval, 4: ventricular refractory period. The lower rate limit is the AVI + AEI. AEI is reset by an intrinsic atrial complex (P). ARP is reset by an intrinsic ventricular complex (R). AVI is reset by an intrinsic ventricular complex (R).

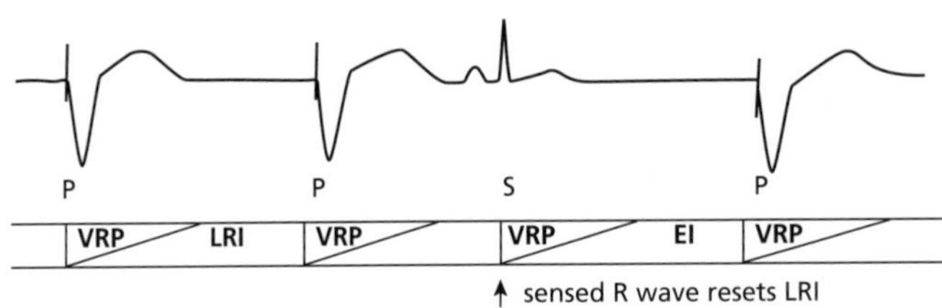

Figure 16.4 VVI pacing intervals. **EI**: escape interval. **LRI**: lower rate interval. **P**: paced. **S**: sensed. **VRP**: ventricular refractory period.

of the native rhythm and prolongs pacemaker battery life.

The atrial escape interval (AEI) is initiated by any ventricular event. If no atrial or ventricular activity is sensed before the end of the atrial escape interval, the pacemaker releases an atrial stimulus. The AEI is calculated by subtracting the AV interval from the lower rate interval.

In DDD pacemakers a sensed event in one channel can initiate a refractory period in both channels. The atrial channel operates in *dual mode*, inhibited or triggered according to the presence or absence of intrinsic atrial beats.

Pacemakers can be programmed to respond to increased physical activity by firing at a more rapid rate, a feature known as *rate-adaptive pacing*. These pacemakers detect body motion, respiratory rate, or other parameters of physical activity.

Pacemaker malfunction

There are three basic forms of pacemaker malfunction: undersensing, oversensing, and failure to capture.

Undersensing occurs when the pacemaker fails to sense normal cardiac electrical activity that falls outside the refractory period. The result is overpacing due to inappropriate discharge. Undersensing can be caused by (1) sensitivity that is too low, (2) lead displacement, (3) intrinsic signals that are too low to be sensed even with appropriate sensitivity, (4) anti-arrhythmic drugs, and (5) pulse generator malfunction.

Low-amplitude signals can be caused by infarction or fibrosis at the point of contact between the pacemaker lead and the myocardium, or can be due to bundle branch block or signal origin from an ectopic focus. The pacemaker lead may lie in the null plane of an ectopic impulse and may therefore fail to sense the impulse owing to low amplitude of signal. Intrinsic signals may also exhibit a low slew rate. *Slew rate* refers to change in voltage per second: a high-voltage, narrow QRS complex has a higher slew rate than a low-voltage, wide QRS complex. Wide, low-voltage complexes with a poor slew rate may escape detection.

Possible solutions to the problem of undersensing include: (1) increasing the sensitivity of the pulse generator, (2) repositioning the lead, (3) changing bipolar sensing and pacing to unipolar sensing and pacing, and (4) correcting metabolic disturbances and serum drug levels. Acidosis, hypoxia, hyperkalemia and hyperglycemia may alter both pacing and sensing thresholds.

Functional undersensing occurs when an intrinsic event falls within a refractory period. A premature atrial extrasystole that falls within the PVARP will not be sensed. Some DDD pacemakers perform *mode switching*, automatically switching from one mode to another in the event of atrial tachyarrhythmia. Mode switching prevents the pacemaker from tracking atrial events until the tachycardia reverts to sinus rhythm.

Oversensing occurs when signals other than P waves or QRS complexes are sensed. The result is underpacing due to inappropriate inhibition. Causes include (1) sensing of physiologic voltage such as T waves or skeletal muscle potentials, (2) electromagnetic interference, (3) static electricity, (4) after-potentials from the pulse generator itself, and (5) lead fracture. Placing a magnet over the pulse generator inactivates the sensing mechanism, causing the pacemaker to fire asynchronously at a fixed predetermined rate called the *magnet rate*, which may help uncover the source of oversensing.

Possible solutions to the problem of oversensing include: (1) temporarily converting the pacemaker to asynchronous pacing, (2) prolonging the refractory period of the pulse generator, (3) increasing the sensitivity, or (4) decreasing the pulse width. If lead fracture is the cause of oversensing, magnet application will result in regularization of the pacemaker spikes. Failure to capture during magnet application will confirm the presence of lead fracture.

Failure to capture occurs when pacemaker impulses fail to elicit depolarization. This may be due to (1) lead displacement, (2) increase in the pacing threshold, (3) myocardial necrosis or fibrosis at the interface between the lead and the heart muscle, (4) anti-arrhythmic drugs, (5) lead fracture, (6) inappropriate programming such as inadequate pulse width, current or voltage, or (7) battery depletion.

Possible solutions to failure to capture include (1) increasing the pacemaker's output, (2) repositioning the pacing lead, and (3) correcting metabolic and/or serum drug levels. Pacer malfunction may occur if the patient fondles or manipulates a subcutaneously implanted pacemaker ('pacemaker twiddler's syndrome').

Pacemaker-related complications

Pacing from the right ventricle produces a precordial pattern of left bundle branch block because depolarization moves sequentially from right to left. Pacing from the right ventricular apex will move the mean QRS axis superiorly. Pacing from the right ventricular outflow tract will result in normalization of the QRS axis and the appearance of QR complexes in the lateral leads (I and aVL) and a dominant R wave in the inferior leads.

Right bundle branch block morphology during right ventricular pacing is abnormal. This finding occurs owing to (1) inadvertent pacing from the coronary sinus, (2) lead movement from the right to the left ventricle due to septal perforation, (3) endocardial pacing of the left ventricle due to inadvertent cannulation of the subclavian artery instead of the subclavian vein, or (4) endocardial pacing of the left ventricle due to passage of the pacemaking lead through a patent foramen ovale or atrial septal defect.

Transvenous pacemaker implantation can cause a number of complications including pneumothorax, air embolism, inadvertent arterial puncture, arteriovenous fistula, thoracic duct injury, subcutaneous emphysema, brachial plexus injury, infection, hematoma formation, thrombosis, and cardiac perforation with tamponade. Following placement, pocket erosion through the skin may occur.

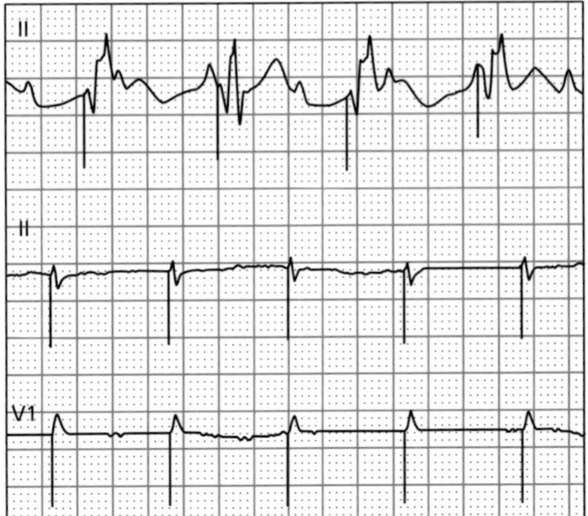

Figure 16.5 Electronic decay curves: third-degree atrioventricular block with a ventricular pacemaker (upper strip). After the patient's demise, pacemaker spikes continue to produce deflections (lower two strips). *These are not QRS complexes*!

Electronic decay curves are small deflections that follow the pacing spike (Figure 16.5). They are most commonly noted during failure to capture or during asystole. It is imperative to distinguish electronic decay curves from QRS complexes. Decay curves, which may be mistaken for responses to pacing, are not followed by T waves.

Implantable cardioverter–defibrillators

The *implantable cardioverter–defibrillator* (ICD) is an anti-arrhythmic device used in conjunction with a pacemaker. It is typically implanted subcutaneously in the anterior chest. All ICD systems incorporate overdrive anti-tachycardia pacing (ATP) and ventricular pacing for bradycardia (Figure 16.6).

The following are well-recognized indications for ICD implantation: (1) ejection fraction of less than 35%, (2) cardiac arrest due to ventricular fibrillation or ventricular tachycardia not due to a reversible cause, (3) sustained ventricular tachycardia with structural heart disease, (4) syncope or hemodynamically significant ventricular tachycardia inducible at electrophysiologic study, (5) nonsustained ventricular tachycardia in subjects with coronary artery disease, prior myocardial infarction, an ejection fraction less than 40% and inducible ventricular fibrillation or tachycardia, and (6) familial or hereditary conditions with a high risk for tachyarrhythmias (long QT syndromes, hypertrophic cardiomyopathy).

The ICD may be programmed to deliver a shock when the heart rate exceeds a set limit or delivers ventricular pacing impulses at a rate faster than the patient's tachycardia. If the interval between paced beats is constant, the technique is called *burst pacing*; if the interval shortens, it is called *ramp pacing*. If the pacing interval decreases from one pacing sequence to the next, but remains constant during that sequence, it is called *scan pacing*.

External defibrillation can be safely performed on a patient with an ICD provided the external paddles are kept at least 4 inches away from the pulse generator. An anterior-posterior paddle position is preferred. The pacemaker should be interrogated

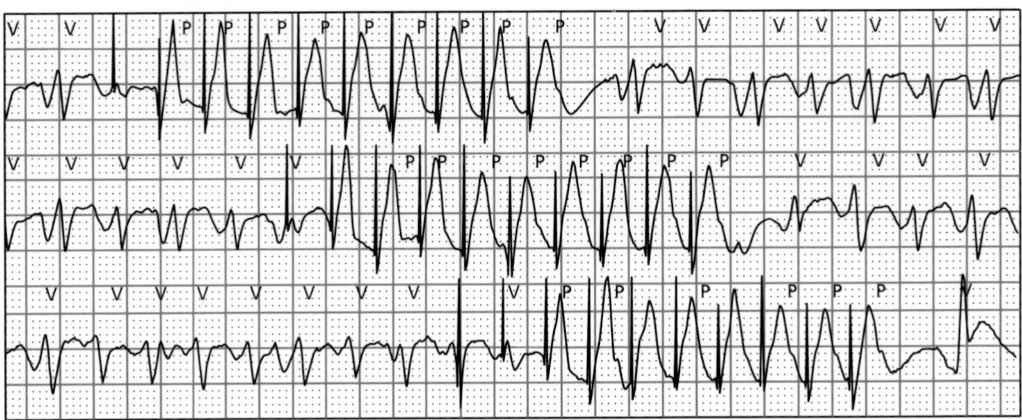

Figure 16.6 Overdrive pacing of ventricular tachycardia. Three bursts of overdrive pacing are delivered before the tachycardia abates.

after cardioversion or defibrillation. ICDs should be deactivated prior to the use of electrocautery. If the patient is pacemaker dependent, the device can be reprogrammed into asynchronous mode. The device should be interrogated and reprogrammed postoperatively.

Magnetic resonance imaging (MRI) scans are relatively contraindicated in patients with ICDs. Flecainide and propafenone may increase pacing and sensing thresholds and increase the defibrillation threshold (DFT). Amiodarone can also increase the DFT. Metabolic abnormalities such as hyperkalemia, acidosis, alkalosis, hypoxemia, hypercapnia and hyperglycemia can change thresholds.

Multiple ICD shocks can be caused by (1) frequent tachycardia or fibrillation ('electrical storm'), (2) failed therapy due to inappropriately low-output shocks or an increase in the defibrillation threshold, (3) lead fracture or displacement, (4) detection of supraventricular arrhythmias, particularly atrial fibrillation, and (5) oversensing of far-field events such as P or T waves or electromagnetic interference.

Self-Assessment Test Six

6.1. Identify the abnormality in the following tracing.

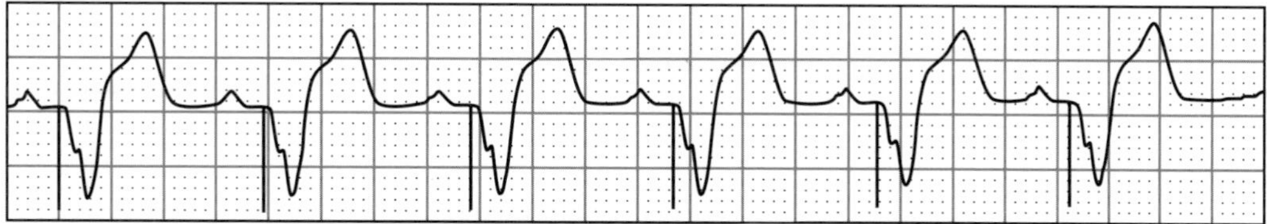

6.2. Identify the abnormality in the following tracing.

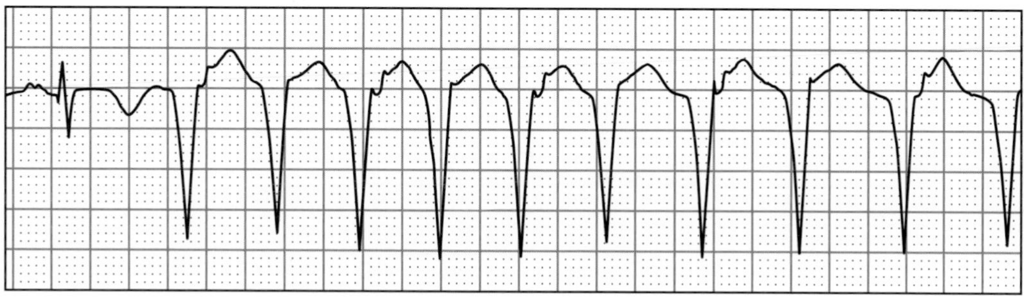

6.3. What is the deflection marked by the arrow? What is its mechanism?

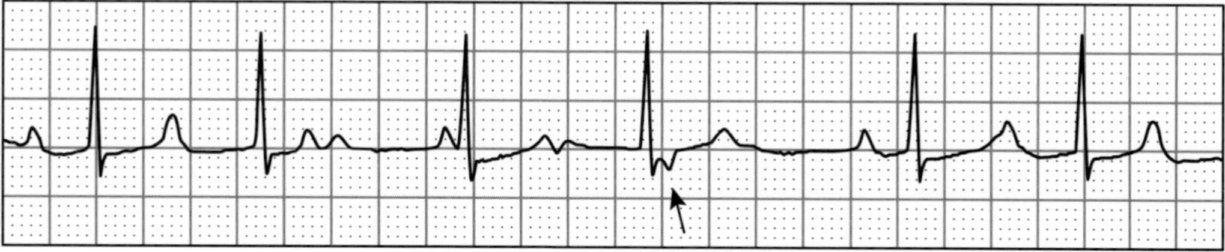

6.4. Identify the abnormality in the following tracing.

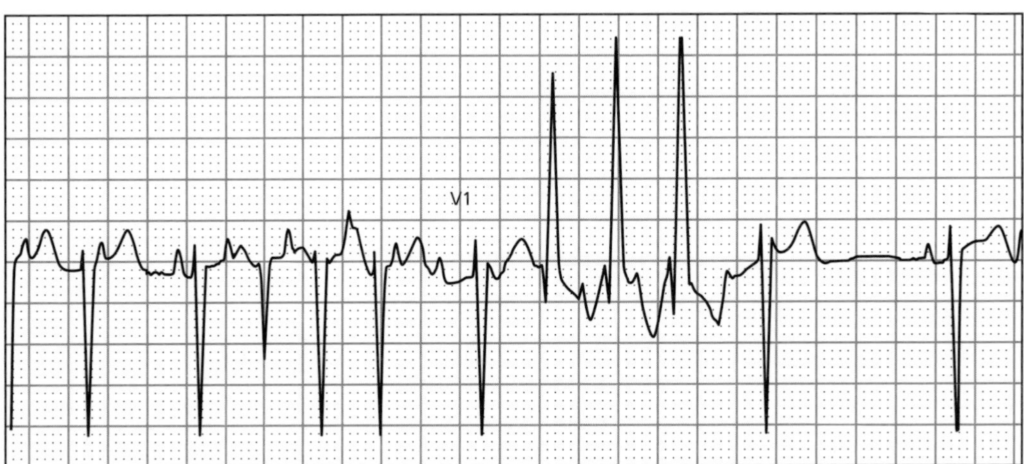

6.5. The inserts show the patient in sinus rhythm. What is the mechanism of the tachycardia?

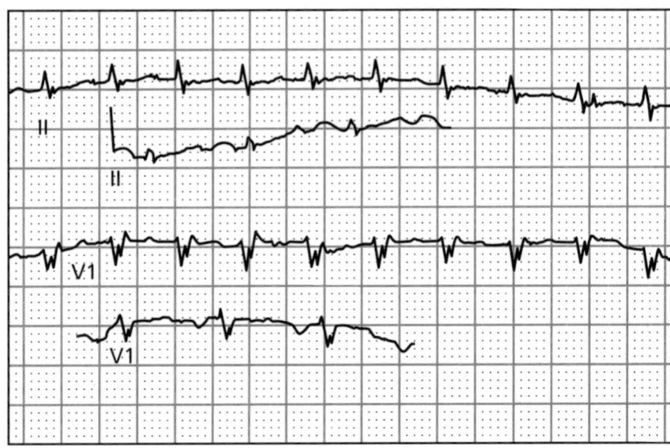

Identify the abnormalities in the following three tracings.

6.6.

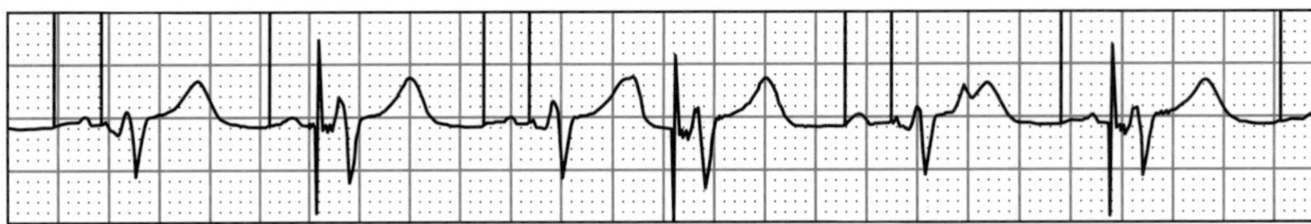

6.7.

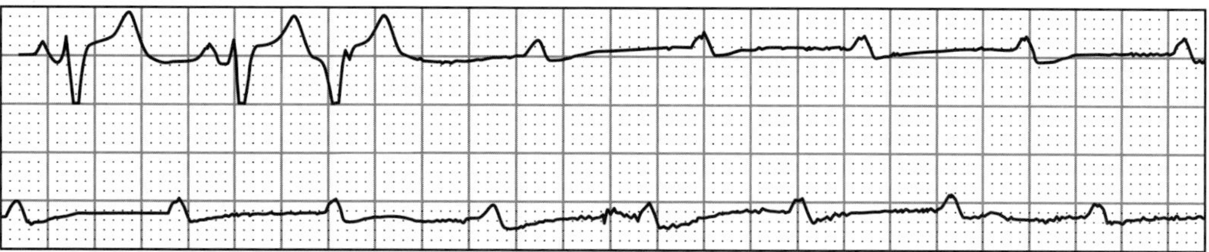

6.8.

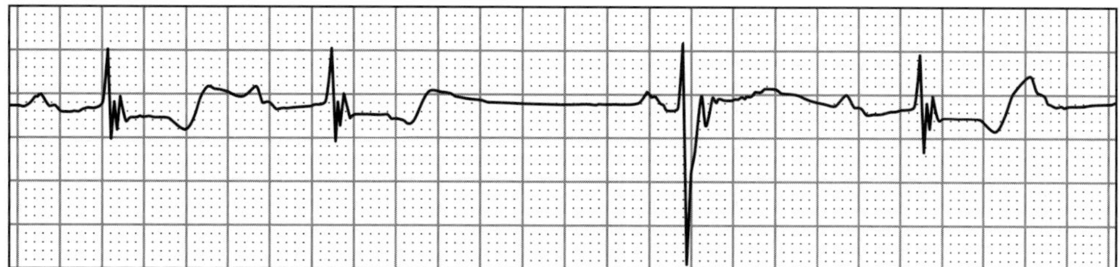

6.9. Ventricular tachycardia that utilizes the left posterior fascicle for antegrade conduction will exhibit . . .

a. left bundle branch block morphology with superior axis
b. right bundle branch block morphology with inferior axis
c. right bundle branch block morphology with superior axis

6.10. Polymorphic ventricular tachycardia in subjects with Brugada syndrome is most likely to be triggered . . .

a. during sleep
b. during exercise
c. by loud noise

6.11. To increase the sensitivity of a pacemaker the setting in . . . must be . . .

a. millivolts . . . decreased
b. milliamperes . . . increased
c. millivolts . . . increased

6.12. Right ventricular outflow tract (RVOT) ventricular tachycardia typically exhibits . . .

a. right bundle branch block morphology with inferior axis
b. left bundle branch block morphology with inferior axis
c. left bundle branch block morphology with superior axis

6.13. Catecholaminergic polymorphic ventricular tachycardia is triggered by . . . and is implicated in death due to . . .

a. loud noises, startle reactions
b. exercise, drowning
c. sleep, apnea

6.14. 'VAT' means the pacemaker . . .

a. senses the atrium and responds to an atrial impulse by pacing the ventricle
b. senses the ventricle and responds by pacing the ventricle if no intrinsic impulse is sensed
c. will overdrive ventricular tachycardia

Identify the abnormalities in the following three tracings.

6.15.

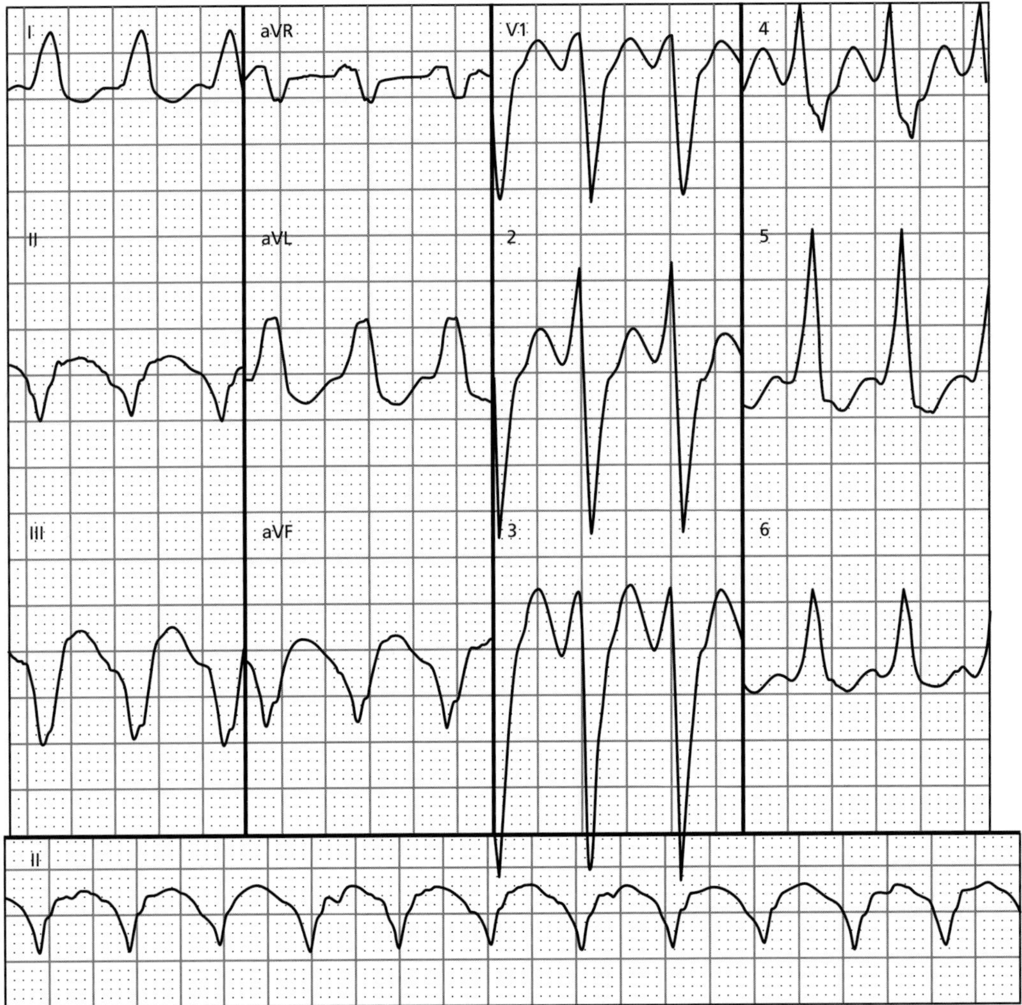

6.16.

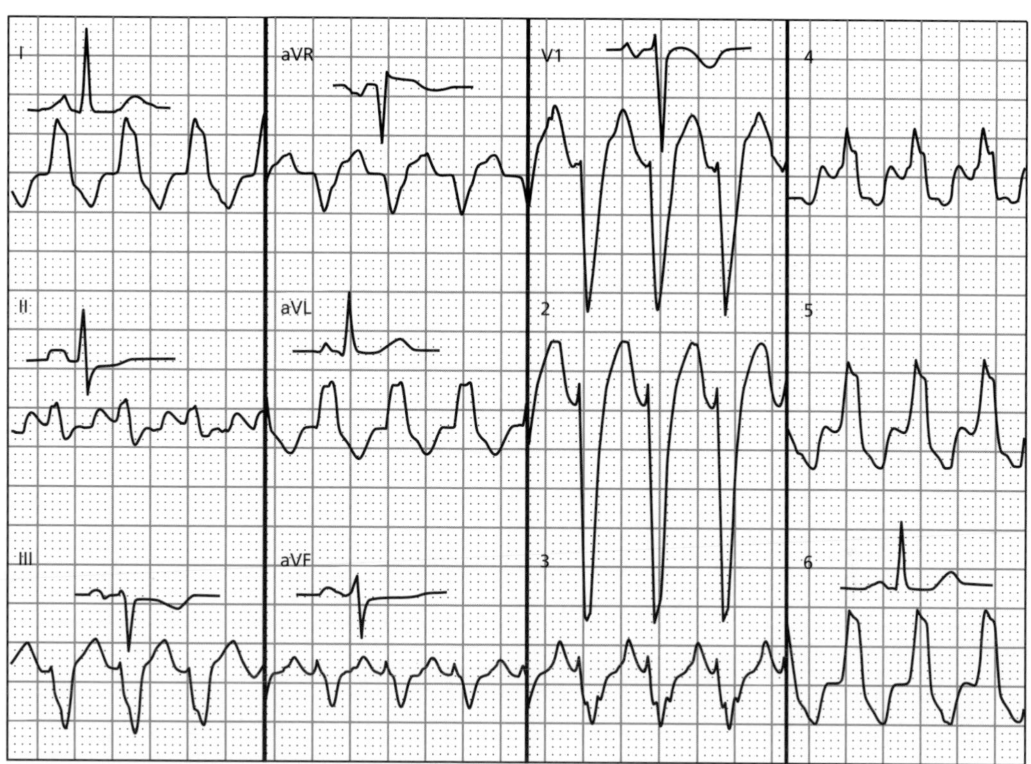

6.17.

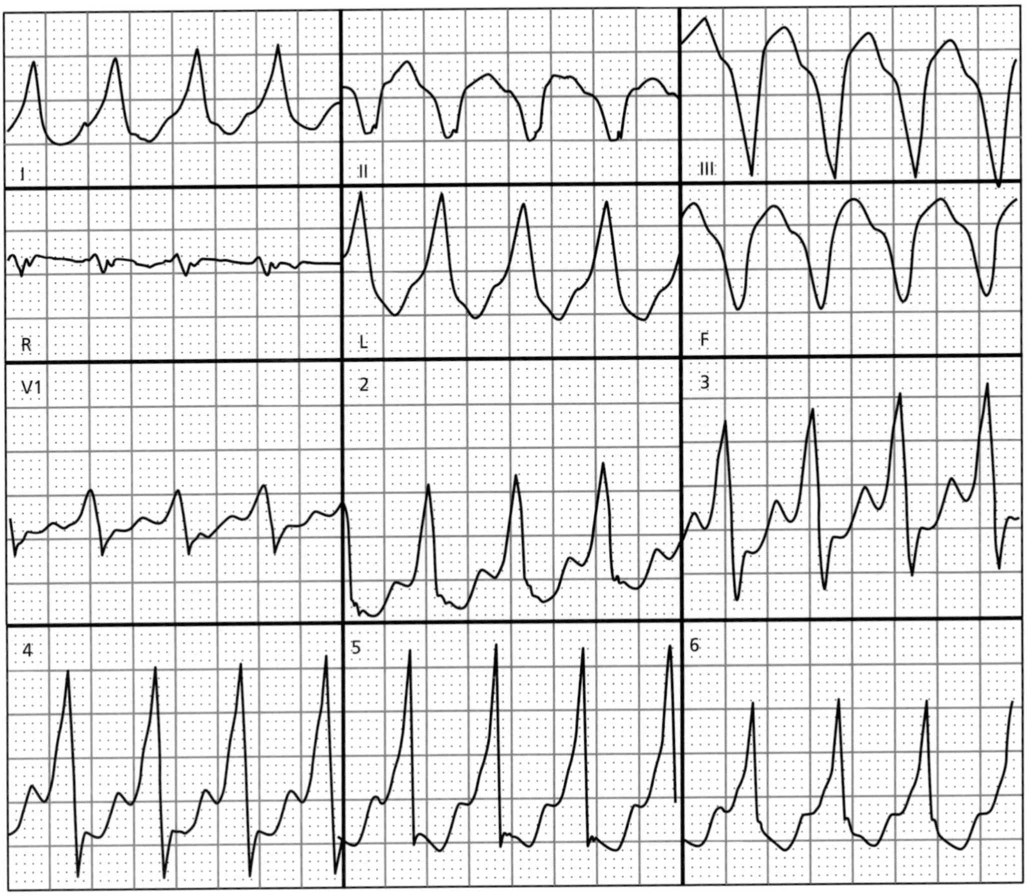

6.18. A 42-year-old female with repetitive polymorphic ventricular tachycardia is seen in the emergency department. This is her ECG in lead II:

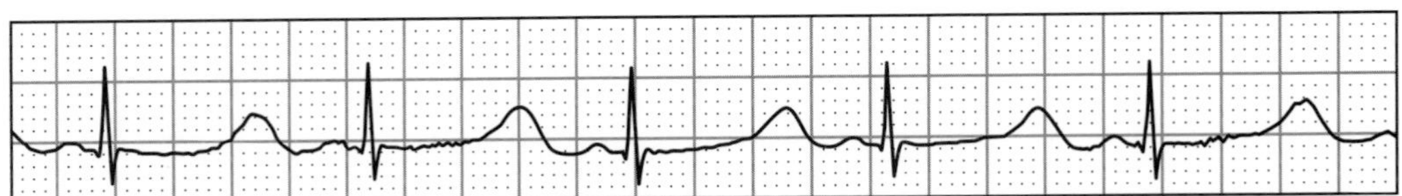

The drug of choice for her arrhythmia will be . . .

a. procainamide
b. amiodarone
c. magnesium sulfate

Identify the abnormalities in the following eight tracings.

6.19.

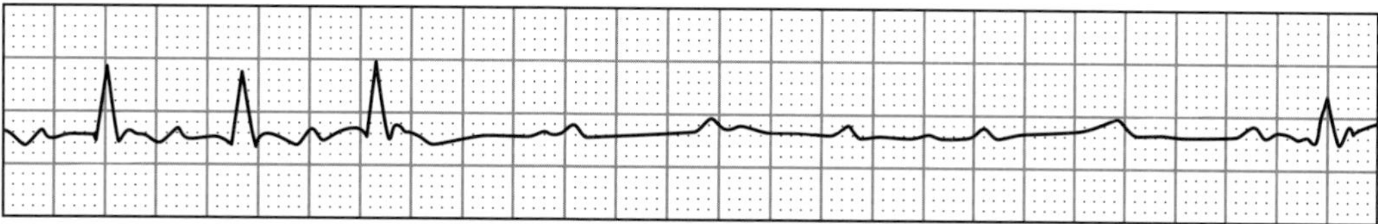

6.20.

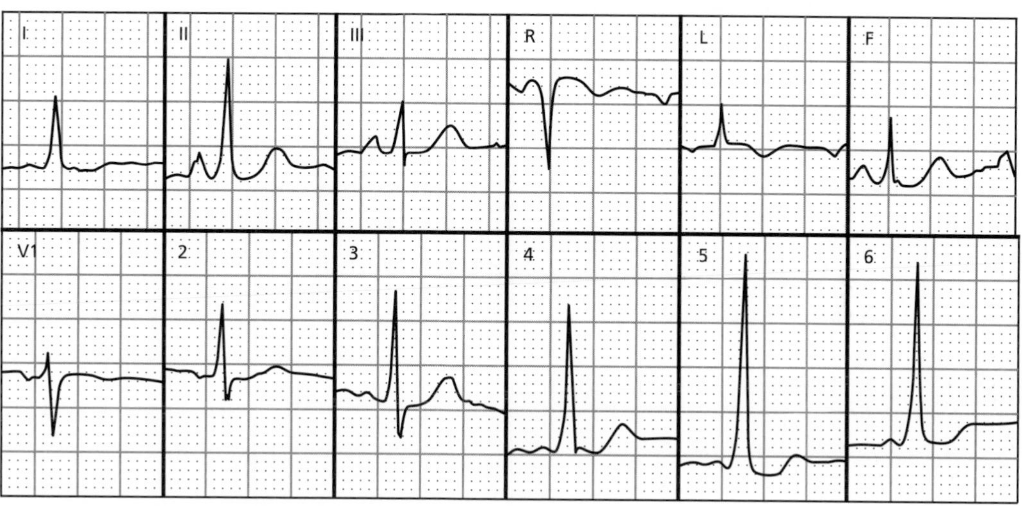

6.21.

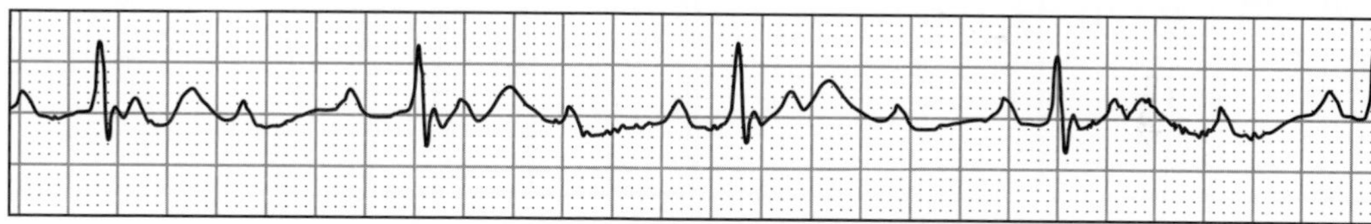

6.22.

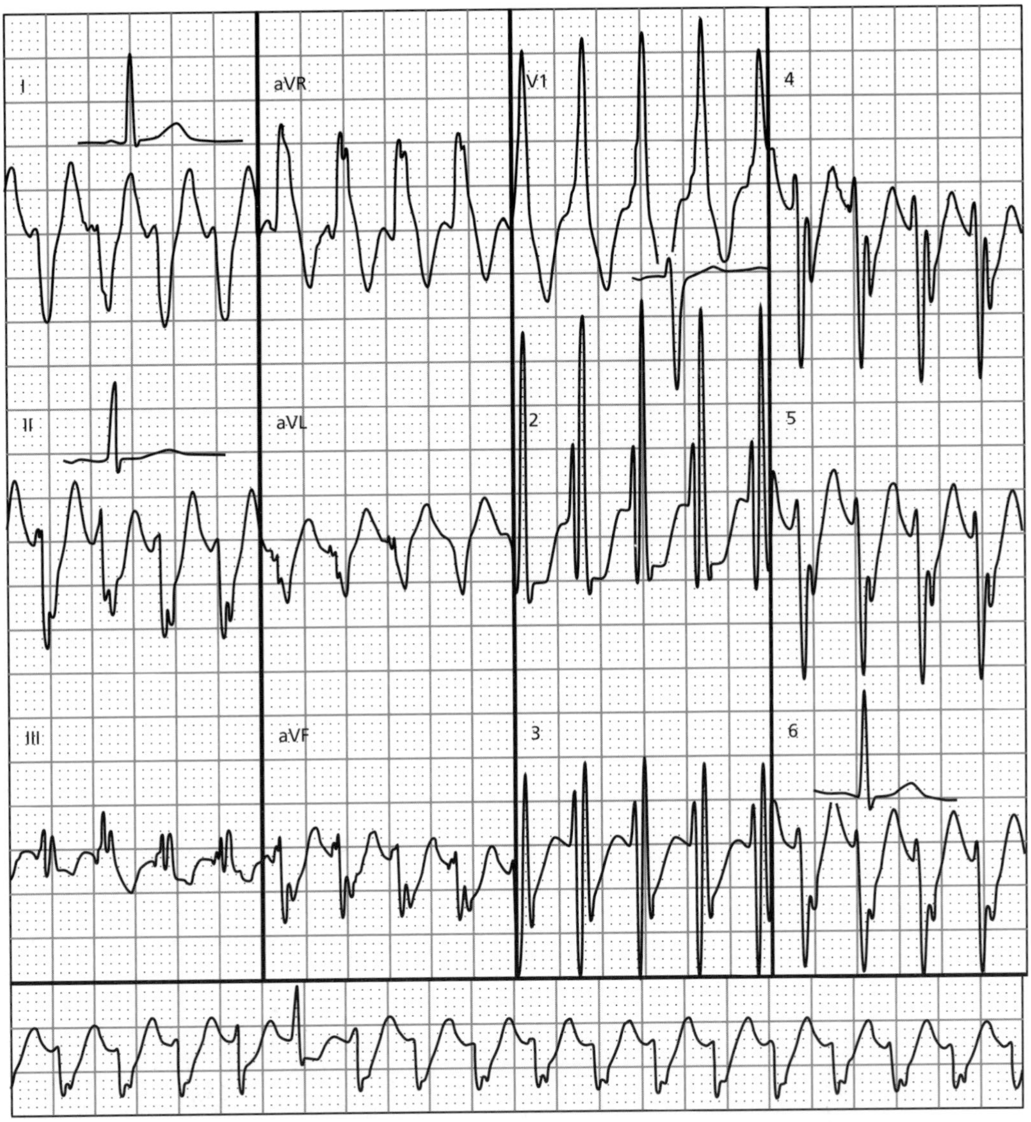

6.23.

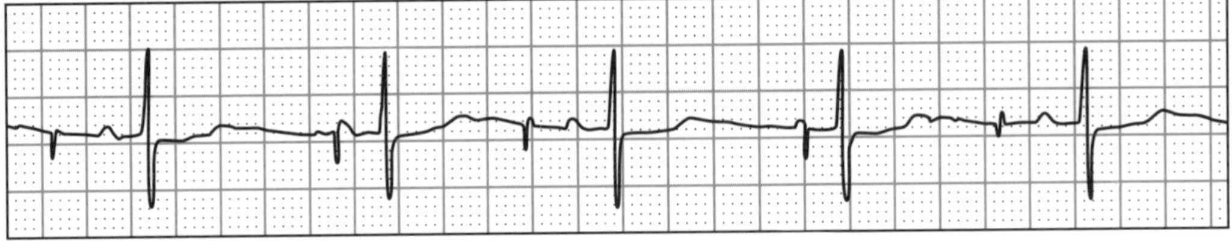

6.24.

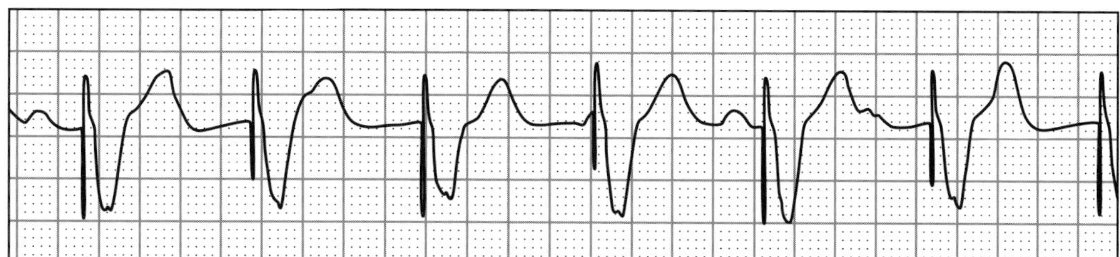

6.25.

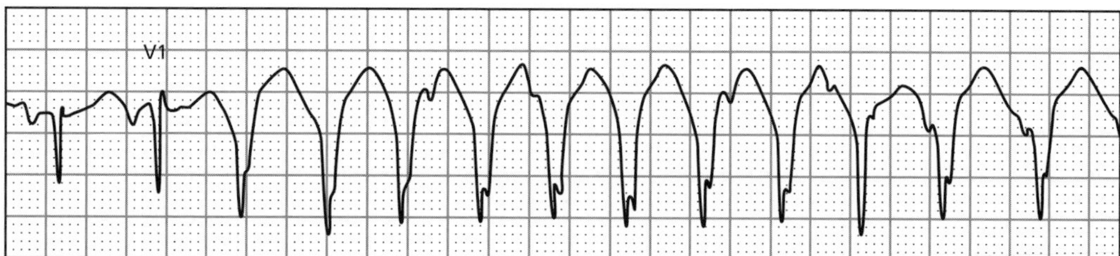

6.26.

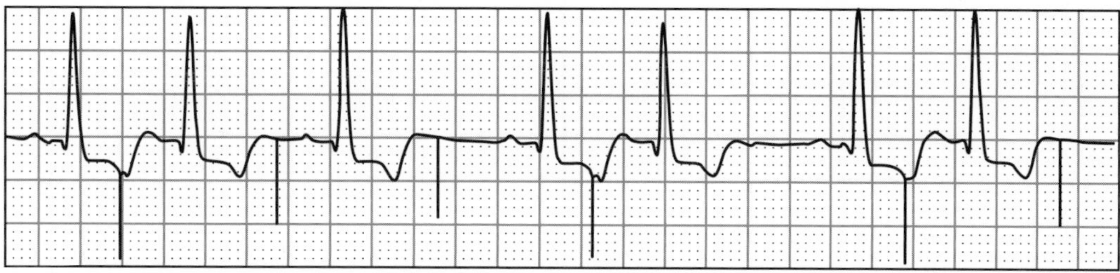

6.27. A supraventricular tachycardia with RP > PR (lead II) is shown. How many possible mechanisms for this arrhythmia can you list?

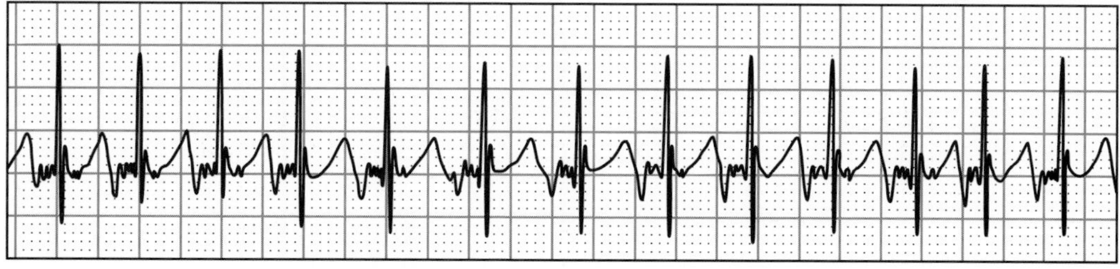

6.28. Variable coupling intervals, interectopic intervals that are multiples of a common denominator, and fusion beating are signs of . . .

a. concealed junctional extrasystoles
b. parasystolic rhythm
c. exit block

6.29. Right bundle branch block morphology, J point elevation greater than 2 mm, and ST segment coving in leads V1–V3 constitute . . .

a. Wellen's sign
b. an Osborne wave
c. Brugada's sign

6.30. Apparent second-degree type I and type II block in the same tracing or random variation of PR intervals is consistent with a diagnosis of . . .

a. concealed junctional extrasystoles

b. parasystolic junctional rhythm

c. concealed atrioventricular re-entry

6.31. You are given a tracing that shows a wide QRS complex tachycardia with left bundle branch morphology. Which observation is **not** suggestive of ventricular tachycardia?

a. The interval from the beginning of the QRS complex to the nadir of the S wave is 20 milliseconds.

b. There is notching on the downslope of the S wave.

c. The initial R wave is greater than 30 milliseconds in duration.

Identify the abnormalities in the following eight tracings.

6.32.

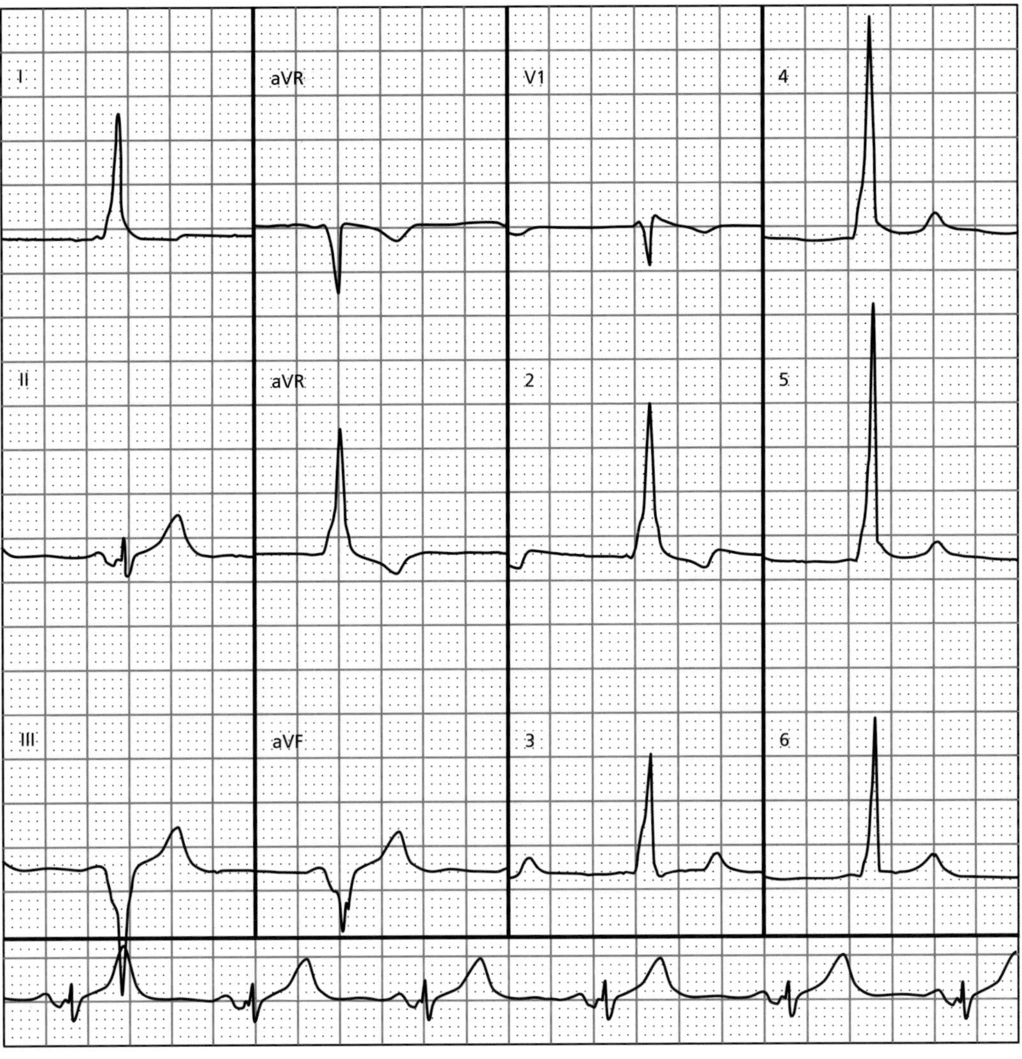

6.33.

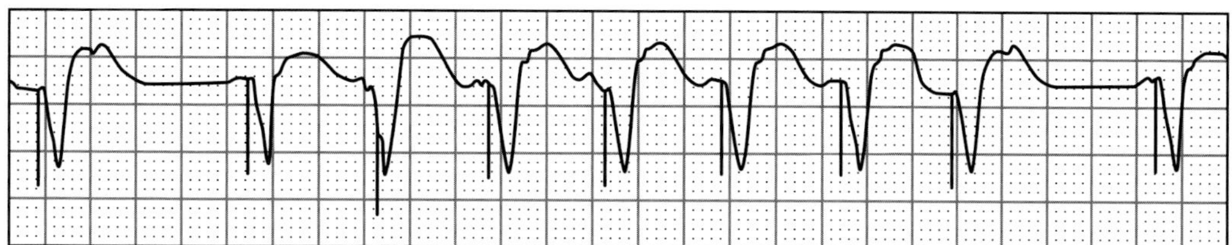

6.34.

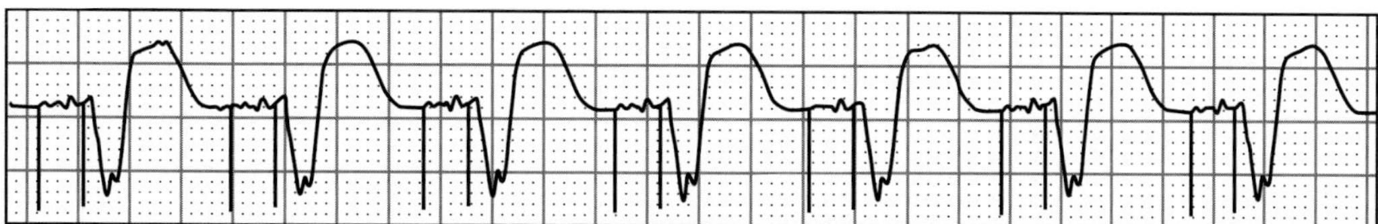

6.35.

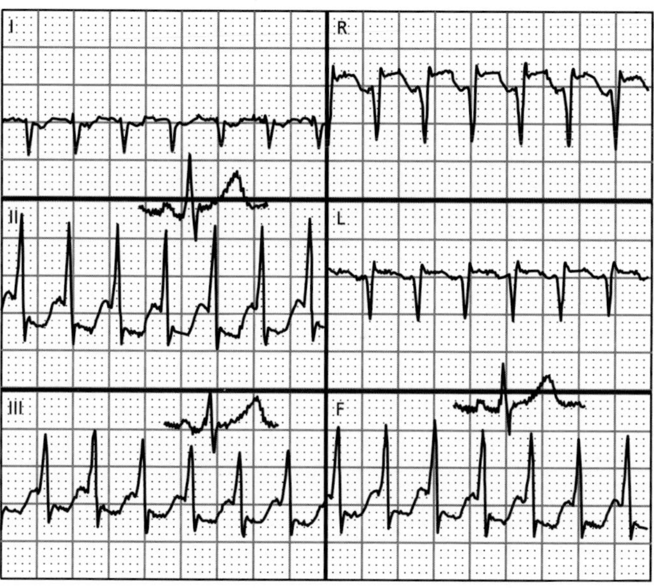

6.36.

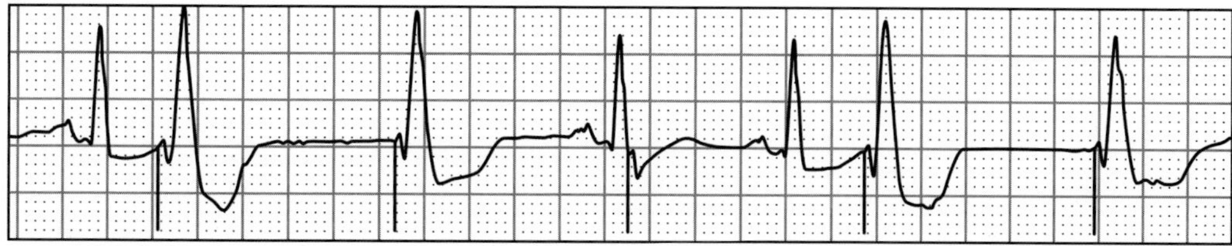

6.37.

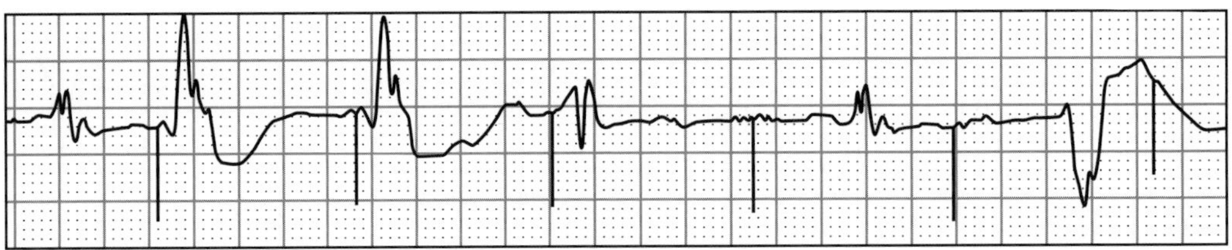

6.38.

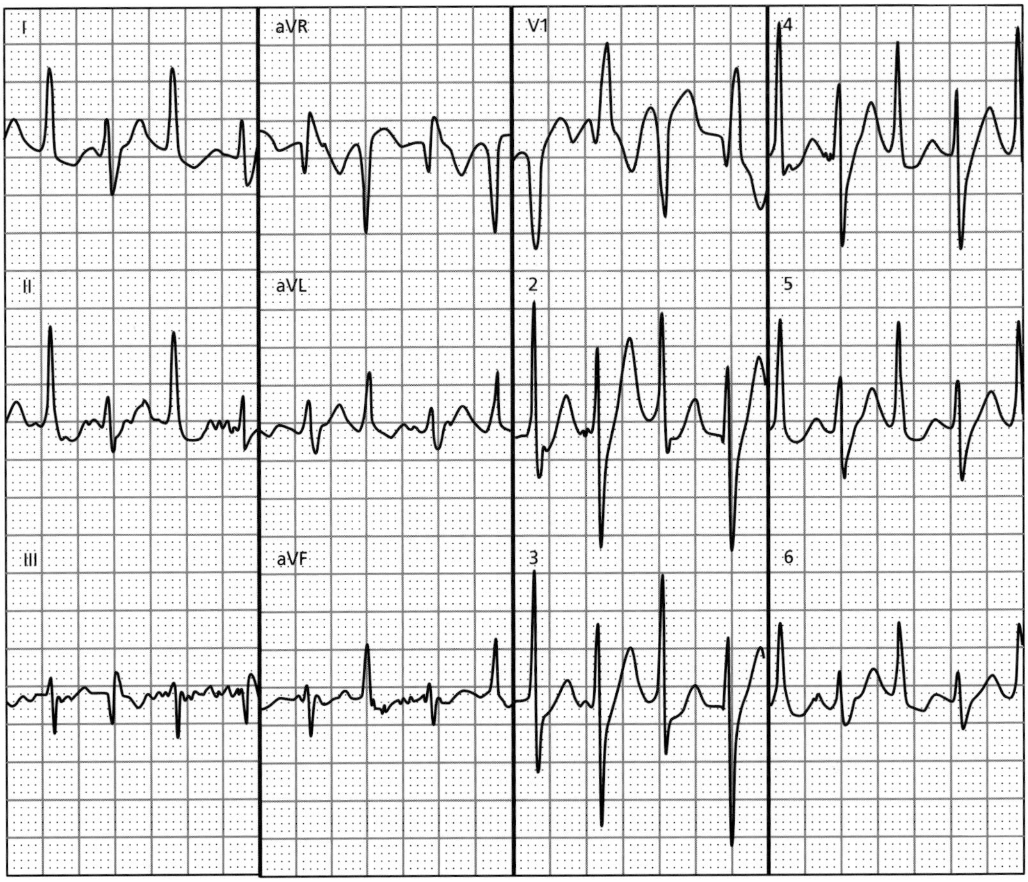

6.39.

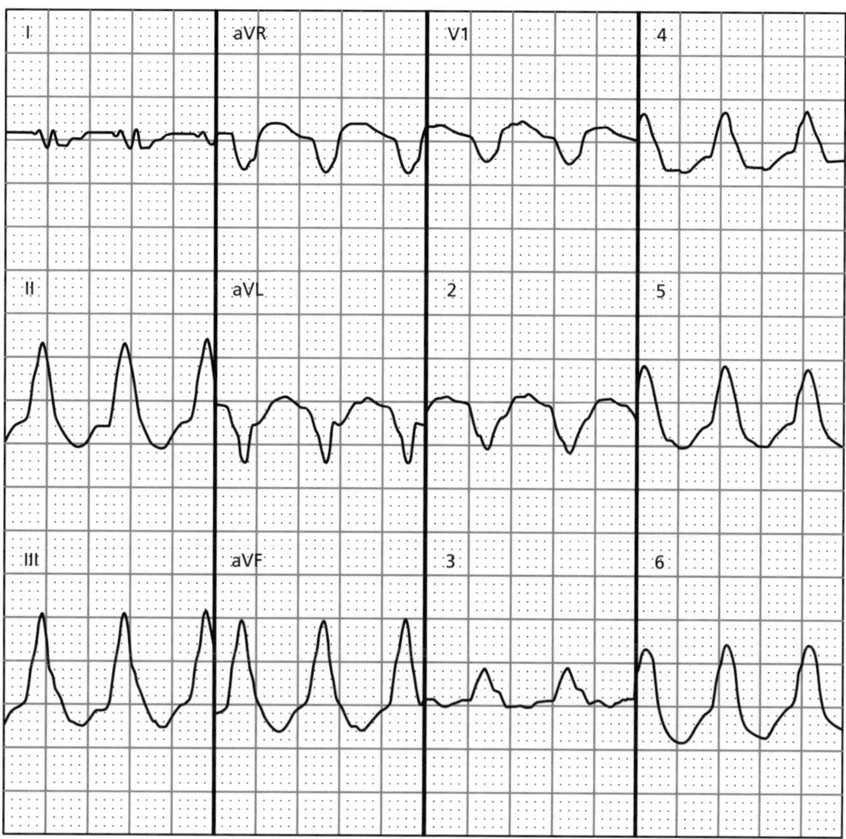

6.40. A 74-year-old male admitted three days ago with an anteroseptal infarction developed third-degree atrioventricular block requiring emergency placement of a transvenous pacemaker. The routine electrocardiogram obtained this morning shows paced ventricular rhythm at 70 per minute with right bundle branch block morphology in lead V1. Which of the following conclusions is **least** likely?

a. The pacing electrode is in the right ventricle
b. The pacing electrode was placed into the coronary sinus
c. The pacing electrode has eroded through the septum into the left ventricle

6.41. Identify the abnormality in the following tracing.

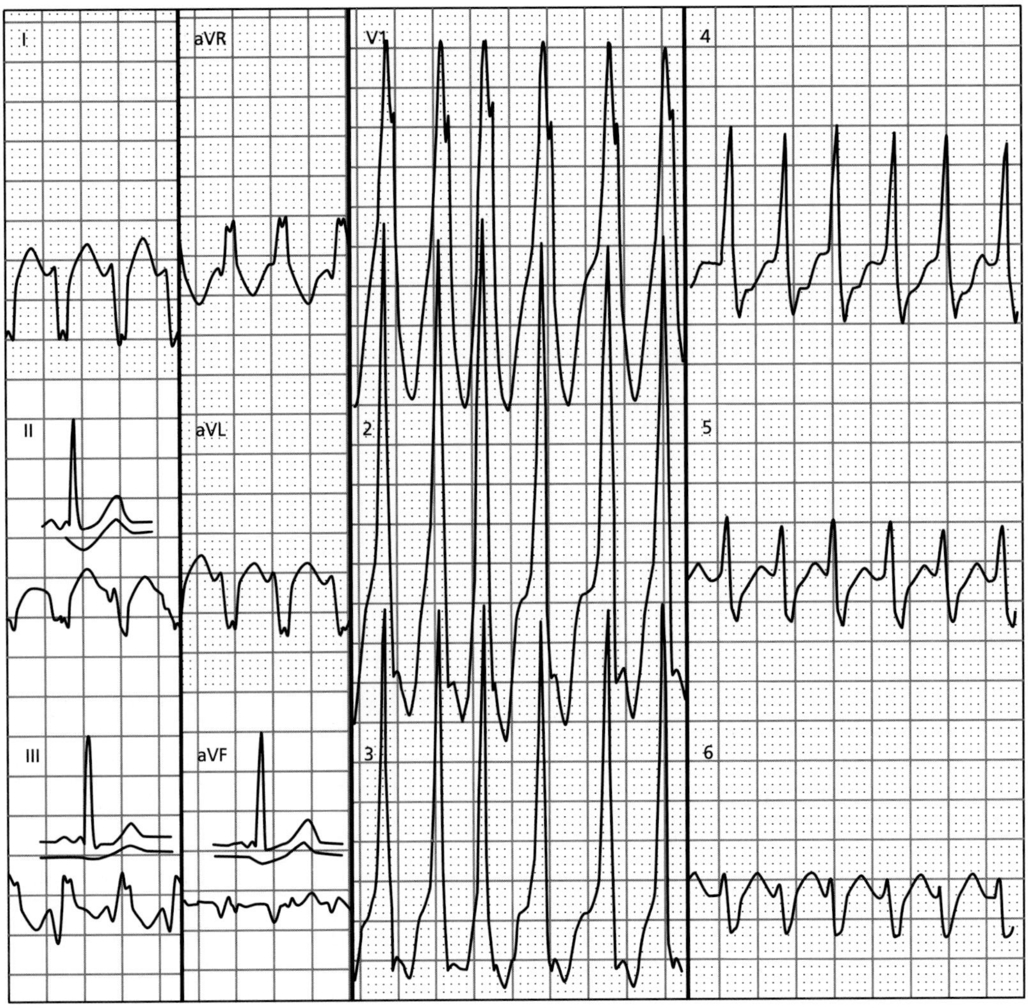

6.42. Identify the pacemaker in use in the following tracing.

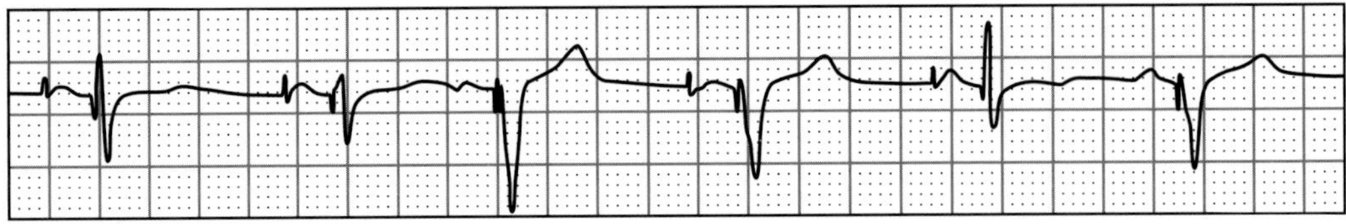

6.43. A 32-year-old woman presents with congestive failure and cardiomyopathy. A section of her ECG tracing is reproduced below. What is the most likely diagnosis?

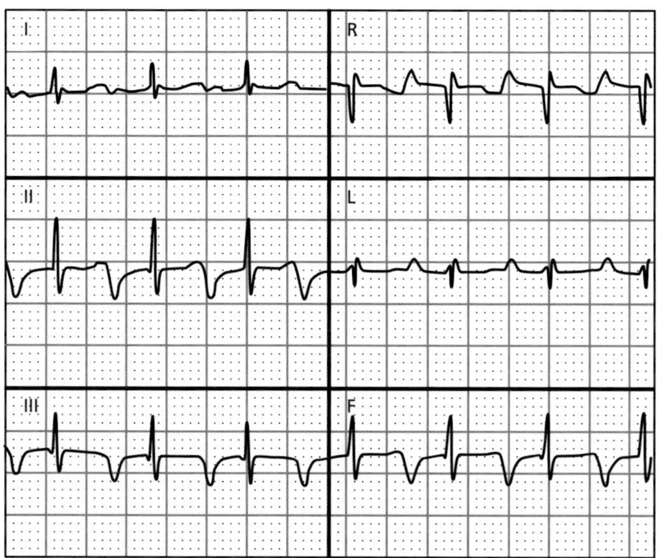

Identify the abnormalities in the following seven tracings.

6.44.

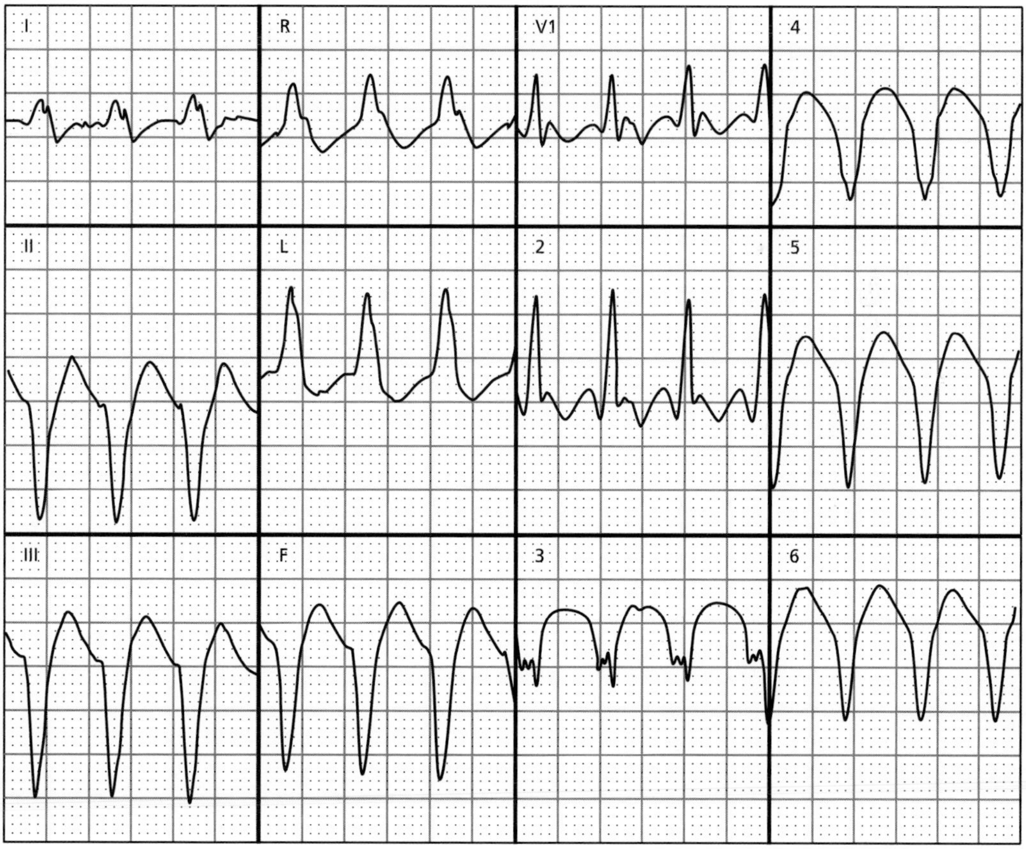

6.45.

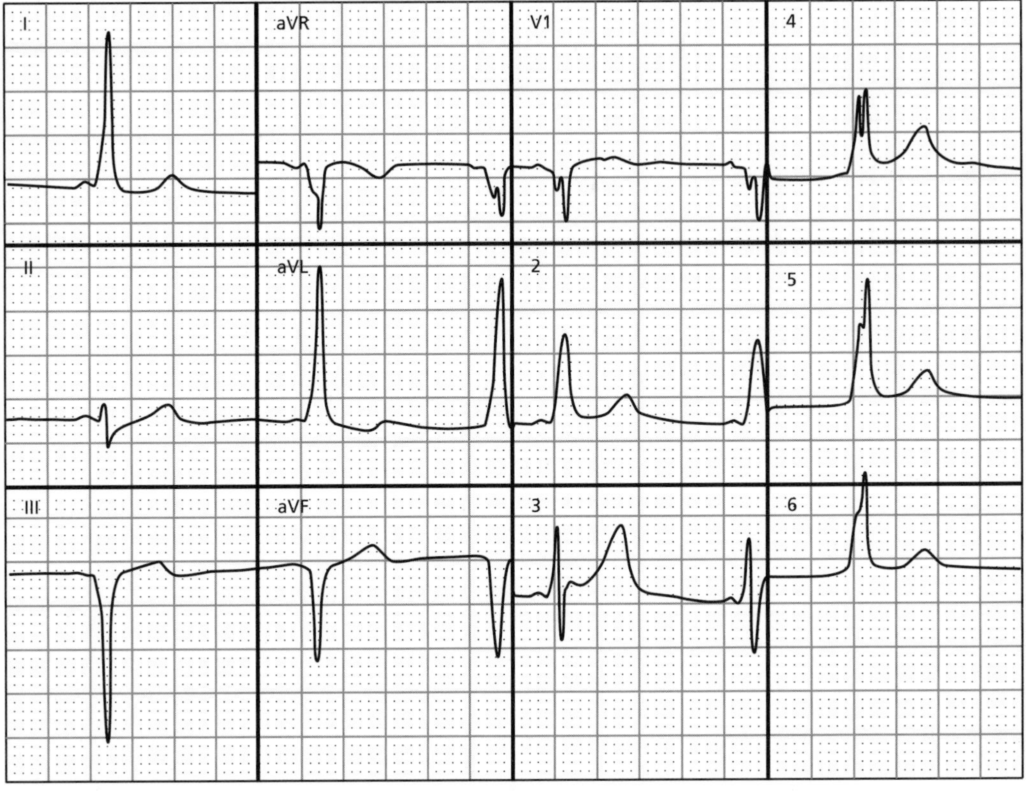

6.46.

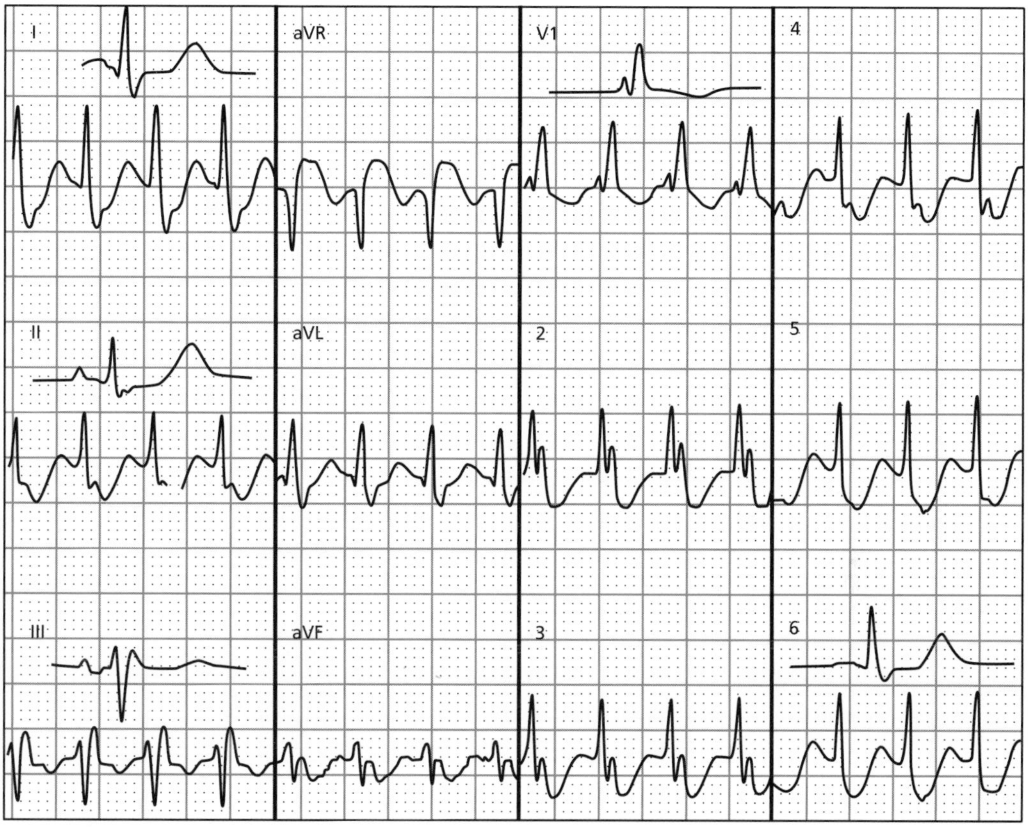

6.47.

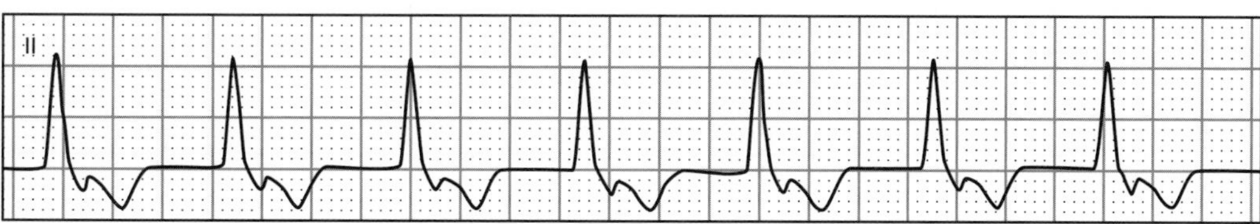

6.48.

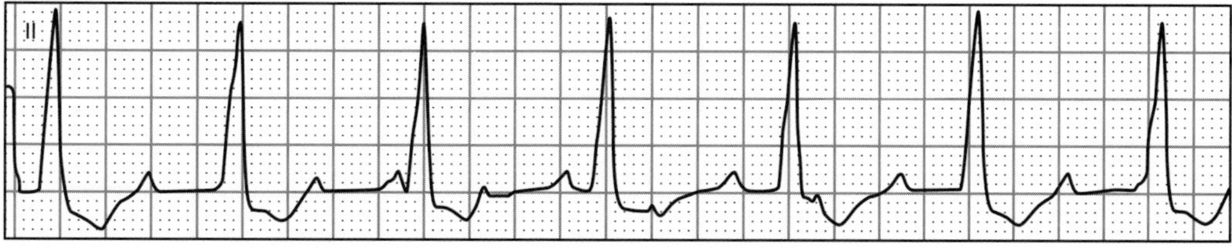

6.49.

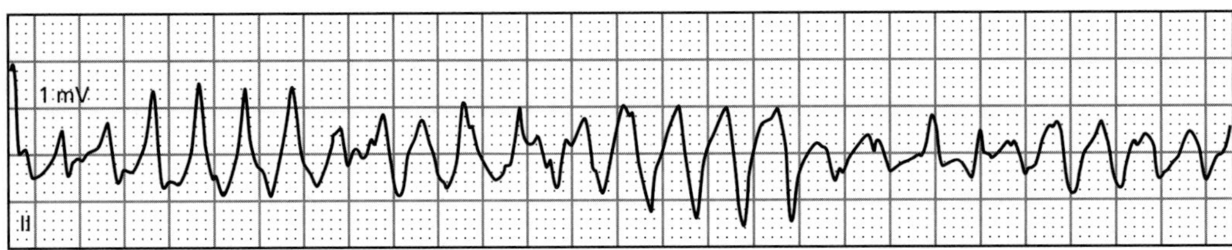

6.50.

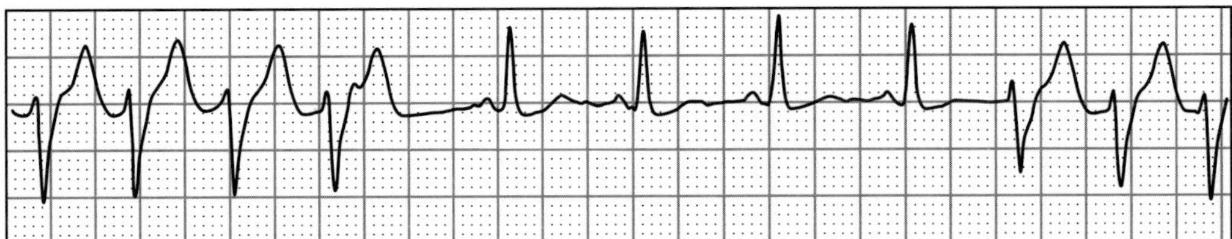

6.51. Three conduction abnormalities are present (lead II). Can you identify them?

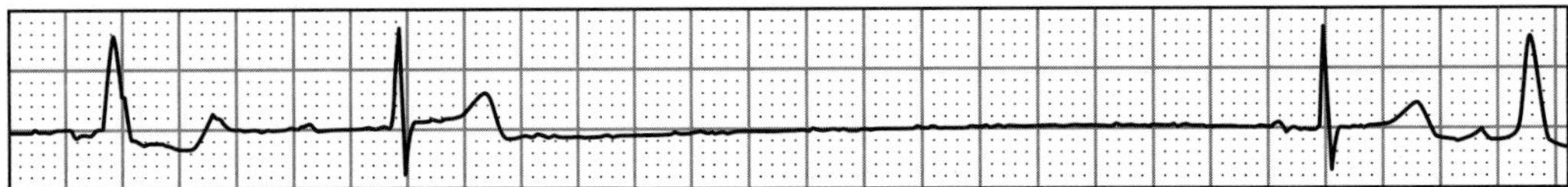

6.52. What are the atrioventricular conduction ratios of the flutter shown below?

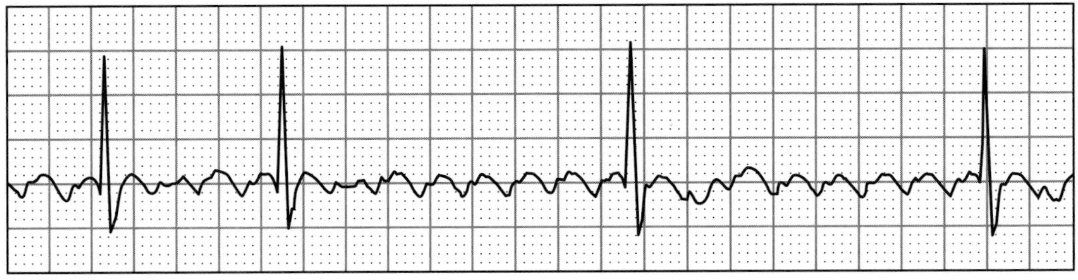

Identify the abnormalities in the following three tracings.

6.53.

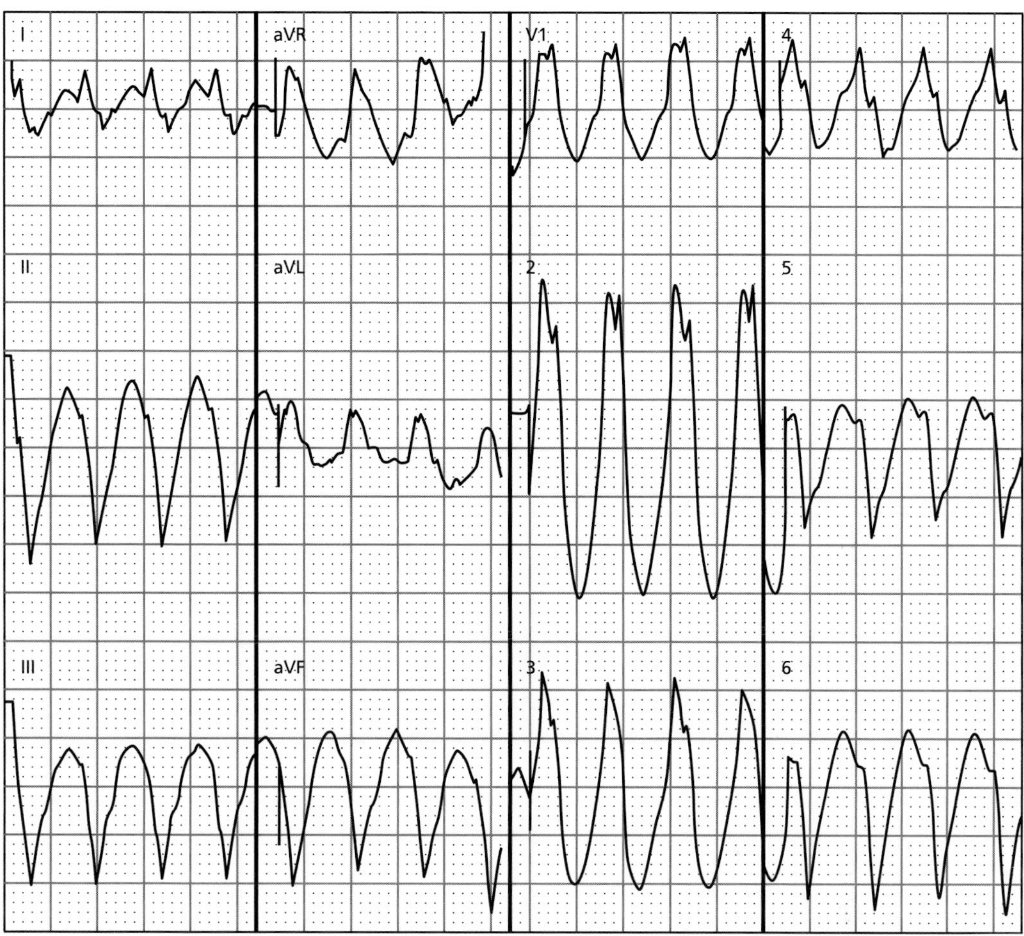

6.54.

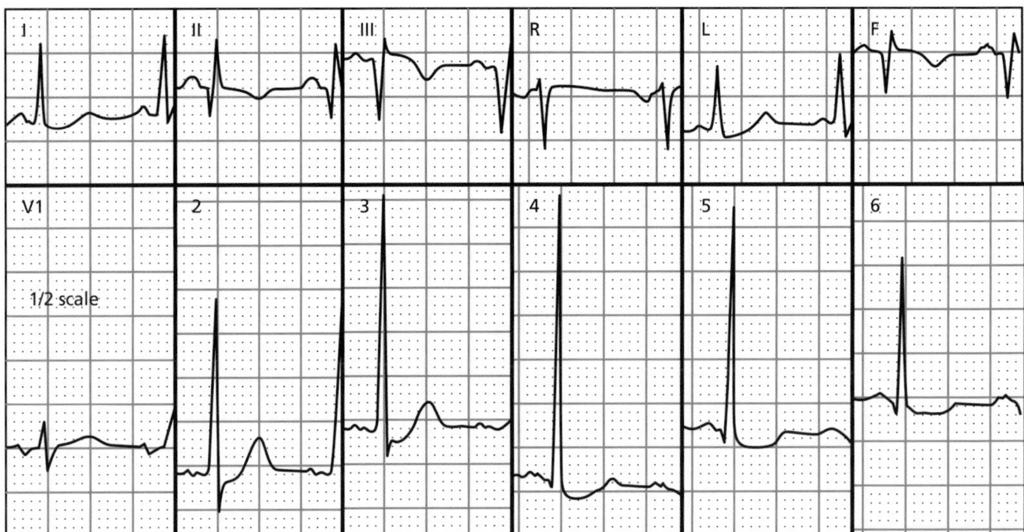
I
II
III
R
L
F
V1
1/2 scale
2
3
4
5
6

6.55.

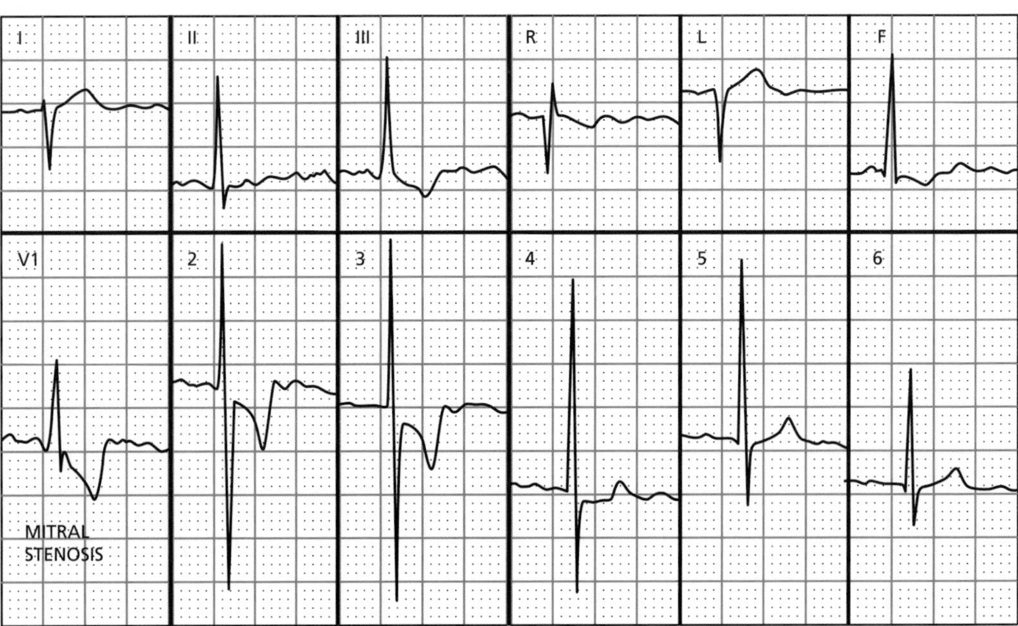
I
II
III
R
L
F
V1
MITRAL
STENOSIS
2
3
4
5
6

6.56. What causes the R–R intervals in the rhythm strip to shorten?

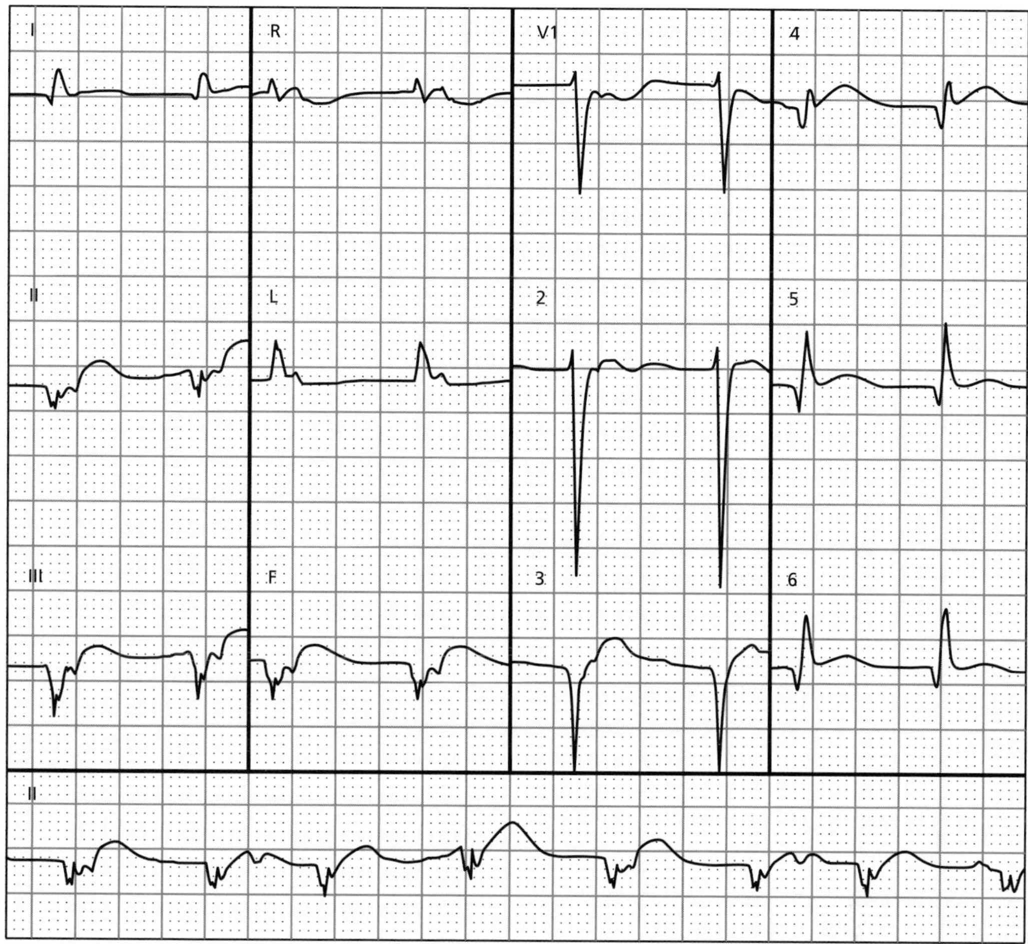

Identify the abnormalities in the following four tracings.

6.57.

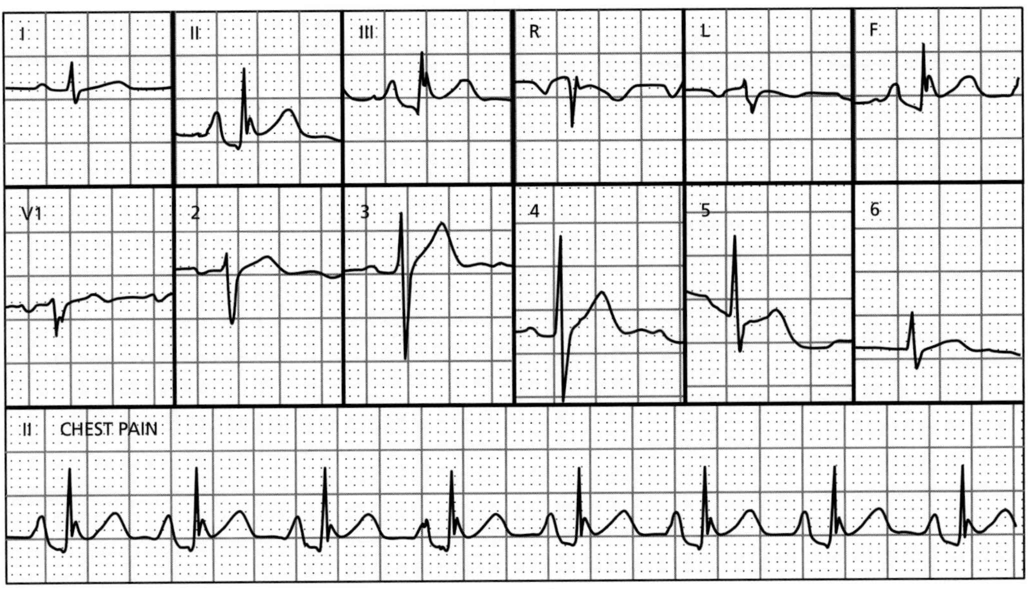

6.58.

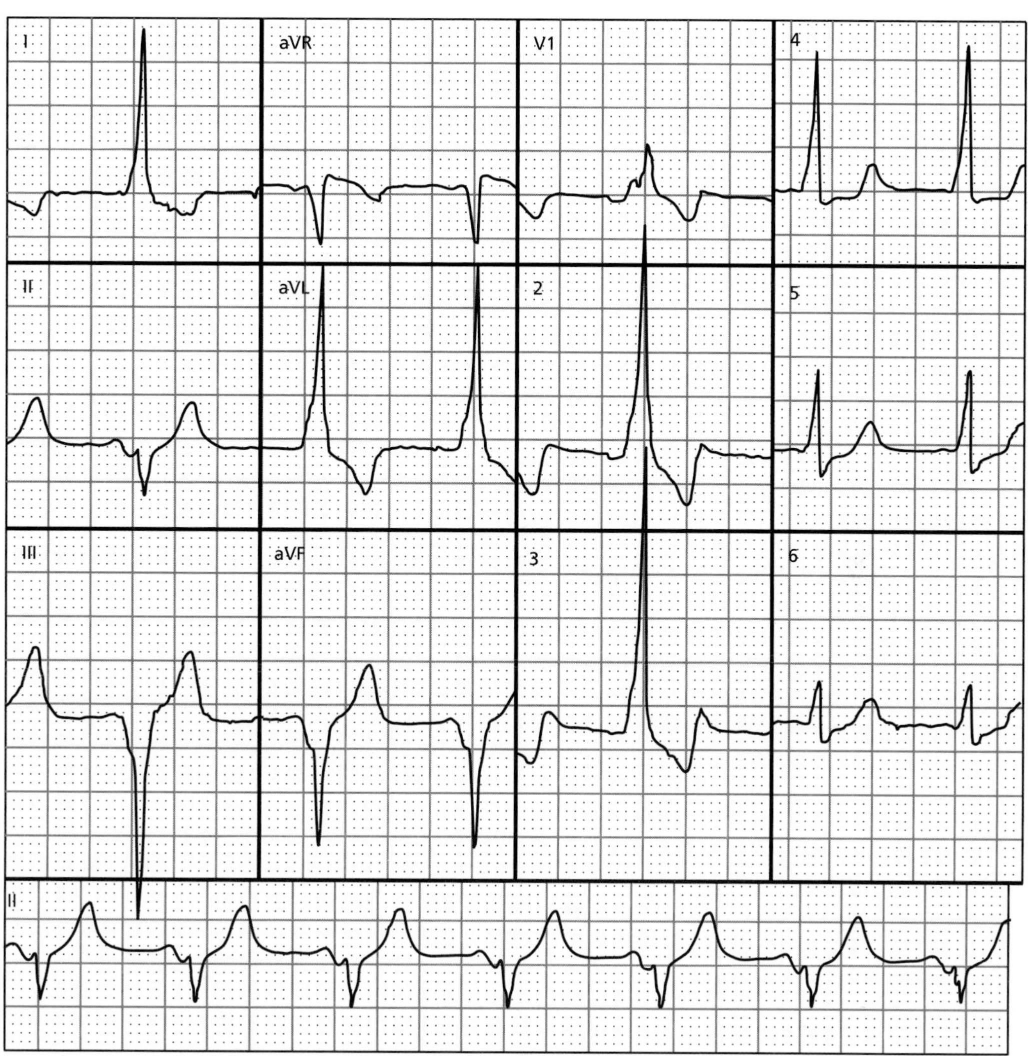

6.59.

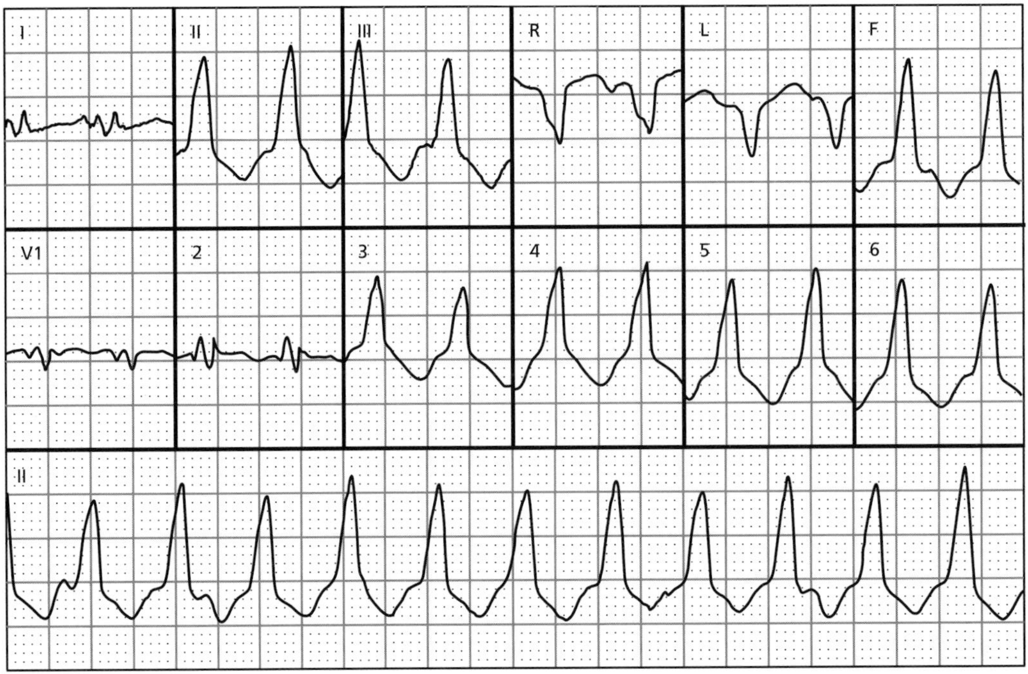

6.60.

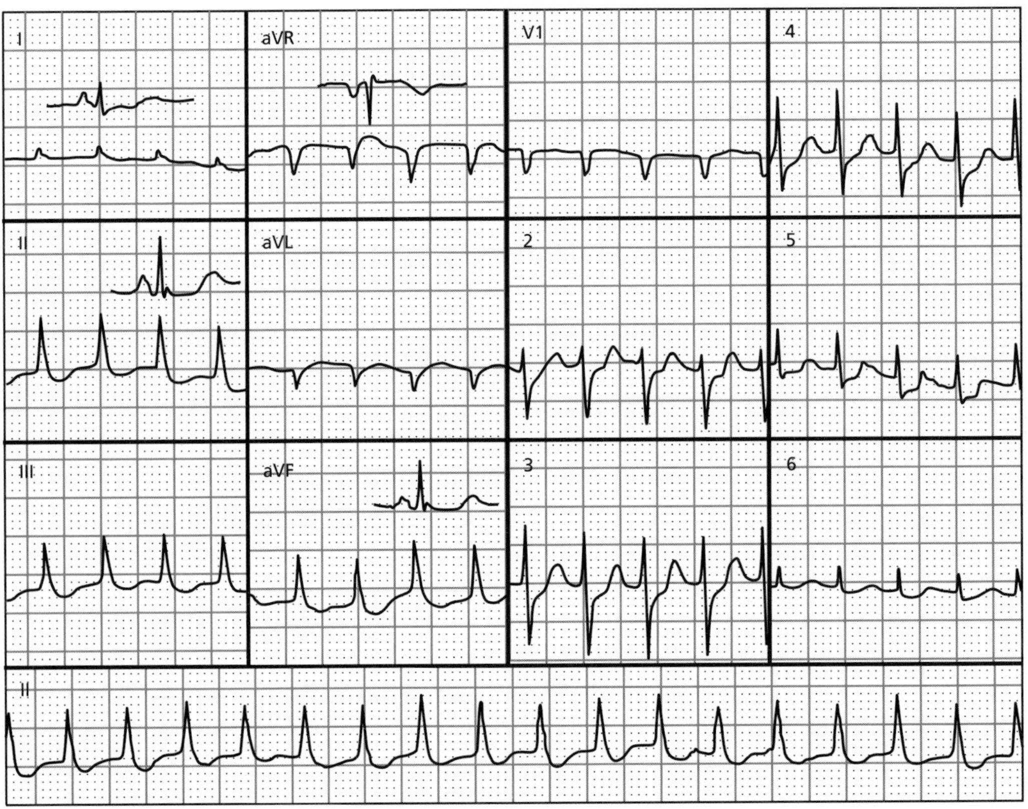

Further reading

Bernstein AD, Daubert JC, Fletcher RD *et al.*, North American Society of Pacing and Electrophysiology/British Pacing and Electrophysiology Group. The revised NASPE/BPEG generic code for antibradycardia, adaptive-rate, and multisite pacing. *Pacing Clin Electrophysiol* 2002; **25**: 260.

Bernstein NE, Sandler DA, Goh M, Feigenblum DY. Why a sawtooth? Inferences on the generation of the flutter wave during typical atrial flutter drawn from radiofrequency ablation. *Ann Noninvasive Electrocardiol* 2004; **9**: 358–361.

Brugada P, Brugada J. Right bundle branch block, persistent ST segment elevation, and sudden cardiac death: a distinct clinical and electrocardiographic syndrome. A multicenter report. *J Am Coll Cardiol* 1992; **20**: 1391–1396.

Buxton AE, Marchlinski FE, Doherty JU *et al.* Hazards of intravenous verapamil for sustained ventricular tachycardia. *Am J Cardiol* 1987; **59**: 1107–1110.

Coumel P. Catecholaminergic polymorphic ventricular tachyarrhythmias in children. *Card Electrophysiol Rev* 2002; **6**: 93–95.

Coumel P, Leclercq JF, Attuel P, Maisonblanche P. The QRS morphology in postmyocardial infarction ventricular tachycardia. A study of 100 tracings compared with 70 cases of idiopathic ventricular tachycardia. *Eur Heart J* 1984; **5**: 792–805.

Fenichel RR, Malik M, Antzelevitch C *et al.* Drug-induced torsades de pointes and implications for drug development. *J Cardiovasc Electrophysiol* 2004; **15**: 475–495.

Haïssaguerre M, Jaïs P, Dipen C Shah *et al.* Spontaneous initiation of atrial fibrillation by ectopic beats originating in the pulmonary veins. *N Engl J Med* 1998; **339**: 659–666.

Josephson ME, Callans DJ. Using the twelve-lead electrocardiogram to localize the site of origin of ventricular tachycardia. *Heart Rhythm* 2005; **2**: 443–446.

Kerr C, Gallaghar JJ, German L. Changes in ventriculoatrial intervals with bundle branch block aberration during reciprocating tachycardia in patients with accessory atrioventricular pathways. *Circulation* 1982; **66**: 196.

Kindwall KE, Brown J, Josephson ME. Electrocardiographic criteria for ventricular tachycardia in wide complex left bundle branch block morphology tachycardias. *Am J Cardiol* 1988; **61**: 1279–1283.

Marriott HJL. Differential diagnosis of supraventricular and ventricular tachycardia. *Geriatrics* 1970; **25**: 91–101.

Olshansky B. Ventricular tachycardia masquerading as supraventricular tachycardia: a wolf in sheep's clothing. *J Electrocardiol* 1988; **21**: 377–384.

Priori SG. Inherited arrhythmogenic diseases: the complexity beyond monogenic disorders. *Circulation Res* 2004; **94**: 140–145.

Schamroth L, Dove E. The Wenckebach phenomenon in sino-atrial block. *Br Heart J* 1966; **28**: 350–358.

Wellens HJ, Bar FW, Lie KI. The value of the electrocardiogram in the differential diagnosis of a tachycardia with a widened QRS complex. *Am J Med* 1978; **64**: 27–33.

Zeltser D, Justo D, Halkin A. Drug-induced atrioventricular block: prognosis after discontinuation of the culprit drug. *J Am Coll Cardiol* 2004; **44**: 105–108.

Answers to self-assessment tests

NB: Values for axis are given within a ten-degree range. Any value within that range should be considered correct. Starting with Test Section 3, axis is given only in support of diagnoses.

Self-Assessment Test One

1.01. a.
1.02. b, a.
1.03. The PR interval is prolonged (260 msec). Otherwise normal. Normal axis, +25 to +35°.
1.04. b.
1.05. Left axis deviation, –35 to –45°.
1.06. b.
1.07. Right axis deviation, +105 to +115°.
1.08. c.
1.09. a.
1.10. Early transition (V2). Otherwise normal. Normal axis, +55 to +65°.
1.11. Normal axis, +60 to +70°.
1.12. Borderline left axis, 0 to –10°.
1.13. Left axis deviation, –55 to –65°.
1.14. Normal axis, +70 to +80°.
1.15. Right axis deviation, +115 to +125°.
1.16. Normal axis, +55 to +65°.
1.17. Early transition (V2). Otherwise normal. Borderline left axis, 0 to –10°.
1.18. Right axis deviation, +160 to +170°. The S1S2S3 sign is present (see Chapter 6).
1.19. Normal. Normal axis, +55 to +65°.
1.20. The QRS complex is abnormal. It exhibits a positive delta wave.

Self-Assessment Test Two

2.01. Left bundle branch block. Axis: –5 to –15°.
2.02. Right bundle branch block and left posterior fascicular block. Axis: +205 to +215°.
2.03. Hyperacute phase of anteroseptal wall myocardial infarction (V1–V5). Reciprocal ST segment depression noted in the inferior leads.
2.04. c.
2.05. b.
2.06. a.
2.07. Acute infero-lateral wall infarction (II, III, aVF, V#–V6).
2.08. Left anterior fascicular block, acute anteroseptal infarction (V1–V6). Axis: –55 to –65°.
2.09. Acute inferior wall infarction (II, III, aVF) with reciprocal changes (I, aVL). Right bundle branch block, prolonged PR interval (240 msec). Axis: +145 to +155°.
2.10. b.

2.11. b.
2.12. ECG of 6/6: the tracing is within normal limits. Axis: +40 to +50°.
ECG of 6/7: anteroseptal hyperacute changes are now present (V2–V5).
2.13. c.
2.14. ECG of 8/19: hyperacute changes in V1–V5. Axis: +50 to +60°.
ECG of 8/21: acute non-Q wave anteroseptal infarction (V2–V5). Axis: +55 to +65°.
2.15. Left anterior fascicular block. Axis: –55 to –65°. Remote lateral wall infarction (I, aVL), anterior wall infarction (V2–V6).
2.16. Recent posterior infarction: reciprocal changes V1–V3 with voltage drop-off in V5–V6. Axis: +40 to +50°.
2.17. ECG of 11/29: probable left anterior fascicular block. Axis: –30 to –40°. Hyperacute anteroseptal infarction (V2–V5).
ECG of 11/30: left anterior fascicular block. Axis: –55 to –65°. Acute anterior wall infarction (V2–V5).
2.18. ECG of 1/25: left anterior fascicular block. Axis: –50 to –60°. Hyperacute anteroseptal infarction.
ECG of 1/26: bifascicular block: left anterior fascicular block and right bundle branch block. Axis: –70 to –80°. Acute anteroseptal infarction (V1–V5). Loss of R wave amplitude is noted in the lateral precordial leads.
2.19. Recent inferior wall infarction (II, III, aVF). Recent posterior wall infarction (reciprocal changes in V1–V3 with voltage drop-off in V5–V6).
2.20. Acute ST segment elevation in the precordial leads (V1–V4) consistent with angina. Axis: +35 to +45°.
2.21. Acute evolving inferior wall infarction (II, III, aVF). Posterior wall infarction (reciprocal changes V1–V3 with voltage drop-off V5–V6). Axis: 0 to –10°.
2.22. Left anterior fascicular block. Axis: –35 to –45°. The PR interval is prolonged (240 msec).
2.23. Remote inferolateral wall infarction (II, III, aVF, V5, V6). Probable remote posterior wall infarction (tall R waves V1–V3). Axis: +210 to +220°. The low voltage and extreme right axis probably reflect loss of left ventricular myocardium.
2.24. Remote inferior wall infarction (III, aVF). Anterior myocardial ischemia (ST depression in V2–V5). Axis: –10 to –20°.
2.25. Left anterior fascicular block. Axis: –55 to –65°. Recent anteroseptal infarction (V1–V3).

Self-Assessment Test Three

3.01. Sinus tachycardia, 136/minute.
3.02. b.
3.03. Sinus bradycardia, 48/minute. Sinus arrest (3.06 sec).
3.04. Sinus arrhythmia, 60–90/minute.
3.05. SET A: Right bundle branch block. Left posterior fascicular block. Axis: +205 to +215°.
SET B: Left bundle branch block. Axis: +55 to +65°.
3.06. Sinus rhythm, 81/minute. Second-degree sinoatrial block, 4:1 conduction ratio. The pause is a multiple of the sinus cycle length. The third QRS complex is a junctional escape beat.
3.07. Sinus rhythm, ±70/minute. Second-degree, type I (Wenckebach) sinoatrial block, 3:2 sinoatrial conduction ratio.
3.08. Left ventricular hypertrophy. Axis: +15 to +25°.
3.09. Right ventricular hypertrophy. Probable right atrial abnormality. Axis: +150 to +160°.
3.10. a.
3.11. a.
3.12. ECG of 11/15: left ventricular hypertrophy. Axis: +45 to +55°.
ECG of 11/16: left bundle branch block. Axis: –10 to –20°.
3.13. Acute pericarditis. Axis: +55 to +65°.

3.14. c.
3.15. Acute pericarditis. Or early repolarization. Axis: +55 to +65°.
3.16. Early repolarization syndrome. Axis: +55 to +65°.
3.17. a.
3.18. ECG of 12/19: acute anterolateral wall myocardial infarction. Left anterior fascicular block. Axis: −70 to −80°.
ECG of 12/21: acute anterolateral wall myocardial infarction. Right bundle branch block. Left anterior fascicular block. Axis: −55 to −65°.
Rhythm strip #1: normal interventricular conduction alternates with right bundle branch block.
#2: normal conduction alternates with left anterior fascicular block.
#3: normal conduction alternates with both left anterior fascicular block and right bundle branch block.
3.19. b.
3.20. c.
3.21. a.
3.22. b.
3.23. Right ventricular hypertrophy. Right atrial abnormality. Axis: +115 to +125°.
3.24. Sinus tachycardia, 107/minue. Sinus arrest.
3.25. Sinus rhythm, 65/minute. Second-degree, type II (Mobitz II) sinoatrial block.
3.26. Sinus rhythm. Second-degree, type I (Wenckebach) sinoatrial block with 4:3 sinoatrial conduction ratio.
3.27. Right bundle branch block. Left posterior fascicular block. Axis: +130 to +140°.
3.28. Acute anteroseptal myocardial infarction. Left anterior fascicular block. Axis: −40 to −50°. Rhythm strip: sinus rhythm, 99/minute, with premature atrial extrasystoles triggering atrial fibrillation.
3.29. Right ventricular hypertrophy. Axis: +115 to +125°. The S1S2S3 sign is present.
3.30. Probably early repolarization syndrome vs. acute pericarditis. Recent inferior wall myocardial infarction. Left ventricular hypertrophy.
3.31. Recent inferior wall myocardial infarction. Probable posterior wall infarction. Acute pericarditis.
3.32. Right ventricular hypertrophy. Axis: +115 to +125°. Rhythm strip: atrial fibrillation.
3.33. Acute pericarditis. Axis: +55 to +65°.
3.34. Left ventricular hypertrophy. Recent inferior wall myocardial infarction. Axis: +5 to −5°.
3.35. Probable subarachnoid hemorrhage with 'neurogenic' T waves. Axis: +25 to +35°.
3.36. Right ventricular hypertrophy. Axis: +115 to +125°.
3.37. Left bundle branch block. Axis: −10 to −20°. Rhythm strip: sinus rhythm, 100/minute. Interventricular conduction intermittently normalizes (narrow QRS complexes).
3.38. Early repolarization syndrome. Axis: +55 to +65°.
3.39. Left ventricular hypertrophy. Axis: +55 to +65°.
3.40. Right bundle branch block. Left posterior fascicular block. Axis: +150 to +160°.
Rhythm strip: second-degree atrioventricular block, type II (Mobitz II).

Self-Assessment Test Four

4.01. Right bundle branch block. Left posterior fascicular block. Axis: +150 to +160°. Rhythm strip: atrial bigeminy.
4.02. Acute anterior wall infarction. Right bundle branch block. Left posterior fascicular block. Axis: +120 degrees. Rhythm strip: paroxysmal atrioventricular block.
4.03. Sinus rhythm, 94/minute. Second-degree, type I (Wenckebach) atrioventricular block (6:5).
4.04. Multifocal atrial tachycardia, ±125/minute.
4.05. Atrial flutter, 4:1 conduction ratio. Ventricular rate: 71/minute.
4.06. Hyperacute phase, anteroseptal myocardial infarction. Rhythm strip: atrial flutter, 6:1 conduction ratio.

4.07. Right bundle branch block. Left anterior fascicular block. Axis: –70 to –80°. Rhythm strip: sinus rhythm, 94/minute. Second-degree atrioventricular block, type II (Mobitz II).
4.08. Recent inferior wall myocardial infarction. Posterior wall myocardial infarction. Rhythm strip: sinus tachycardia, 105/minute. Second-degree atrioventricular block, type I (Wenckebach), 4:3 conduction ratio.
4.09. Multifocal atrial tachycardia, ±150/minute. Probable right ventricular hypertrophy. Axis: indeterminate.
4.10. Sinus rhythm, 78/minute. Right bundle branch block. Sinus arrest.
4.11. Sinus tachycardia, 106/minute. Third-degree atrioventricular block. Escape rhythm, 37/minute.
4.12. Right ventricular hypertrophy. Axis: indeterminate.
Rhythm strip: atrial tachycardia with variable Wenckebach conduction changing to 2:1 conduction.
4.13. Acute anteroseptal myocardial infarction. Low atrial (junctional) rhythm.
Rhythm strip: sinus rhythm, 83/minute. An atrial extrasystole triggers atrial fibrillation.
4.14. Sinus tachycardia, 105/minute. The first pause is due to a nonconducted premature atrial beat. A second premature atrial beat is conducted with aberrancy (QRS 7).
4.15. Right bundle branch block. Probable right ventricular hypertrophy. Axis: +115 to +125°. Atrial fibrillation.
4.16. Sinus rhythm, 81/minute. Second-degree atrioventricular block with 2:1 conduction.
4.17. Sinus rhythm, 94/minute. Second-degree, type I (Wenckebach) atrioventricular block. Second-degree, type II (Mobitz II) sinoatrial block. An example of double nodal disease.
4.18. Sinus tachycardia, 102/minute. Right bundle branch block. Left posterior fascicular block. Axis: +150 to +160°. 2:1 AV block.
Rhythm strip: second-degree atrioventricular block with 2:1 conduction. Lengthening of the R–R interval allows interventricular conduction to momentarily normalize.
4.19. Acute inferior wall myocardial infarction. Sinoatrial block, type I (Wenckebach), with 3:2 to 4:3 conduction ratios.
4.20. Sinus rhythm, 86/minute. Second-degree atrioventricular block, 2:1 conduction ratio.
4.21. Sinus rhythm. Third-degree atrioventricular block. Junctional escape rhythm, 36/minute.
4.22. Sinus rhythm, 73/minute. First-degree atrioventricular block (PR 420 msec).
4.23. Atrial bigeminy.
4.24. Third-degree atrioventricular block. Sinus tachycardia, 125/minute is dissociated from a junctional escape rhythm, 37/minute.
4.25. Sinus rhythm, 88/minute. Second-degree atrioventricular block, type II (Mobitz II) with 4:3 ratio of conduction.
4.26. Sinus rhythm, 94/minute. Third-degree atrioventricular block. Junctional escape rhythm, 36/minute.
4.27. Clockwise atrial flutter, 2:1 atrioventricular conduction ratio (320:160).
4.28. Sinus rhythm. A premature atrial extrasystole initiates atrial tachycardia, 156/minute.
4.29. Sinus rhythm, 71/minute. Second-degree sinoatrial block, type II (Mobitz II).
4.30. Sinus rhythm, 65/minute. Second-degree sinoatrial block, type II (Mobitz II).
4.31. Sinus rhythm, 94/minute. Right bundle branch block. Left anterior fascicular block. Axis: –75 to –85°.
Rhythm strip: third-degree atrioventricular block. Escape rhythm, 45/minute.
4.32. Acute inferior wall infarction. Second-degree, type I (Wenchebach) atrioventricular block.
4.33. Sinus rhythm, 88/minute. A premature ventricular extrasystole triggers paroxysmal atrioventricular block. Two escape beats from different foci are noted.
4.34. Counterclockwise atrial flutter with 3:1 atrioventricular conduction. The ventricular response is about 100/minute.

4.35. Left bundle branch block. Rhythm strip: second-degree atrioventricular block. Escape-capture bigeminy.
4.36. Sinus rhythm, 64/minute. Second-degree atrioventricular block, 2:1 to 3:1 conduction ratio.
4.37. Left anterior fascicular block, QRS axis −55°. Right bundle branch block. Left ventricular hypertrophy.
4.38. Left bundle branch block. Sinus tachycardia, 115/minute. Second-degree atrioventricular block, 2:1 atrioventricular conduction ratio progressing to high-grade atrioventricular with slow escape rhythm (23/minute). The second QRS complex in the last strip results from momentary sinus capture.
4.39. ECG of 9/10: hyperacute anteroseptal wall myocardial infarction.
ECG of 9/11: acute anteroseptal wall myocardial infarction.
4.40. Right ventricular hypertrophy. Axis: +130 to +140°.
4.41. Sinus rhythm, 83/minute. First-degree atrioventricular block (PR 440 msec). Nonconducted premature atrial beats result in escape-capture bigeminy.
4.42. ECG of 12/19: acute pericarditis.
ECG of 12/23: resolving pericarditis. The T waves invert as the ST segment returns to the baseline.
4.43. Left bundle branch block.
4.44. ECG of 5/03: Left bundle branch block.
Rhythm strip: sinus tachycardia, 105/minute. Third-degree atrioventricular block. Junctional escape rhythm, 61/minute.
ECG of 5/04: right bundle branch block. Left anterior fascicular block. Axis: −55 to −65°. The rhythm is now atrial fibrillation.
4.45. Left bundle branch block. Rhythm strip: sinus rhythm, 71/minute. Second-degree, type I (Wenckebach) atrioventricular block, 3:2 to 5:4 conduction ratios. Interventricular conduction partially normalizes owing to longer R–R intervals.

Self-Assessment Test Five

5.01. Sinus tachycardia, 106/minute. Wolff–Parkinson–White syndrome (posterior septal accessory pathway).
5.02. d.
5.03. b.
5.04. ECG of 3:31 pm: atrial fibrillation pre-excited tachycardia, 273/minute.
ECG of 5:18 pm: Wolff–Parkinson–White syndrome.
5.05. Atrioventricular nodal re-entrant tachycardia (AVNRT), 176/minute.
5.06. Atrioventricular re-entrant tachycardia (AVRT), 181/minute. Note precordial ST segment depression. P waves in ST segment.
5.07. Right ventricular hypertrophy. Axis: +125 to +135°.
5.08. ECG of 8/2, 12:47 am: orthodromic tachycardia, 214/minute.
ECG of 8/2, 12:50 pm: minimal pre-excitation.
ECG of 8/3, 05:53 am: Wolff–Parkinson–White syndrome (right anterior accessory pathway).
5.09. Atrioventricular nodal re-entrant tachycardia (AVNRT), 215/minute.
5.10. Wolf–Parkinson–White syndrome (left lateral accessory pathway).
5.11. Atrioventricular nodal re-entrant tachycardia (AVNRT), 167/minute.
5.12. Sinus rhythm, 83/minute. First-degree atrioventricular block (PR 320 msec). An atrial premature beat triggers paroxysmal atrioventricular block. The third QRS complex represents a junctional escape beat.
5.13. Sinus rhythm, 84/minute. Nonconducted premature atrial extrasystoles.
5.14. Atrioventricular re-entrant tachycardia (AVRT), 150/minute.
5.15. Wolff–Parkinson–White syndrome (posteroseptal accessory pathway).

5.16. Wolff–Parkinson–White syndrome. Orthodromic tachycardia, 230/minute. Right bundle branch block aberrancy.
5.17. Atrioventricular nodal re-entrant tachycardia (AVNRT), 190/minute.
5.18. Sinus rhythm, 75/minute. Second-degree, type I (Wenckebach) atrioventricular block.
5.19. Sinus tachycardia, 106/minute. Atrial tachycardia, 136/minute.
5.20. Atrioventricular re-entrant tachycardia (AVRT), 187/minute. Note the ST segment depression in the precordial leads and P waves in ST segment.
5.21. Atrioventricular re-entrant tachycardia (AVRT), 190/minute. Note P waves in the ST segment.
5.22. Atrioventricular nodal re-entrant tachycardia (AVNRT) with alternating cycle lengths. Electrophysiologic study (EPS) revealed that antegrade conduction alternated between two slow pathways with retrograde conduction over a single fast pathway.
5.23. SET 1: sinus tachycardia, 107/minute. Wolff–Parkinson–White syndrome.
SET 2: orthodromic tachycardia, 215/minute.
SET 3: atrial fibrillation pre-excited QRS complexes. The shortest pre-excited R–R interval is ±160 msec, making the potential ventricular rate ±330/minute.
5.24. Atrioventricular re-entry tachycardia (AVRT), 214/minute. Note the subtle QRS alternans in lead V1.
5.25. Counterclockwise atrial flutter, 2:1 variable conduction.
5.26. ECG of 1/13: Wolff–Parkinson–White syndrome (left lateral accessory pathway).
ECG of 1/19: orthodromic tachycardia, 197/minute.
5.27. Atrioventricular re-entrant tachycardia (AVRT), 214/minute.
5.28. Left ventricular hypertrophy.
5.29. Wolff–Parkinson–White syndrome (right anterior accessory pathway).
5.30. Atrioventricular nodal re-entrant tachycardia (AVNRT), 158/minute.
5.31. Atrioventricular re-entrant tachycardia (AVRT), 187/minute.
5.32. Wolff–Parkinson–White syndrome (right posterior accessory pathway).
5.33. Remote anterior wall myocardial infarction. Left posterior fascicular block. Axis: +115 to +125°.
5.34. Wolff–Parkinson–White syndrome (posteroseptal accessory pathway).
5.35. Early repolarization syndrome.
5.36. Wolff–Parkinson–White syndrome (posterior accessory pathway).
5.37. Atrioventricular nodal re-entrant tachycardia (AVNRT), 172/minute.
5.38. Atrioventricular re-entrant tachycardia (AVRT), 217/minute.
5.39. Atrioventricular re-entrant tachycardia (AVRT) with left bundle branch block aberrancy. (Inverted P waves are present in the ST segments in the inferior leads.)

Self-Assessment Test Six

6.01. VAT pacemaker, 75/minute.
6.02. Ventricular tachycardia, 129/minute with 2:1 ventriculoatrial conduction.
6.03. Sinus tachycardia, 107/minute. Second-degree, type I atrioventricular block. The 5th P wave is a premature atrial extrasystole that re-enters to produce an atrial echo beat (*arrow*).
6.04. Atrial tachycardia, variable conduction, with 3 beats of right bundle branch block aberrancy.
6.05. Atrioventricular nodal re-entrant tachycardia (AVNRT), 172/minute. Inserts are sinus rhythm.
6.06. DDD pacemaker. QRS #4 is in response to a premature atrial beat. A premature atrial beat following QRS #5 falls in the PVARP and is not sensed.
6.07. Sinus tachycardia, 103/minute. A premature ventricular beat precipitates paroxysmal atrioventricular block.
6.08. Sinus bradycardia, 57/minute. First-degree atrioventricular block (PR = 400 msec). Second-degree, type II sinoatrial block. QRS #3 is an escape beat. This is an example of 'double nodal disease.'
6.09. b.

6.10. a.
6.11. a.
6.12. b.
6.13. b.
6.14. a.
6.15. Ventricular tachycardia, 152/minute. NB: atrioventricular dissociation.
6.16. Supraventricular tachycardia, 156/minute. Left bundle branch block aberrancy. NB: the atrial rhythm is likely atrial flutter with 2:1 conduction.
6.17. Ventricular tachycardia, 147/minute.
6.18. c.
6.19. Sinus tachycardia, 120/minute. A premature atrial beat precipitates paroxysmal atrioventricular block. QRS #4 is an escape beat.
6.20. Wolff–Parkinson–White syndrome (right anterior accessory pathway).
6.21. Sinus tachycardia, 125/minute. Third-degree atrioventricular block. Junctional escape rhythm, 46/minute.
6.22. Ventricular tachycardia, 202/minute. NB: a capture beat occurs in the rhythm strip.
6.23. Sinus rhythm, 60/minute. Lack of capture and sensing in either chamber is noted.
6.24. Sinus rhythm, 91/minute. Atrioventricular dissociation. VVI pacemaker, 75/minute.
6.25. Sinus tachycardia, 129/minute. Ventricular tachycardia, 151/minute. NB: QRS #2 and #11 are fusion beats. Atrioventricular dissociation is present.
6.26. Sinus rhythm, 62/minute. Premature atrial beats. Pacer spikes without capture. Intermittent appropriate sensing.
6.27. There are five possibilities: (1) ectopic atrial tachycardia, (2) fast–slow atrioventricular nodal re-entrant tachycardia (F–S AVNRT), (3) slow–slow atrioventricular nodal re-entrant tachycardia (S–S AVNRT), (4) atrioventricular re-entrant tachycardia (AVRT) with ventriculoatrial conduction over a slowly conducting accessory pathway, or (5) permanent junctional reciprocating tachycardia (PJRT).
6.28. b.
6.29. c.
6.30. a.
6.31. a.
6.32. Wolff–Parkinson–White syndrome (posteroseptal accessory pathway).
6.33. VVI pacer (QRS #1), probable atrial tachycardia, 215/minute with 2:1 paced response (upper rate tracking).
6.34. DDD pacemaker, 82/minute.
6.35. Wolff–Parkinson–White syndrome (insets). Orthodromic tachycardia, 230/minute.
6.36. VVI pacemaker, 60/minute. Failure to sense. QRS #4 is a pseudofusion beat.
6.37. VVI pacemaker, 68/minute. Intermittent failure to sense and capture.
6.38. Bidirectional ventricular tachycardia, 167/minute.
6.39. Ventricular tachycardia, 160/minute.
6.40. a.
6.41. Wolff–Parkinson–White syndrome. Atrial fibrillation intermittently conducted over an accessory pathway. The shortest pre-excited R–R interval is 220 msec.
6.42. DDD pacemaker, 62/minute.
6.43. Permanent junctional reciprocating tachycardia, 131/minute.
6.44. Ventricular tachycardia, 168/minute.
6.45. Wolff–Parkinson–White syndrome (posteroseptal accessory pathway).
6.46. Atrioventricular nodal re-entrant tachycardia (AVNRT), 187/minute. Pre-existing right bundle branch block.

6.47. Accelerated ventricular rhythm, 86/minute.
6.48. Probable atrial tachycardia, 174/minute. AV dissociation. Escape rhythm, 73/minute.
6.49. Polymorphic ventricular tachycardia.
6.50. Ventricular tachycardia, 131/minute, 6:1 exit block. NB: atrioventricular dissociation is present.
6.51. First-degree atrioventricular block, left bundle branch block, second-degree type II sinoatrial block with 4:1 conduction.
6.52. Atrial flutter, 4:1 to 8:1 conduction ratios.
6.53. Ventricular tachycardia, 231/minute. Superior axis.
6.54. Recent infero-posterior myocardial infarction. Left ventricular hypertrophy.
6.55. Atrial fibrillation, right ventricular hypertrophy. Axis: +115 to +125°.
6.56. Accelerated junctional rhythm, 95/minute. Retrograde conduction produces ventricular echo beats.
6.57. Acute pericarditis. NB: PR segment depression in the inferior leads.
6.58. Wolff–Parkinson–White syndrome (left posterior accessory pathway).
6.59. Ventricular tachycardia, 137/minute. NB: atrioventricular dissociation in the rhythm strip.
6.60. Atrioventricular nodal re-entrant tachycardia (AVNRT), 216/minute.

Index

Page numbers in *italics* represent figures, those in **bold** represent tables